Comfort to the Sick

Comfort
to the Sick

by
Brother Aloysius

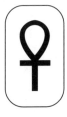

SAMUEL WEISER, INC.

York Beach, Maine

First published in 1992 by
Samuel Weiser, Inc.
Box 612
York Beach, Maine 03910

Library of Congress Cataloging-in-Publication Data
Aloysius, Brother.
     [Troost der zieken.   English]
     Comfort to the sick / Brother Aloysius.
          p.   cm.
     Includes index.
     1. Herbs—Therapeutic use.   I. Title.
     RM666.H33A4613   1992
615′.321—dc20   91-22826
                                                                   CIP
     ISBN 0-87728-525-X
     MV

Translated by Jane Meijlink-Green.

Cover art is entitled "Tea Time,"
© 1991 Beverly Duncan. Used by kind
permission of the artist.

Typeset in 11 pt. Baskerville
Printed in the United States of America

The paper used in this publication meets the minimum requirements of the
American National Standard for Permanence of Paper for Printed Library
Materials Z39.48-1984.

CONTENTS

PUBLISHER'S NOTE

Comfort to the Sick was originally published in Holland in 1901. It was written by Brother Aloysius, who was a member of a monastery headed by Monseigneur Savelberg in Heerlen. He came to be interested in the study of herbs and the water cure because he had healed himself of consumption using the Kneipp Water Cure. This brought him to study with Mgr. Kneipp, and eventually to work with common herbs—plants found in the local woods and fields—to help people maintain health when the energies of the body are out of balance. This book is the culmination of his study, and was issued in several editions in Dutch at the turn of the century.

Brother Aloysius wrote two cautions in regard to his original publication. Readers should work with fresh herbs. All herbs should be gathered new every year as old herbs do not have the healing effects he describes in this book. He also wants readers to know that most of the recipes could be made with approximate measurements. We could use a handful, or a pinch of an herb. He mentioned that 3 grams usually meant a full tablespoon, or a small handful, of a finely chopped herb. We think that he wanted readers to develop a warm feeling for working with the herbs in order to get the best from them for health changes.

Because this book was originally published in Europe, with metric measurements, we have added American measures so readers can measure herbs in tablespoons and cups, pints and quarts. The less common herbs and more pharmaceutical ingredients are measured in ounces. Readers should also note that we are using 1 quart/1 liter liquid combinations even though this is not an exact conversion, because these are easier to work with in both the American and European household.

Brother Aloysius was clear about working "easily" with the herbs—our reasoning in this decision.

Brother Aloysius also made references to the changes necessary when working with adults and children. For example, if an adult would drink tea made from ¼ cup (15 grams) of an herb per 2 cups (½ liter) water, the dose would have to be less for a child. Children from 1 to 2 years would be given about 1 teaspoon (1¼ grams) of the herb to 2 cups (½ liter) of water, children from 3 to 4 years would use 2 teaspoons (½ gram) and so on, according to age, adding a little more of the herb for each additional year. Of course, we also are most clear that parents should not use this herbal as a medical device; they should consult a physician when a child needs to have a health problem diagnosed.

In the process of editing this book, we discovered that some herbs are not easily available, or only available in Europe, or that Brother Aloysius worked with substances other than herbs and these substances are no longer used today. Some readers will probably want to try making their own herbal recipes, just to see if they work; others will find the recipes very practical and helpful. Sometimes ingredients can be obtained from the local pharmacy. A number of ingredients listed in this book are available over the counter if you ask for them. Americans tend to buy over-the-counter combinations and it doesn't occur to us that we can buy certain ingredients without a prescription. If your local herb store or health food store doesn't stock the materials that you need, you can contact Aphrodisia at 264 Bleecker St., New York, NY 10014 (telephone (212) 989-6440) or ask for their mail order catalog ($2.00). They may be able to help supply herbs that are not carried locally.

This book has been years in the making. We thank the translator, Jane Meijlink-Green, for the great work that she has done in bringing this book into English. Because this material is so interesting, we wanted to make it accessible to American readers and in doing so found ourselves tracking down definitions of various ingredients. We learned that some ingredients are difficult to obtain today and that the names of some herbs vary from Europe to England to the United States.

We do not intend that this book be used as a medical textbook; it is simply an informative documentation of herbal remedies, and is of interest to herbalists and anyone seeking to know more about alternative health, as well as being a valuable contribution to the history of medicine. Some of the recipes are included for curiosity or for their folk value to give readers the idea of the medicines used at the turn of the century. Certain recipes are very dated, and should be regarded as historical, while other recipes are common household remedies still in use today by people familiar with friendly herbs. We have enjoyed the time it has taken to prepare this book for publication, especially since it seems to us to be both historically interesting and a modern guide to good health. The various people hunting for herbal remedies during the editorial process have developed a new relationship with plants previously considered weeds. No longer is the plantain taken from the lawn. No longer are the dandelions dug up and thrown away. We have developed a new set of friends!

INTRODUCTION
TO THE FIRST EDITION

Having been called by divine Providence to the monastic life, I had a very wonderful opportunity to fulfill my ardent wish of being able to help suffering humanity. From my youth, I had been keen to learn about medicinal plants and their virtues; and now taking advantage of very favorable conditions, and with the approval of my reverend Superior, I set to work with joy. Tabermontanae, Dodonaeus, Lobel and other old authors, read and compared with various more recent ones, soon gave me a good grasp of the subject.

In 1889, I came across "Meine Wasserkur" (*My Water Cure*) by Monseigneur Kneipp. As I myself was very unwell due to a family complaint (phthisis), I began to practice on myself what I had been learning in *My Water Cure*, even though I shrank from using cold water. This was on the 7th November of the above-mentioned year. After 1½ years of braving the Cure, I was healed of the disease, to everyone's surprise. Four years ago, on the occasion of a visit to a university, a professor specializing in chronic diseases expressed amazement after giving me a thorough examination.

For some years now, poor patients from the environs of Heerlen have been coming here to seek help for their families and themselves. One evidence of the good results achieved was the increase in the number of visitors, who began at length to be so numerous that they had to be turned away, because they were making it almost impossible for me to perform my monastic duties.

Three times we stopped and tried to prevent any more being admitted, but the afflicted defeated us by ruses and entreaties, and God's holy will had to be seen in this. So, in 1891, my reverend Superior dispatched me to Woerisholen to study hydrotherapy under Mgr. Kneipp, after I had already employed it on the sick with good success for almost a year. On the occasion I was away for five months, and immediately on my return so many people came to consult me that I obtained permission to devote myself entirely to their suffering. In spite of the fact that arrangements were initially very primitive, the poorest of the poor rubbed shoulders with sick folk from the highest ranks of society—all looking for relief. Not content with the treatment itself, people kept urging me after my return from Woerisholen to set down my experiences in print. Some people are not easy to deny.

For many years I had been keeping records of tried and tested remedies, and (especially at Woerisholen) had made a collection of most of them, so that I had a big stock of remedies of all sorts for rich and poor alike. I would quite willingly have fulfilled long ago the urgent wishes of patients that I should write about these remedies for publication, but I did not feel I was in a position to do so. Finally, however, with the approval of my reverend Superior and with an invocation to the Holy Spirit, I took my pen and summoned up the courage to set to work.

In describing the plants, I have made full use of the beautiful work by Prof. C.A.J.A. Oudemans, and have borrowed many details from it. I hope that readers will give me their kind indulgence.

On the occasion of my second visit to Monseigneur Kneipp, the latter said, after a short conference on the Heerlen Water Cure and in the presence of certain noblemen such as the Archduke Jozel of Oostenrijk, Prince van Arenberg and other distinguished persons: "Carry on with your herbs; you are doing almost as much good with your herbs as I am doing with my water."

This was an incentive to pursue my work with medicinal plants even more vigorously, and to build on what I had already achieved. Everyone who has seen our fine botanical dispensary has been quite amazed. It is always such a delight and satisfaction to me that we are now able to supply each individual so easily with the herbs they require. Not only can people find the dried

herbs in our dispensary, but botanists and those who wish to get
to know the medicinal plants mentioned in our little book find
ample scope for their studies in our so-called Kneipp garden.

Described in this work are some 300 medicinal plants with
a great compilation of domestic remedies of all sorts; in addition, there are the symptoms of various diseases together with
their treatments and a list of useful remedies. Most of the plants
mentioned in this book are widely available, and are to be found
in fields and gardens, in woods and meadows. A note is made
in the description if the species is rare.

Most medical works are too technical for the general
reader, so I have tried to make myself understood by everyone.
The preparation of the tisanes and the quantities to employ are
accurately given, so that even the simplest person can prepare
his or her medicine without difficulty. The reader will also
discover in the work a list of herbal compounds with indications
for their use.

Plants do need to be gathered at just the right time; and
this is stated for every species. What is more, the plants should
be carefully dried in a warm, dry place; a loft or garret is best
for this purpose. The plants must never be dried in the sun.
They keep best in a dry place, in paper sacks or bags. Roots,
which usually are gathered in spring or autumn, must be carefully dried in the oven, after being sliced or cut up into small
pieces if they are thick. To ensure good results, fresh herbs
should be gathered each year. Stale herbs, more than a year
old, which no longer smell fresh, have lost their virtue; they
are more likely to be harmful than beneficial. The prejudice
many people have against herbs is very likely due to the use of
old and musty specimens.

The following example will show what I mean: a gentleman
was suffering from a severe nosebleed; none of the measures
taken seemed to help him, and there was fear for his life. Not
knowing what to do, his anxious family came to me. I recommended shepherd's purse; but nobody believed that it would
do any good, because it had already been tried without success.
Immediately suspecting that stale material had been employed,
I had a strong infusion prepared; this the patient sniffed up
his nose. He also drank a cupful. The nosebleed stopped almost
instantaneously.

A gentleman from Friesland who was already under treatment here, started spitting a quantity of blood. The doctor, who happened to be present, feared for his life. We gave him a tablespoon of the infusion of shepherd's purse and purple loosestrife every ten minutes. After taking the first spoonful cold, he did not expectorate another drop of blood. And yet these two plants are only weeds.

A university professor stayed with us for a few days to find out about the Kneipp Cure. He was suffering from gastric trouble. Soon noticing the herbal dispensary, he said, "I certainly believe in water, but not in the power of these herbs; they are nothing more than cattle fodder."

I asked "Professor, are you familiar with herbs?" and was answered in the affirmative. Then I quoted some examples which seemed to convince him: and I followed this up with, "Professor, if you don't take herbs, there is no reason to expect that you will be cured here."

I had an infusion of an herbal compound prepared for him and on a number of occasions after he had taken it, I heard him say, "That bitter juice does me good." Seldom have I received more gratitude than I received from that professor.

A lady had been crying day and night for a period of some weeks because of a pain in the liver region. None of the medical treatments she tried seemed to help. Her father came and begged me to help her. I prescribed hot compresses of a decoction of hayseed to be laid on the painful place, that goosegrass (clivers) boiled in milk should be given as hot as possible to the patient. The lady was out and about cured in three days.

I cite these examples by way of encouragement and as evidence that God has placed healing plants within reach of the sick. I could fill a book with similar examples.

Finally, I hope that all who read this book can recognize the good intentions with which it has been written, and that they will see it for what it is: an attempt to answer the urgent pleas of the suffering.

May its title, *Comfort to the Sick*, prove by God's grace to be a true description of the book, and may what I have written bring consolation to all who need consolation and comfort. I send *Comfort to the Sick* into the world, for the greater glory of God and for the welfare of my fellow humans.

Brother Aloysius
Heerlen, January 1901

INTRODUCTION TO THE SECOND EDITION

On the occasion of the issue of this new edition it is necessary for us, in the first place, to record our thanks to Almighty God, who has permitted our work however incomplete it may be, to be used for the blessing and healing of many. We are also grateful to the large numbers of people who seem to have approved of it so heartily.

The new edition differs in many respects from its predecessor. Above all the contents have been noticeably expanded; the number of diseases it treats and the number of herbs described have both been considerably increased, and (in response to popular demand) the classification has been altered in several important respects. In the first part, there is a description of diseases, the treatment to adopt for them and the means required for a cure. In the second part are listed the medicinal plants with their characteristics and use, together with a long register of tisanes, remedies, ointments, etc. In the third part, there has now been included a brief account of the water cure: douches, baths, compresses, wet sheets and so on. The index has been altered too, and there is an alphabetical list of diseases with indication of suitable herbs.

We flatter ourselves that this new edition will appeal to readers as improved and expanded, while still begging that they will treat it with indulgence. At the same time we pray for God's blessing on it. May He, the great Lord of healing, Lord of the living and the dead, indeed impart curative power to the indicated remedies, and may He grant comfort and healing, relief and recovery to poor suffering humanity. May these pages contribute to His further honor and glory and to a deeper recognition of His infinite love for suffering men and women.

Brother Aloysius
Heerlen, Spring 1912

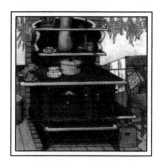

Part I

The Treatment of Disease

ILLNESSES AND REMEDIES

ABSCESSES

Since abscesses are the result of some kind of illness, one should try to diagnose and cure the illness; the abscesses will then disappear.

1) Anyone who is severely plagued by abscesses should boil stinging nettles in milk and drink this decoction throughout the day.

2) A daily cup of sassafras tea is also a good remedy.

3) Two hay-shirts and four whole washes are highly recommended; depurative tea should also be taken.

4) Soak white bread in hot milk, add a little saffron and apply this poultice.

ABSCESSES AND ULCERS

1) If there is burning, apply a poultice of white bread and milk; if there is much pain, add a little nightshade (belladonna); this quickly alleviates the pain.

2) A plaster of fenugreek is always one of the best remedies for ulcers or abscesses.

3) Thoroughly mix together 1 tablespoon rapeseed oil, 1 egg yolk and 1 tablespoon of wheat flour. Apply this mixture to the ulcers and renew when it begins to dry. This stills the pain, brings it quickly to a head and heals it.

4) The application of grated or scraped comfrey is a very potent remedy.

5) Anyone who suffers greatly from ulcers should drink stinging nettles boiled in milk throughout the day until the ulcers have gone. A daily cup of sassafras tea can also be taken.

6) A plaster of Mother Ointment can be applied twice daily. This ointment is prepared by slowly melting the following ingredients in a double boiler:

> ¼ cup (62 grams) unsalted butter
> 2 tablespoons (32 grams) lard
> ⅓ cup (62 grams) mutton fat
> ½ cup (125 grams) olive oil

When everything has melted, slowly add 2 ounces (60 grams) lead oxide,[1] stirring continually. Mix well, keep stirring until the ointment turns brown and remove it from the fire.

7) In addition, a short compress of hayseed decoction should be used on alternate days.

ANXIETY/CRAMPS/CONGESTION OF THE BLOOD

Take ¾ cup (24 grams) of yarrow, ¾ cup (24 grams) sage, 1½ cups (24 grams) lemon balm, and 1 cup (24 grams) spearmint; ½ cup (15 grams) common chamomile and ¼ cup (15 grams) lime blossom; 3 tablespoons (8 grams) blessed thistle seed; 3 teaspoons (4 grams) caraway seed, 3 teaspoons (4 grams) aniseed and 2 teaspoons (4 grams) fennel seed. Pound all the seeds to a coarse powder and boil everything together in 8 cups (2 liters) of water. Take 1 tablespoon every hour on the first day, and 1 tablespoon every two hours on the second day. In addition apply a hot compress of hayseed decoction on the abdomen for one hour daily. This compress should be renewed every half-hour.

ARTERIOSCLEROSIS (HARDENING OF THE ARTERIES)

This complaint occurs particularly in older people, but may also arise in young people through wanton living, gout, obesity,

---

[1]Lead oxide: used in the preparation of plasters; taken internally it is poisonous. This ingredient may be found at some pharmacies.

misuse of alcohol and tobacco, lack of physical excercise, or syphilis. The arteries lose their elasticity through calcium deposits which collect on the artery walls, making them hard and lumpy to the touch, more or less twisted and visible to the eye. The consequences are: enlargement of the left heart-ventricle, indigestion, constipation, piles, bursting of smaller blood-vessels (in the brain) causing cerebral hemorrhage or a stroke. Old people should take care to refrain from excessive eating and drinking, and over-strenuous work; they should ensure regular, soft bowel movements—never forcing it by exerting great pressure.

The following advice is recommended for people with a tendency to obesity: plenty of exercise, and moderation in food and drink. Meat, spices, coffee, tea, and spirits should be avoided, while vegetables, milk and farinaceous foods are recommended. A raw onion and 1 cup ash leaf tea should be taken daily, or 1 cup comfrey tea daily, four whole washes and three upper body washes weekly.

ABDOMINAL DROPSY (ASCITES)

Ascites is generally caused by a heart, liver, or kidney condition, or by anemia. It is also known that most drunkards suffer from dropsy. Dropsy can also be caused by too many purgatives, by drinking when sweating, by living in damp houses or marshy places, etc. Dropsy sufferers are usually very thirsty, and the more they drink, the greater the thirst; for this reason it is better to drink with a spoon. If the dropsy is at an advanced stage, there is usually nothing more to be done on account of the extensive anemia; if it remains constant, it can still be cured.

1) In cases of dropsy, hot water should never be used, i.e., hot compresses or vapor baths; this would cause even greater weakness. Suitable cold water applications have an invigorating, dissolving, expelling action. Such patients should present themselves in person to the physician so as to obtain a suitable prescription for water baths.

2) Tea from meadowsweet is a very good remedy to drive out the water.

3) Dwarf elder root, rosemary, knotgrass are also efficacious.

4) Inner rind of elder wood with licorice (see elder flowers) can help.

5) Every morning and evening take 2 sugarspoons unbruised white mustard seed.

6) The following mixture is very good:

> ⅓ cup (30 grams) juniper berries
> 1 cup (30 grams) young juniper twigs

Leave to steep for four days in 1 quart (liter) of Rhine wine (or other sweet white wine), then add:

> ¼ cup (30 grams) sugar
> 5 tablespoons (15 grams) common wormwood
> 4 teaspoons (15 grams) radish

Take 3 to 4 tablespoons daily.

7) Boil ⅓ cup (15 grams) rue and ⅓ cup (15 grams) common centaury in 1 quart (liter) of Rhine wine until reduced by a third; keep it hot near the fire and take 1 tablespoon every two hours.

8) Every morning and evening rub the abdomen well with warm olive oil.

9) Boil ¼ cup (20 grams) juniper berries with 2 cups (½ liter) of water and drink 3 cups daily.

•   •   •

The following remedy is particularly efficacious; I have experienced its excellent curative powers many times when all else failed:

10) Take half a handful of haricot beans (kidney beans) and an equal quantity of inner rind of elder wood; boil in 1 quart (liter) water until reduced by half; later, as it cools, add ½ sugarspoon saltpeter and drink this quantity throughout the day.

11) 2 cups goldenrod tea daily has also helped many people.

12) 5 Dutch Drops (see page 18) taken in milk every other day, or 2 cups daily of meadowsweet or pellitory or broom tea.

13) If the ascites is caused by a heart condition, take, in addition to one of the above mentioned remedies, 5 drops tincture of false hellebore three times a day.

PIMPLES (ACNE VULGARIS)
1) Apply twice daily one of the following: a poultice of clay mixed with half water and vinegar, a poultice of unsalted soft cheese, or apply scraped comfrey.

2) Mix honey with a little flour, smear this on a linen cloth and apply this plaster twice a day.

3) Apply hot compresses of heartsease boiled in milk; renew the compresses as soon as they begin to dry.

4) Hot compresses of goosegrass (*Galium aparine*) are also highly recommended.

5) Apply a plaster of Mother Ointment twice a day. (See recipe on p. 4).

ANEMIA
For anemia, use the following treatments: a daily upper body wash; on alternate days, a hot compress of hayseed decoction on the abdomen for half an hour; after one week a whole body wash every day, a compress on alternate days, and three knee waterings per week. The third week take four whole washes, three knee waterings, and three cold hip-baths for thirteen to fifteen seconds.

With the water applications, take a daily cup of tea made from common centaury, white horehound and thyme with sugar. In addition, twice a day take a bowl of Kneipp's tonic soup and pinch (or half a sugarspoon) of bone-dust. Children should take a small pinch of bone-dust twice daily; adults half a sugarspoon twice daily. (See also Green Sickness.)

APPENDICITIS (TYPHLITIS)

This illness, which occurs more in men than in women, is mostly caused by constipation. The appendix lies on the lower right side of the abdomen. Some time before the onset of inflammation, the following symptoms may occur: sometimes severe colic, constipation or diarrhea, the intestinal wall gradually loses its elasticity, food residue remains in the same place and hardens, causing infection and ulceration of the intestinal wall. The slightest pressure on or near the affected part causes the patient acute pain; some people vomit at the onset of the complaint; the abdomen is swollen, there is a lack of appetite and great thirst due to fever. If the fever subsides (which may frequently happen in more fortunate cases), the patient is on the way to recovery, pain and vomiting stop and bowel movement gradually follows.

As soon as one becomes aware of the above-mentioned symptoms, a doctor should be consulted as he, alone, is in a position to make a diagnosis. It is important to ensure regular bowel movement by the application of several cold enemas until the bowels move. Purgatives are not advisable in this case; only 1 or 2 tablespoons castor oil may be tried. The patient should remain quietly in bed, applying cold poultices of clay with equal quantities of water and vinegar, to be renewed every two hours, sometimes earlier if they become too warm. The patient can also apply a poultice of soft cheese and drink 2 cups blackberry leaf tea daily. If there is no sign of recovery, a physician should most definitely be consulted; he will probably have to perform a small operation to remove the pus.

ASTHMA (BREATHLESSNESS AND WHEEZING)

By asthma, one means a feeling of difficulty, tightness and distress when breathing, as though the chest is being constricted. From time to time, usually in the evenings or at night, there are heavy attacks which pass of their own accord.

The causes of this complaint are very varied. Sometimes it occurs from a sudden feeling of chilliness, anger, from internal skin disorders and gout, at other times from stubborn constipation, bad air in a room due to the presence of too many people; from carbon monoxide, chills, misuse of strong, over–

heating drinks, too much physical stress, as a consequence of pneumonia, etc. Asthma is generally accompanied by coughing. In the case of a dry cough, it is called dry asthma; with a mucous cough, humid asthma. Asthma is, in fact, an infection of the nerves. It frequently occurs in hypochondriacs or hysterical people, sometimes to a very high degree, so that the sufferers fall down, as though suffocated, in a state of suspended animation. Not withstanding the severity of these attacks, there is little danger involved; they disappear as quickly as they arise. You can treat as follows:

1) The patient must abstain from heavy, indigestible food, alcoholic drinks, beer, vinegar and coffee. He or she should avoid damp cold, likewise strong smells, dust etc; he or she should be moderate and always ensure good bowel movements. The following herbs are highly recommended: valerian, sage, plantain, Aaron's rod (mullein), common St. Johnswort, lime blossom, chamomile flowers, or a cup of brambleleaf (blackberry leaf) tea in the morning and evening.

2) Mix 5 teaspoons (3 grams) each of sage, Aaron's rod (mullein) and plantain (ribwort) steeped in 2 cups (½ liter) boiling water and strained makes, with the addition of 2 tablespoons honey, an excellent tea for asthmatics. Take 1 tablespoon every hour. In addition, a hot compress of water and vinegar may be laid on the chest for half an hour every day. If the patient cannot lie down, the compress may be applied to the abdomen (belly).

If the patient does not need to lie in bed, twice weekly upper body waterings, two or three knee waterings with three half-baths, and one minute treading water daily are highly recommended (see Part III, The Water Cure, p. 401).

When an attack occurs, it is good to rub the back hard with a dry woolen cloth, then to give it a quick rinse with cold vinegar and water and wrap the patient up warm; the attack usually quickly subsides.

Although, generally speaking, coffee is forbidden, a strong cup of coffee often gives immediate relief from an attack. Keeping the arms in hot water also frequently helps to dispel an attack.

3) If the asthma is caused by internal skin complaints, one should try to draw out the rash by wearing hot hay-shirts in bed for an hour-and-a-half two or three times a week. In addition, drink 1 cup elder tea with 1 sugarspoon of purified flowers of sulphur every evening before retiring.

4) If coughing up phlegm alleviates the patient, it is beneficial to take a sugarspoonful of the following mixture from time to time: 1 tablespoon wine vinegar mixed with 2 tablespoons honey. This remedy is particularly recommended for dry wheeziness.

5) Vapor baths (see The Water Cure, p. 407) are very efficacious in the treatment of asthma. Inhalation of vapor from Aaron's rod (mullein) is highly recommended for dry asthma.

6) Let 7½ teaspoons (4 grams) of hyssop steep for fifteen minutes in a covered pan containing 1 cup boiling water, strain it and add 2 tablespoons honey and 1 tablespoon wine vinegar; bring this to the boil again and take 1 tablespoon of the mixture every two hours.

7) Aniseed tea is also very effective.

8) Another very potent tea is the following:

> 5 teaspoons (3 grams) coltsfoot
> 5 teaspoons (3 grams) plantain
> 5 teaspoons (3 grams) sage
> 2 tablespoons (1 gram) Aaron's rod (mullein)

Leave this to steep for fifteen minutes in 2 cups (½ liter) boiling water. Then strain and add 2 tablespoons honey and briefly boil again. Take 1 tablespoon every two hours.

ATROPHY OF THE MUSCLES/INFLAMMATION (ATROPHIA MUSCULORUM)

See Part III, Water Cures, p. 401 and use the following treatments: a daily whole body wash, three half-baths a week for 5 seconds, gradually adding arm and knee waterings, then thigh and back waterings. Add a wineglass of arnica tincture to a bottle of old white wine and twice a day rub this mixture in well with a flannel cloth, especially from the arm to the spine.

Also take a pinch of powdered eggshell with a spoon of milk daily, and a sugarspoon of white mustard seed three times a day.

BACKACHE/PAIN IN THE CROTCH

There arc so many different causes of backache that it is advisable to consult a physician, especially if the remedies which have been applied have not brought about any improvement. It may be caused by rheumatism, sciatica, female complaints, piles, nerves, cancer sores, or the rectum. One should refer to those illnesses. Remedies that can be tried are:

1) Mix 1 part spirits of ammonia with 8 parts olive oil; gently rub the back with this twice a day. This is a particularly good palliative remedy and may be used in all cases of backache.

2) It also sometimes helps to rub with camphorated spirits or camphorated oil. A mixture of ¼ cup (50 grams) camphorated spirits with ¼ cup (50 grams) spirits of turpentine can also be used and rubbed on the back twice a day.

BAD BREATH

1) Take 1 sugarspoon of black bone-dust,[2] mixed with sugar or chocolate, in a small amount of milk four times a day.

2) Mix equal quantities of charcoal powder and chocolate powder (cocoa, etc); take ½ a sugarspoonful every evening in a small amount of milk.

3) Drink a cup of spearmint tea mixed with ½ sugarspoon of caraway seed daily.

BASEDOW'S ILLNESS (MORBUS BASEDOWII)

Basedow's Illness, so called after Doctor Basedow from Maagdenburg, who was the first to describe it, is a singular disease

---

[2]Bone-dust is chalk, specifically, black bone-dust was made from the ashes of the bones of a healthy ox.

of the nervous system. It usually begins with strong palpitations, agitated pulse, internal uneasiness, distention of the eyeballs, and severe swelling of the thyroid glands. It is also called scrofula and often occurs in women and particularly in chlorotic girls—seldom in men. Treatments are as follows:

1) Many people unable to find relief anywhere have been radically cured by a mild water cure, such as whole body washes, neck waterings, neck compresses, sometimes cold half-baths and various herbal mixtures (see Water Cures, p. 401).

2) Herbal tea, such as 2 cups of speedwell tea daily, may be highly recommended.

3) Holding a bag of warm salt against the throat can provide relief.

4) Fill a bag made of fine linen or muslin cloth with the following mixture: ¼ ounce (4 grams) ammonium chloride, ¾ ounce (16 grams) slaked lime (calcium hydroxide) which must first be allowed to dry a little, and ¼ cup (32 grams) powdered oak bark. Grind all these ingredients to a powder and place it round the throat. The contents should be renewed every fourteen days.

5) A nun who had tried all possible remedies in vain soon fully recovered by means of the following breathing exercises:

Breathe deeply ten times. Breathe deeply ten times with the mouth closed and breathe out with the mouth open. Breathe deeply outside lying on the ground or in front of an open window with the head a little raised. Follow this by breathing in seven times with the fingers pressing on the lungs just as one would press the keys of a piano, and breathing out while beating on the chest with the fists. The patient should begin these exercises with care; to begin, he or she should breathe in only two or three times and gradually increase the number, otherwise the strain will exceed the patient's strength.

BEDSORES (DECUBITUS)
To avoid bedsores, rub the red patch twice a day with half a lemon. If you have bedsores, do the following:

1) Fry some sage in unsalted butter and smear on the open sore.

2) Smear the sores with melted candle fat mixed with Bordeaux wine twice a day.

3) Let pips or seed from the quince steep in French brandy and wipe the red patches with this twice a day.

4) Take 3 cups (600 grams) olive oil and 2 tablespoons (15 grams) yellow wax; let the wax melt in the olive oil in a double boiler, then add 17 ounces (500 grams) white lead, let it boil thoroughly, remove from the fire, leave to cool, add 3 tablespoons (31 grams) camphor and apply a plaster of this daily.

5) Melt ¼ cup (30 grams) white wax in ⅓ cup (60 grams) olive oil, cool a little and stir in a well-beaten egg yolk. Smear the affected area with this three times a day, or liberally smear the ointment on lint and apply this.

6) Mix well-beaten egg white with an equal quantity of French brandy; smear the place with this twice a day.

7) The following is a very potent remedy against bedsores: let 8 spoons olive oil boil in a new glazed earthenware pot. As soon as it begins to boil, add 5 teaspoons (10 grams) white wax. When this has melted, add 1 tablespoon white zinc. Allow it to boil a little longer, remove from the fire and keep stirring until the ointment is cold. Smear this on twice a day.

BED-WETTING (ENURESIS NOCTURNA)
1) This simple remedy may be employed to break children of this habit. When the child goes to bed, a towel should be tied around him with the knots at the back. Should there be an impulse to urinate, the child will want to lie on his back, but this will be prevented by the knots and the child will wake up.

2) If the bed-wetting is caused by over-sensitivity of the bladder, goats' or sheeps' milk with sugar is an excellent remedy.

3) A good tea against bed-wetting is:

>6 teaspoons (2 grams) horsetail
>3 teaspoons (3 grams) tormentil
>7 teaspoons (4 grams) plantain

Leave this to steep for twenty minutes in 2 cups (½ liter) boiling water. Give 3 tablespoons three times a day.

4) Tread water (up to the calves) twice a day, two to five minutes each time. This has cured not only many young children but also older ones age 16 to 18. (See Part III, Water Cures, p. 411.)

5) A successful remedy is a sugarspoon of powdered agrimony in a glass of Bordeaux wine in the evening before retiring; this remedy is also excellent for urinary incontinence in older people.

6) Tea made from equal quantities of yarrow and chamomile flowers strengthens a weak bladder in children. Drinking oak leaf tea every evening may also help this condition.

7) The following very old recipe is most efficacious: boil a good handful of parsley with an equal equantity of houseleek (*Sempervivum tectorum*) in 8 cups (2 liters) milk and 4 cups (1 liter) buttermilk until only 1 quart (1 liter) remains; remove it from the fire, strain through a cloth and add 2½ tablespoons (30 grams) of tartar. This quantity must be used in one day. It is not usually necessary to use this remedy more than three times, but while it is being taken, nothing else should be drunk.

8) Place the foot of the bed higher than the head.

BILIOUS COLIC

With bilious colic there is severe pain beneath the ribs and heart, particularly at night. There is also sometimes nausea, belching, a very bitter taste in the mouth, and bilious vomiting. You can try one of the treatments:

1) A recommended remedy is chicory tea. Drink 2 cups a day, for four or five days. Common wormwood tea is also good.

Bilious colic can be avoided by taking 1 teaspoon (3 grams) of tartar daily or:

2) Let 1⅓ cups (20 grams) fresh greater celandine (*Chelidonium majus*) steep in a bottle of white wine; take 3 to 4 tablespoons daily. This remedy should not be used if there is much burning.

3) Tea made from chamomile flowers, especially common chamomile, is still one of the best remedies.

4) Compresses of hayseed (or hot water and vinegar) are also highly efficacious here.

5) If there is also constipation, 1 to 2 tablespoons of castor oil should be taken.

BILIOUS VOMITING

1) A remedy for this complaint is to take an egg yolk with a little sugar and 1 tablespoon of French brandy.

2) Drink a large quantity of lemon water or simply cold water.

3) Steep 2 teaspoons (3 grams) aloe, 2 teaspoons (3 grams) myrrh and 2 teaspoons (3 grams) jalap in ⅓ cup (100 grams) gin for two days. Take 2 tablespoons (25 grams) in the mornings on an empty stomach. This acts as a purgative and purifies the gall.

4) Drinking large quantities of sour buttermilk and eating dry rusks is also an excellent remedy.

5) To avoid bilious vomiting, fresh herring is highly recommended.

BITE FROM A MAD DOG

Before the doctor arrives, immediately and constantly apply compresses of chemically pure soda water as hot as possible, renewing them every ten to fifteen minutes. Even better, bathe the limb, if possible, in strong soda water. If no chemically pure soda is available, common soda (baking soda) may be used, two handfuls to every quart (liter) of water.

BLADDER CATARRH/BLADDER COMPLAINTS/URINARY INCONTINENCE

In old people this is mostly a paralysis of the bladder—very difficult to treat and very seldom cured. In children, the water escapes without their being aware of it. This ailment often cures itself as the children grow older.

1) Cold baths for three seconds, treading water, and common St. Johnswort tea can be highly recommended. In addition, three times a week use hot compresses of hayseed decoction placed on the lower part of the body for half an hour. (For a definition of decoction, see footnote 25 on p. 136.)

2) Before retiring in the evening, take a glass of Bordeaux wine with a sugarspoon of powdered agrimony (see also Goldenrod).

BLADDER INFLAMMATION

Inflammation of the bladder causes a burning pain in the area around the bladder, external swelling, burning, and pain on contact. The urine burns and is red; there is stoppage of the water, constipation, fever, strong pulse rate, sometimes vomiting.

Hot compresses of horsetail are highly recommended, also hot poultices of linseed meal on the lower part of the body. A probe is usually necessary here. One should not fail, therefore, to consult a physician.

In the case of stoppage of the urine, a decoction of wild rosehips is highly beneficial. With stoppage, however, one should not be confused by the absence of the urine which is, above all, accompanied by a desire to urinate without the patient being able to achieve it. This stoppage can be a weakening or paralysis of the bladder, or an obstruction of the prostate (in males) caused by inflammation as described above. Most of these complaints must be opened by means of a probe.

1) A hip vapor bath of horsetail decoction may be tried, especially if the obstruction is due to a chill; a hot bath of oatstraw decoction is sometimes of great value.

2) An excellent and unusually potent remedy is to take 2 cups goldenrod tea daily.

3) Another very potent remedy is the following mixture:

> ½ cup (15 grams) cherry, laurel
> ¾ cup (15 grams) dead-nettle
> 3 tablespoons (15 grams) calamus
> ⅓ cup (30 grams) juniper berries
> ¼ cup (30 grams) hempseed
> ¾ cup (30 grams) rosemary
> ⅓ cup (30 grams) licorice
> ¼ cup (30 grams) black currant skins (*Ribes nigrum*)
> ¼ teaspoon (10 centigrams) saffron

Boil these ingredients together in 4 quarts (4 liters) water until reduced by half. Take 4 to 5 tablespoons *hot* three times a day: in the mornings on an empty stomach, at 11:00 A.M. and before retiring.

BLADDER RASH (PEMPHIGUS FOLIACEUS)
Apply hot compresses of horsetail decoction. In a case when all other possible remedies had been applied in vain for months, this remedy cured a lady within a few weeks.

BLADDER STONES (UROLITHI)
Continual pressure to urinate, often with severe pain; with the stream of water frequently breaking off or stopping completely during the act; external itching, continual mucous deposit in the urine containing grit, sand or small stones, sometimes mixed with blood—these are signs of bladder stones. One can almost certainly conclude that there is a stone present in the bladder, but only a medical investigation can determine this for sure. One of the following treatments may be of help:

1) Oatstraw tea is a potent remedy for expelling stones; in addition a hot compress of oatstraw decoction can be applied to the lower part of the body. 2 to 3 cups knotgrass tea is also very efficacious as I have often experienced.

2) If a person has stones, the pain should first be stilled by drinking a decoction of linseed tea and also by applying hot compresses to the lower part of the body.

3) Steep mistletoe in gin and take 1 tablespoon of this three times a day. The following remedy can also be recommended. Mix together thoroughly ½ cups (100 grams) walnut oil, ½ cup (100 grams) sweet almond oil. Take 3 sugarspoons of this twice a day. Also take 1 cup licorice tea.

4) Take 15 Dutch Drops[3] daily in milk. Goldenrod steeped in wine may also be of help.

BLEEDING

Apply cotton wool dipped in hot water to the place or, if possible, place the limb in hot water. I used this remedy twice when I severely cut my big toe. I placed the foot in hot water and on both occasions the bleeding stopped immediately. I acquired this simple remedy from a French doctor. The following remedies are also useful:

1) Sprinkle charcoal powder on the bleeding wound, or mix wheat flour with an equal quantity of salt and bind this around the wound, or quite simply sprinkle it on the wound and bind a cloth round it.

2) The bleeding can also be stopped by binding Madonna lily petals around the wound. If anyone wishes to preserve these petals, it can be easily done by leaving the freshly picked lily petals to steep for several days in strong gin and then allowing them to dry.

3) Another highly valued remedy is arnica tincture. Diluted arnica tincture should be used. Mix ⅓ water with the tincture in which a piece of cotton wool should be dipped and then placed on the bleeding wound. Not only will the bleeding stop, but the wound will be completely healed very quickly. On sev-

---

[3]A medicine made in Haarlem since 1672 and consisting of a preparation of oil of turpentine, tincture of guaiacum, spirit of niter, oil of amber and oil of cloves; once a popular remedy.

eral occasions I have found that large fresh wounds healed within three days.

One day a boy came along to see me; he had been bitten in the arm by a large dog. I was shocked when I saw the ugly wound; I cleaned it out with diluted arnica tincture, applied a piece of cotton wool dipped in arnica tincture and gave him a little bottle to take along so he could renew it as soon as the cotton wool began to dry. The next day he fetched another bottle and on the third day it had closed up very well. By quoting examples here and there, my intention is to offer encouragement to those who are suffering.

BLEEDING FROM THE NAVEL
Apply compresses of arnica tincture, half diluted with water.

BLEEDING FROM THE NAVEL (IN CHILDREN)
Apply compresses of arnica tincture, diluted with half water.

BLISTERS ON THE FEET FROM WALKING
When you get blisters on your feet from too much walking, you can do the following:

1) Take hot footbaths of horsetail or hayseed decoction for twelve to fifteen minutes.

2) Mix arnica tincture with half water; dip a piece of cotton wool in this and apply to the blister; renew it as soon as it begins to dry.

BLOCKAGE OF LIVER AND GALLBLADDER
1) Drink tea made from parsley, white horehound, angelica, or common centaury. Every day drink 1 cup of tea from one of these herbs.

2) Let 2 handsful box leaves steep in a bottle of gin; take 2 tablespoons daily.

BLOOD POISONING

I have frequently discovered with this complaint that pain and swelling quickly subside if the limb is placed in cold, raw buttermilk, or, if buttermilk is not available, in sour milk, until the pain, swelling, and blue color have quite gone. The milk should be changed as soon as it becomes warm. If neither buttermilk nor sour milk are available, soda water should be used, as hot as possible. Two handfuls of soda, preferably chemically pure, to each quart (liter) of water. The affected limb should be held in this until all danger has passed. After bathing, a hot poultice of fenugreek, or, failing that, a poultice of linseed should immediately be applied. This is particularly good for nighttime use. If the affected limb cannot be bathed, hot compresses of soda water, cold buttermilk, or sour milk should be constantly applied. These compresses should be renewed very frequently.

A butcher came to me with a very painful, extremely swollen arm and hand. The doctor had already opened up his hand twice. A bone of a recently slaughtered cow had deeply pierced the ball of the thumb, causing immediate blood poisoning. I advised him to bathe his hand at once in a strong solution of chemically pure soda water for six hours, the water being as hot as possible and renewed every twenty minutes, as the water or the solution should always remain hot otherwise it would not help at all. After the six hours had passed, he should apply a poultice of fenugreek and leave it on the whole night. I told him to return the following morning. The next day the butcher came to thank me for the radical cure.

A baker had been stung by an insect; this first appeared as a small, very painful blister, the size of a pea. I opened it with a needle and applied a poultice of fenugreek. The man was unable to sleep the whole night long from pain; the hand was badly swollen and so painful that I feared the worst. I sent him to the doctor immediately; as the latter could not be reached, I was greatly disturbed and good advice was dear. From sheer necessity, I prepared a poultice of potatoes and buttermilk which I applied very thickly directly to the hand, renewing it as soon as it began to dry; the following day the hand was much better and my fears subsided. I told him to continue to apply the same poultice; the next day the hand was quite back to normal.

I should like to quote a third case so as to show that these two cures were not pure coincidence. A worried, agitated gentleman came to show me his very swollen, painful hand, the cause of which was quite unknown to him. The hand was becoming increasingly painful and swollen, even the arm was beginning to swell. I advised him to bathe the hand immediately in cold buttermilk and to apply a poultice of fenugreek around it at night. Two days later, the happy gentleman returned to inform me delightedly that the pain had immediately decreased on bathing the hand in buttermilk, and when he awoke the following morning the hand was back to normal.

I could quote many more such examples, but it would be unnecessary. If such cases occur, they can be safely treated by means of these remedies.

•   •   •

To avoid blood poisoning, you can do the following: after a cut from some kind of object, or a stab or fall, or sting from a poisonous insect, Peruvian balsam[4] should be immediately applied. This may be purchased from any herbal dispensary or drugstore. It is most advisable to keep a small bottle in stock. Instead of Peruvian balsam, sour milk, buttermilk or soda water can equally well be used, or even better, as described above. Or a poultice of boiled leek can be applied three times a day.

BLOOD-SPITTING (HEMOPTYSIS)
Coughing or spitting blood can have so many varied causes that only a physician can give the reason with certainty. It is therefore essential to submit to an examination by a qualified doctor. If there is no doctor in the neighborhood, one should first ensure that the patient lies flat in bed, remains very calm and refrains from speaking. He or she should be given nothing to

---

[4]Peruvian Balsam: a brown-yellow aromatic balsam, smelling a little like vanilla, comes from the trunk of a Central American tree, *Myroxylon Balsamum var. pepeirae* (Fam. *Papilionaceae*). It has been used as a fixative in the soap and perfume industry and as a remedy for healing wounds. *Tr.*

eat but may be allowed salt water to drink. If the blood-spitting is accompanied by a mild cough, and the blood is bright red and foaming, it comes from the lungs. If the blood comes up without a cough, and is dark red, as thick as coffee, sometimes mixed with food, it comes from the stomach and this indicates stomach disease or ulceration or cancer of the stomach. It can, however, be caused by piles and by excessively heavy or suppressed menstruation. There are a number of possible treatments:

1) The treatment for spitting blood from the lungs is: take cold drinks, salt water, and cold compresses on the stomach region; tea made from a mixture of shepherd's purse and horsetail. In this case one should take 1½ to 2¼ cups (30–50 grams) in 2 cups (½ liter) of water and give it at the onset of blood-spitting. If it is frequently repeated, give 1 tablespoon, cold, every ten minutes. As the blood-spitting diminishes, lessen the dosage of tea.

2) If the blood comes from the stomach, the tea is also good; even better is 1⅓ to 2 cups (20–30 grams) sanicle boiled in 2 cups (½ liter) water to which 2 tablespoons of honey should be added. At the onset, 1 tablespoon should be given every half-hour to every two hours.

3) If the blood-spitting is caused by excessively heavy menstruation, the following medicine is more advisable than the previous one: take 1⅔ cups (50 grams) willow leaves, reduce them in 3 cups (¾ liter) of wine to ⅛; a small wineglass of this should be taken three times a day.

4) Boil 1 cup (30 grams) comfrey in 1½ quarts (1½ liters) water until reduced by half. Strain through a linen cloth and take 1 tablespoon three times a day.

5) Yarrow tea is also an efficacious remedy. At the onset take 2 teaspoons every fifteen minutes, then 1 tablespoon every half hour. If the blood-spitting decreases, the patient may proceed to take 1 tablespoon every hour.

6) See also Part II: Aaron's rod (mullein), comfrey, speedwell, agrimony, stinging nettles, etc.

BONE DISEASE (OSTITIS)

Inflammation of the bones, peristoneum or marrow—which can only be diagnosed by a doctor—generally begins with high fever and severe pain in the affected limb. This part gradually begins to swell—a sign that the bone is inflamed. Chronic inflammation of the bone is mainly caused by tuberculosis and develops much more slowly, is less noticeable, and without much pain; it can sometimes last for years, gradually increasing. Pus collects and seeks an outlet—a fistula.

The finest cures are effected by the following simple remedies; they may be applied without fear since they cannot cause the least harm. I applied them to more than four hundred such patients within three years and nearly always with the best results.

1) Dissolve a good handful of chemically pure soda (*Carbonas natricus*) to each quart (liter) boiling water and bathe the affected limb four times a day for twenty minutes. If the limb cannot be bathed, apply the hottest possible compress of the same solution four times a day for half an hour. Immediately after the bath or compress, apply a hot poultice of fenugreek; in the evening again a poultice which must remain in position the whole night. If a leg or hip is affected, the patient must stay in bed until fully recovered, otherwise the leg will remain twisted or stiff.

After the application of baths for some time, painful swelling sometimes occurs in the infected area; this should not give rise to alarm as the recovery is usually not far off. This swelling and pain will speedily disappear if a poultice of potatoes and buttermilk (see also Sores) is applied around the swollen part three times a day. Baths and compresses should naturally not be taken while the poultice is being applied, but may be taken as soon as the swelling and pain have subsided. Continue with baths or compresses even if there are open sores with much pus, etc.

The chemically pure soda dissolves all waste matter, draws it out and has a power of healing which sometimes surpasses all understanding. It is also antiseptic. But those who suffer from tubercular bone disease should not think that they can be cured in a few weeks; that is quite impossible. They must be patient but the cure is bound to come.

2) Baths or compresses of oatstraw or horsetail infusion have also been found very beneficial. The application of water cures (see pp. 406, 409) is also advisable with this treatment; likewise taking some kind of depurative tea, for example yarrow or meadowsweet, speedwell or heartsease and half a sugarspoon of bone dust twice a day; children only a pinch twice a day. The patients should abstain from coffee, beer, alcoholic drinks, spices, excessive salt, pork, black bread, potatoes and too many vegetables. They must eat nourishing, wholesome food; tonic soup is particularly good. The food should contain protein, much fat, milk, eggs, meat, beef tea. A few examples of water cures are as follows:

• A lady from V. suffered from tubercular ulceration of the elbow. After various medicines had been tried, she was injected for three weeks. The result was a stiff, wasted arm so that amputation was being considered. She was radically cured in six weeks by application of the soda baths described above.

• A lady from the neighborhood of Cologne had six open sores on the hip and abdomen and had sought a cure for years in vain. Hot soda hip baths and a gentle water cure cured her in three months.

• A 10 year old child from Heimsberg was cured of tubercular hip sores in six months.

• A 22 year old lady had been operated on her hip and leg six times in eight years. Her arm was now also affected by inflammation. After taking the soda cure for five months, she was cured; this took place four years ago and she still enjoys good health.

• A girl from a neighboring town lay in hospital for nine months with a tubercular foot which had already been operated on three times; the foot was very enlarged, unnaturally swollen and very painful. Amputation had been decided on when my advice was sought. I advised the soda cure and after nine months the foot had healed so well that she was walking in tight fitting shoes.

· While I was writing this last description, an artist from Dus-
seldorf called on me to thank me for the complete recovery
of his tubercular hand. Exactly one year ago, this same gentleman came to ask my advice; I hardly had the courage to
prescribe a remedy for him. He informed me that his hand
had been operated on two years earlier and since that time
he had been unable to open it. A new tubercular tumor had
now formed. By taking soda baths for a whole year, he was
now—to my great delight—so well healed that he could continue with his painting once again.

·   ·   ·

These examples, of which I could give numerous others, should
be sufficiently eloquent to encourage acquaintance with this
simple remedy in similar cases.

BREASTS (ULCERATED)

1) Apply a plaster of the following ointment twice a day: Take
½ cup (100 grams) of fat from a male swine (boar); ⅛ cup (50
grams) burgundy tar, ½ cup (100 grams) olive oil. Allow these
ingredients to boil together for two hours in the double boiler,
stirring continually with a stick. When the ointment has cooled,
add 2 egg yolks and 1 tablespoon sugar. This ointment is also
very good for burns.

2) Take a handful of the inner rind of limewood, let this boil
in 2 cups (½ liter) water until slimy, then add 2 teaspoons (10
grams) old butter, 1 teaspoon (2 grams) medicinal soap and
enough wheat flour to make a not too thick paste. Apply this
to the ulcerated breast. The pain will swiftly subside, but will
return after a few hours. Apply a fresh poultice and the breast
will soon open up. When it has opened, apply the following
mixture: Take 2 egg yolks with 2 teaspoons (10 grams) sweet
butter. Part of this mixture should be smeared on the ulcer,
after which the poultice may again be applied. When the ulcer
is no longer burning, ½ teaspoon (2 grams) of Peruvian balsam
may be added to the mixture of egg yolks and sweet butter.

This remedy cured within a few weeks a woman who had
seven holes in her breast and was threatened with removal of
the breast. That was thirty years ago and the woman is still
healthy.

BRONCHITIS

Bronchitis is a severe cold, also called lung and chest catarrh. If it is a mild attack with little fever and a moist cough with phlegm, see Cough.

If the cold is really heavy and the cough dry with constriction on the chest, great care should be taken; if such a cold is neglected, it can become chronic and is very difficult to cure. The following prescription is highly recommended:

1) A daily whole wash, three upper body waterings three times a week and three hot compresses of vinegar and water on the chest for half an hour each week. Every two hours take 1 tablespoon of tea made from angelica, plantain, fennel seed and stinging nettles. Or every two hours take 1 tablespoon tea made from hop flowers or coltsfoot with ground ivy or moneywort. (See also Chest and Lung Catarrh.)

BRONCHITIS (CHEST CATARRH)

The easiest way of curing this complaint is by taking the following every week: four whole washes, applying three cold water and vinegar compresses on the chest for half an hour, and taking 1 tablespoon tea made from the following mixture every two hours: coltsfoot, ground ivy and angelica—equal quantities of each mixed together. Steep 1 tablespoon of this for twenty minutes in an ordinary cup of boiling water, then strain it and add 1 tablespoon honey to the infusion, bringing it briefly to the boil again.

Before retiring also take a cup of hot tea made from elder and chamomile flowers with sugar.

BRUISES/SWELLINGS/DISLOCATIONS

1) Apply compresses of arnica tincture mixed with an equal quantity of water.

2) Apply clay compreses mixed with arnica tincture.

3) Powdered fenugreek mixed to a paste with honey and placed on the bruised or swollen area is an excellent remedy.

4) Dissolve 2 ounces (60 grams) green soap in 1¼ cups (270

grams) French brandy (or 1 quart (liter) 50% alcohol). Apply compresses of this, or use a rapeseed oil compress.

5) Smear the following mixture on a linen cloth and apply twice a day: 4 tablespoons (32 grams) alum powder, ¼ cup (60 grams) gin, and the white of 2 eggs, beaten well together.

6) Rub three times a day with the following mixture: 1 tablespoon (10 grams) camphorated oil, ½ teaspoon (1 gram) spike oil, ¼ cup (50 grams) turpentine and 1½ cups (350 grams) gin; this is also an excellent remedy for cramps in the legs.

7) Rub 3 times a day with this mixture: ½ ounce (15 grams) camphorated spirit, ½ ounce (15 grams) opodeldoc (camphorated soap liniment) and 2 teaspoons (5 grams) juniper oil.

8) Boil a quantity of vervain in vinegar; apply compresses which should be renewed as soon as they begin to dry.

9) Place the limb in heavily salted cold water; the inflammation or swelling will quickly disappear.

10) For lumps on the feet from shoes or clogs, apply a poultice of fenugreek, alernated with hay compresses.

11) For knotty swelling, apply mashed houseleek or hay compresses. If this is continued for some time, the knotty swelling will disappear.

BULIMIA

Those who have occasional attacks of bulimia are advised to carry a lump of sugar to be used in case of an attack. It is also helpful to chew some plant or other.

BURNS

1) In the case of a burn, the affected limb should immediately be plunged into cold water and kept there for six hours, with renewal of the water. Or cold compresses should be constantly applied. After six hours, the burns will be completely cured.

2) A good cure for burns is the following: beat the white of an egg until stiff, add 1 tablespoon uncooked linseed and sufficient

chalk powder to make a not too thick ointment; smear this very thickly on cotton wool and place it on the wound. This should be renewed before the ointment is dry.

3) Take 5¾ cups (300 grams) common St. Johnswort flowers, 1 cup (200 grams) olive oil, 1 cup (200 grams) gin. Allow these ingredients to steep and apply in the form of compresses. This remedy is also good for fresh wounds.

4) Mix equal quantities of cream, olive oil and egg white; apply compresses and renew them as soon as they begin to dry. (See also Hemorrhoid Ointment.)

5) Mix an egg yolk with unsalted butter; smear this liberally on linen cloths and apply.

6) Compresses of sweet milk are also helpful.

7) One of the best and easiest remedies is lanolin (wool fat); it should be generously smeared on linen and applied as a plaster two or three times a day.

8) If a child has been burned and it has been possible to plunge the burned limb immediately into cold water for six hours and to renew the water from time to time, no blisters will form and the child will be unaware of any pain. I myself have used this remedy with optimal results.

9) The following most efficacious remedy is very well known: beat 3 to 4 eggs into 2 cups (½ liter) of uncooked linseed oil and smear the wounds with this four times a day.

10) An excellent ointment for burns: take 2½ cups (500 grams) olive oil and a small handful of the inner rind of elder wood, let this boil thoroughly for half an hour. Squeeze it out and then add white wax, stirring continually until it begins to cool. Apply a plaster of this twice a day. (See also St. Johnswort oil.)

CALLUSES (CORNU CUTANEUM)
1) Apply poultices of fenugreek or hay compresses.

2) Mix 1 part arnica tincture with 10 parts glycerine; rub with this twice a day, or apply it as a compress.

CANCER (CARCINOMA)

Cancer-like ulcerations can sometimes be treated successfully by means of the following remedies:

1) Boil together in 1 quart (liter) water:

⅛ cup (15 grams) oak bark
⅓ cup (10 grams) sage
2 tablespoons (5 grams) common wormwood
⅓ cup (15 grams) tormentil
½ cup (10 grams) horsetail

When these ingredients have boiled for fifteen minutes, strain through a cloth. Then add ½ pound (¼ kilo) honey and bring to a boil again briefly. Wipe the sores with this twice a day. The herbs can also be steeped in alcohol and the honey added later.

2) Place a fairly thick layer of carrot scrapings on the sores and renew it as soon as it begins to dry.

3) Put live (male) lobsters in the oven to dry in an earthenware pot; pound them to a fine powder; take some of the powder and mix with an equal quantity of finely chopped garlic. Place this mixture in a very fine linen bag, sew up the bag, tightly bind it to the cancerous area by means of a bandage so that it cannot slip. Leave for twenty-four hours, then remove it and bury it forthwith in the ground as it spreads a pestilential air. Before removing the bag, it is advisable to tie a cloth with some kind of perfume, camphorated spirit or simply vinegar over the nose. The bag should not be removed with bare hands. Immediately after removal of the bag, a quantity of elder flowers drawn in buttermilk, or boiled in it, should be bound over the cancerous area. The patient should drink a little buttermilk and rest in bed for twelve hours. The elder flowers should then be removed.

If the cancer is not cured, the last remedy should be repeated. As long as the bag of lobster powder, etc., remains on the cancerous area, the patient should be kept awake. A priest, who had cancer on the tongue, informed me that he was cured in twenty-four hours by means of this remedy. The scar could be clearly seen. It should be noted that this remedy is for closed cancer.

4) Drink tea made from goosegrass. In addition, place the freshly crushed herb on the sores, or use compresses of the decoction of dried goosegrass.

5) Mix together fresh comfrey crushed with rye bread and place this on the cancerous sores.

6) It is also recommended to apply crushed fresh chervil mixed with honey.

7) It is most efficacious to drink three cups agrimony tea daily and to use powdered agrimony root in all food.

8) Crushed fresh green leaves of agrimony, mixed with lard, applied as a plaster, is very beneficial for cancer or fistulas.

9) Bruised cinquefoil with the root, mixed with old lard (pork fat) applied as a plaster is a very effective remedy.

10) Crush fresh stinging nettles, add a little salt, and apply on the cancer sores.

11) Make a strong decoction of leaves, stalks and seeds of the white dead-nettle (*Lamium album*), and apply throughout the day as compresses.

12) According to Mathiolus, there is no remedy more splendid for curing cancer than the herb of the blessed thistle (*Cnicus benedictus*). A woman with cancer of the breast, eaten nearly through to the bone, was cured by a decoction of the blessed herb. The sores should be washed four times a day with the decoction and, after each wash, powder from the dried leaves should be sprinkled on them. This remedy is also excellent for old sores.

13) The sap of common toadflax (*Antirrhinum linaria*) with the sap of greater burnet saxifrage cannot be praised highly enough for cancer sores.

14) Apply wine-yeast mixed with an equal quantity of alum to the cancerous place.

15) Juniper wood oil is praised for both internal and external cancer.

16) The following cancer ointment has been most highly recommended to me and used for more than thirty years by a brother in the monastery:

1¼ cup (250 grams) old pork fat
3⅓ pounds (1½ kilos) yellow wax
⅝ cup (125 grams) olive oil
½ cup (15 grams) sage
½ cup (150 grams) white lily bulbs
⅔ cup (250 grams) black tar
½ cup (100 grams) sugar candy
¼ ounce (7½ grams) lead oxide
14 ounces (400 grams) red lead
4 ounces (100 grams) white vitriol (zinc sulphate)
3 teaspoons (5 grams) spirits of white vitriol

Fry the well-chopped pork fat, sage and lily bulbs together; firmly squeeze it through a cloth, place in a glazed earthenware pot, add tar, wax, oil and sugar, leave to boil slowly, stirring continually, until the water in the lily bulbs and sage has evaporated. Remove from the fire, allow to cool a little, then add, while still stirring, the lead oxide, the red lead, the white vitriol, and the vitriol spirits and keep on stirring until the ointment is stiff and cold. During the boiling process scum will form from the tar; this should be skimmed off.

The ointment should be smeared on chamois leather, applied and renewed once a day. The cancer sores should be kept really warm while this ointment is being used. This cancer ointment may be applied to both open and closed cancer. In addition, the patient should drink three cups of tea made from walnut leaves picked halfway through June.

17) Take equal quantities of figs, garlic and leaven; pound them together in a china mortar. With open cancer or cancer sores, apply a fresh poultice daily, preferably in the morning.

18) Pound some garlic and place between two thin linen cloths on open or closed cancer. With open cancer renew every hour, with closed cancer as soon as it begins to dry. (Pub. note: this will burn the skin and form scar tissue.)

19) For cancer of the womb, take walnut blossom tea.

20) For internal cancer, or stomach cancer, tea made from the leaves of the marigold (*Calendula officinalis*) is most efficacious.

21) For cancer of the tongue, a recomended remedy is to sprinkle camphor powder on the affected area a few times daily and to take mouth washes of horsetail tea and salt. It is also good to give the tongue a daily cold watering, if the cancer is near the tip of the tongue.

22) A lady from Brussels was cured in six months of a bleeding cancer, which had been treated unsuccessfully for a long time, by using the following remedies. Throughout the day, use as many compresses of horsetail decoction as possible, alternating now and then with compresses of alum water. In addition, each week use two short compresses of hayseed decoction and a few washes. The lady, who is now about 80, still enjoys good health.

23) To remove the putrid smell of cancer, try using finely pounded cloves that have been boiled in vinegar to keep the air pure. Or place ground coffee in the room. You could also mix 100 parts gypsum with 3 parts coal tar and place in the room.

CARBUNCLE

1) Boil the following ingredients for half an hour to make a not too thick poultice:

  1 quart (1 liter) brown ale
  16 oz. (500 grams) rye bread
  ¾ cup (25 grams) elder flowers
  1 cup (25 grams) chamomile flowers (matricaria)
  3 tablespoons (38 grams) tallow
  3 tablespoons (38 grams) fresh sweet butter

This mixture should be applied thickly five times a day. Before applying the poultice, apply compresses of marshmallow for half an hour. If the poultice is too thick, brown ale should be added. This poultice cures carbuncles, whitlows, plague botches, ulcers and abscesses. I cured a whitlow with this in four days. I also tried this poultice for caries and found it excellent:

the pus burst out, the swelling subsided and even the small bones which were affected came to the surface. It is quite harmless and cannot be recommended highly enough in such cases.

2) Apply fenugreek poultices.

3) The application of basilicum ointment brings it quickly to a head.

CARE AND NOURISHMENT OF INFANTS

The care and nourishment of our little ones is—especially nowadays with the extremely high figures for the death rate in children—a most important topic. A few important directions are as follows: the best and most efficacious nourishment is mother's milk. If the infant cannot have this, weak children should be given 1 part cow's milk mixed with 2 parts boiled water for the first month; the second and third months they should get 1 part water and 1 part milk. From the fourth month onward, 1 part water with 2 parts milk; later on, 3 parts milk and 1 part water, eventually giving undiluted milk. About 2 tablespoons (20 grams) sugar may be added per 4 cups (1 liter) of mixture. Instead of sugar, 3 tablespoons (25 grams) of the best milk-sugar (lactose) may be used per quart (liter) of milk; ordinary sugar turns it sour.

With strong infants it is not so important to pay attention to thinning the milk with boiled water. There are plenty of examples, particularly in the country, of children who take undiluted cows' milk in the very first month. But for weak infants it is essential to follow strictly the dilution as prescribed above.

Before use, the milk must be boiled, that is, well boiled, as harmful germs will only be killed in this way. The milk pan or milk jug must always be kept covered. One should particularly avoid giving sour milk; the use of this will cause very serious digestive disorders. Bottles and sucking apparatus must be scrupulously clean.

Around the seventh or eighth month, the milk can be made into a paste-like consistency with the addition of a little rusk, tonic flour, etc., gradually building up to ordinary solid food. If feeding with milk alone is continued for more than a year, infants frequently suffer from anemia, bone disease, scrofulous complaints, etc. Their teeth do not come so quickly, they stand and walk later and the legs grow crooked. It is very injurious for both infant and mother if the child sucks too long; the mother becomes anemic and weak, with nervous debility; this is later followed by indigestion, pallor, palpitations, attacks of giddiness, etc.

It is a mistake to cover the child with too many hot blankets and very bad to keep it continually swaddled, particularly if the arms are also swaddled. The infant should simply be laid in bed, well-covered, with the blankets securely tucked in so that the child cannot kick them off. A warning should also be given against cradles, since they not only cause vomiting but the organs are rocked and jolted too much.

Always ensure plenty of fresh air; accustom the child at an early age to the fresh air, as soon as there is summer warmth and no wind. One should take care not to let the child stand and walk too early; if it starts too young, the legs grow crooked. Cutting teeth is often a difficult business. When the teeth break through, the pain causes cerebral irritation which is sometimes dangerous. The infant is often restless, refusing food; there is sometimes constipation, other times hot diarrhea. The cerebral irritation frequently causes convulsions, and in that case it is necessary to call the physician, since cerebral disturbance can result in permanent paralysis of the limbs. While awaiting the doctor, apply the following remedies: keep the head cold and place hot rue compresses on the abdomen.

It is advisable and laudable always to keep an eye on the child; one should particularly take care that it does not come into contact with painted or colored objects which it can lick or even swallow. In doing so, it can be exposed to great danger.

CARIES

In the case of caries, one should apply compresses of horsetail, oatstraw or yarrow or, better still, freshly crushed yarrow herb or leaves and also drink a cup of yarrow tea daily. It is beneficial to apply a poultice of fenugreek, alternating with compresses of a mixture of clay, water, and vinegar. Instead of water and vinegar, a strong decoction of yarrow mixed with clay may be recommended. (See also Bone Diseases.)

CHANGE OF LIFE (MENOPAUSE)

Drink tea made from 4 tablespoons (3 grams) common centaury, 3 tablespoons (3 grams) horsetail, and 4 teaspoons (3 grams) vervain; let steep in 2 cups (½ liter) boiling water and take 3 tablespoons three times a day.

CHAPPED HANDS

Rub the hands twice a day with olive oil, sweet almond oil, glycerine, or lanolin.

CHEEKS (SWOLLEN)

The best and simplest remedy is to apply a plaster or poultice of unsalted soft cheese.

CHEST HERBS

1) Take 1 tablespoon (4 grams) each of marshmallow root and coltsfoot, 1½ teaspoons (2 grams) licorice and 1 teaspoon (1 gram) aniseed. Let these ingredients steep together for twenty minutes in 2 cups boiling water, and take 1 tablespoon every two hours.

2) Take ½ cup (30 grams) marshmallow, 3 tablespoons (24 grams) fennel, 3¾ cup (125 grams) coltsfoot, 2⅔ cups (125 grams) veronica, 1 cup (60 grams) angelica, ½ cup (60 grams) polypody root and mix together thoroughly. Let 1 cup (10 grams) of this mixture boil for fifteen minutes in 2 cups (½ liter) water and take 1 tablespoon every hour.

3) Take 1 cup (60 grams) of marshmallow root, 2 cups (60 grams) chicory, 2 cups (60 grams) coltsfoot and 2½ cups (60 grams) plantain. Let 2 cups (60 grams) of this mixture boil for half an hour in 2 cups (½ liter) water; then add 3 tablespoons (15 grams) licorice; allow this to steep for fifteen minutes, strain, and take 1 tablespoon every hour.

4) A good chest and depurative tea can be made as follows: Mix 3 tablespoons (8 grams) betony, ½ cup (8 grams) lemon balm, 1 tablespoon (8 grams) veronica, ¼ cup (8 grams) basilicum, 2 tablespoons (10 grams) sassafras, 1 tablespoon (6 grams)

quinine, 4½ teaspoons (6 grams) licorice, 1 tablespoon (6 grams) polypody root, 1 teaspoon (1 gram) aniseed and 2 teaspoons (1 gram) fennel. Let 1 tablespoon of this mixture steep in 1 cup of boiling water and take 1 cup daily with a spoon.

CHEST AND LUNG CATAARH

Let 2 cups (50 grams) of plantain and ⅓ cup (40 grams) of fennel boil in 1 quart (liter) of water until reduced by one third; strain and add ½ cup (150 grams) of honey; let it now boil for another fifteen minutes over a gentle heat and skim well. Take 1 sugarspoon of this three times a day. This remedy is very good for coughs, phlegm, colic, wind, cramps, phlegm cough, throat ailments, chronic colds, asthma, leukorrhea, consumption, and constipation. It facilitates digestion and is an excellent depurative. (See also Bronchitis.)

CHICKEN POX

This belongs to the list of contagious diseases although it is not dangerous. It is an illness which usually rarely affects children over 12. Its course resembles that of measles. The illness begins with shivering, headaches, a little fever, restless sleep and lack of appetite. The fever continues for one to four days. Small red spots, the size of a pinhead, subsequently appear on the body; they cause severe itching and then develop into smaller or larger blisters filled with a watery fluid. Sometimes the whole body is affected, sometimes only a part. They may even appear in the mouth, in the nose and on the palate; this rash is of little significance. The patient should be kept in bed for a few days, but not kept too warm and should be given fluid nourishment only, for example milk, tonic soup, etc. In order to stop the itching, lukewarm washes may be given, or a daily hay-shirt.

CHILDREN'S INJURIES (PAIN)

Wash the affected place two to four times a day with a decoction of chamomile flowers, horsetail, yarrow, marshmallow, or bran water. Ointments or powders containing lycopodium (this is frequently used) can be very injurious to the child. Baths of the prescribed herbs can also be given. After being washed with the plants mentioned, or bran water, the child should be gently dried and smeared with unsalted butter or cream.

CHILDREN'S SKIN RASHES (EXANTHEM)

Skin rashes can be very varied, taking the form of pimples, dandruff, Crusta lactea (milk rash), head rash, Guinea worm or seborrhea. We are concerned here with the latter; the other complaints are discussed elsewhere in this book. In children, seborrhea (dermatitis) may be found on the forehead, face, or other parts of the body. Small blisters filled with yellow fluid appear, and when they burst, they form crusts which then dry. Although this complaint is not dangerous, one should try to free the child from it as quickly as possible; otherwise it may become more deeply rooted and last for years. I find that the following remedies still give the best results:

1) Boil a handful of heartsease (*Viola tricolor*) in 4 cups (1 liter) milk and give one cup of this daily with a spoon to the small patient. Throughout the day, apply constant hot compresses of this milk on the rash and renew them as soon as they become dry.

2) In the mornings, apply a poultice of soft cheese for three hours. In the evenings, a fresh poultice should remain in position throughout the night. Instead of cheese, potatoes and buttermilk may be used, alternated now and then with a poultice made from clay, water, and vinegar, which should be renewed as soon as it dries.

3) It is advisable after a few days to smear the rash with sweet butter and then sprinkle it with powdered white beans (haricot beans). This should be done twice a day. Meanwhile no further compresses or poultices should be applied; but the patient should continue to drink the milk described above.

The small patient should also be given two or three hay-shirts weekly for an hour-and-a-half each time.

CHOLERA

Cholera is one of the most dangerous illnesses which can affect us; it is dangerous on account of its rapid course, its wide-spread effect and the innumerable victims it generally claims. Should anyone be attacked by this illness, one should first ensure that the patient is warmed up; to that end the patient should be rubbed hard with bare hands, with a brush or a piece of flannel soaked in camphorated spirit.

If warmth does not speedily follow, the patient's whole body should be massaged; if that does not help either, stinging nettles should be placed on the body. To reduce the vomiting, rather thick starch solutions should be given; this will also counteract the diarrhea, if it is mixed with a little comfrey decoction.

Because the patient is suffering a great loss of fluid, he or she has an acute thirst which burns the throat and chest; for this reason a large glass of fresh water should be placed within reach so that he or she may drink at will. This simple remedy has saved many people from cholera.

1) A remedy for the cramps is to rub the patient hard as described above. The following remedies will also help to fight cholera.

2) Take 1 cup sweet milk, 2 tablespoons olive oil and 2 tablespoons gin; mix this well. The patient should drink this in one dose and go to bed. He or she will soon begin to sweat, and recovery frequently follows.

3) Another remedy is as follows: Take 1 tablespoon ripe plantain seed (*Plantago major*) and a handful of vervain; boil these ingredients together in 1 quart (liter) water and give the patient a cupful every two hours. The plantain seed stops the dysentery; the vervain makes the stiffened blood, causing the coldness, fluid again.

4) This remedy is from Monseigneur Kneipp: The patient feels very shivery, severe cold over the whole body, first in one place, then in another. He or she has acute cramps in the stomach and intestines, cold hands and feet, and loss of energy; the muscles become totally weak; muscles, blood and saps are severely affected. Recovery will follow if rough linen cloths,

folded into six or eight, are quickly soaked in water and vinegar, wrung out and laid as hot as possible on the patient, from the chest to the lower part of the body, even over the knees. After five minutes, this compress must be renewed and again applied as hot as possible. After another five minutes, the patient will become restless and begin to sweat, and the compress is renewed for the third time. The sweating becomes consequently heavier; the compress is renewed yet again and the patient is left to sweat as much as possible. The more he or she sweats the better, and the patient is saved but very weak. He or she should be given complete rest for two days; a hot compress should be laid on the back and he or she should simply be left to sweat.

There is nothing further to do other than three or four whole washes per day. If the patient is again attacked by cold, the compresses should be repeated. Internally the patient should be given 1 tablespoon milk boiled with fennel every ten minutes. This has an affect on urination and wind. After five days, the patient is much better. If there is any sign of appetite, tonic soup is the best food. After fourteen days, the patient will greatly improve and after a month, he or she can return to work.

5) To make a cholera tincture take ¼ cup (32 grams) elecampane, ⅓ cup (32 grams) yellow gentian root, ¼ cup (32 grams) angelica root and 4 teaspoons (10 grams) Simaruba Honduras bark. Place all the ingredients in 1 quart (liter) of gin and let steep for three weeks. Adults should be given 1 liqueur glass daily; children of twelve years a good tablespoon and so on according to age. This remedy is also good against cholerine.[5] It must be taken as soon as the cramp is felt and continued until a full recovery takes place.

COLIC

Most intestinal pain is called colic. It may have different causes; this is why there are different kinds of colic. We shall deal with the most common forms.

---

[5]Cholerine is British or summer cholera, a mild diarrhea; the term has also been used to describe the early stages of cholera.

1) Wind colic is caused by excessive gas in the stomach and intestines. It is usually due to indigestion, weakness and severe gastric irritability, caused by heavy, windy food such as cabbage, peas and beans, but it can also be the result of a nervous condition. That is why colic is found in hysterical people or hypochondriacs and in those whose abdomen has been weakened by numerous purgatives, too much sitting, etc. The treatment of wind colic is very simple: Place hot compresses of hayseed, water and vinegar, or chamomile flowers on the abdomen and renew them very half hour. Drink tea made from aromatic, stimulating herbs or seeds, such as aniseed, fennel, mint, angelica, yarrow, chamomile flowers, lemon balm, hyssop, caraway seed, dill, sage, etc. Volatile oils are also recommended, for example: spike oil, peppermint oil, aniseed oil, fennel oil, etc. Take 4 to 5 drops on sugar two or three times a day; if the colic continues, 4 drops may be taken every hour. They should not, however, be misused. A sugarspoon of salt in half a glass of cold water also brings rapid relief.

2) Nervous colic is a complaint frequently caused by acute anxiety, secret abuse, particularly in those who suffer from nerves and by catching cold. The colic is generally seated near the navel and is easily recognized by pressing a finger on the painful area, whereby the pain noticeably decreases. It is often coupled with nausea and vomiting. During this complaint, the pulse is weak and irregular, the skin cold. The treatment is the same as in wind colic but, instead of using compresses, poultices of linseed meal or fenugreek may be applied, if the basic compresses do not bring about a speedy recovery.

3) Colic Miserere is a complaint that is very dangerous and often fatal. There is severe, unbearable abdominal pain, vomiting of matter which cannot move on account of obstinate obstruction in the stomach and intestines. Symptoms of this illness are as follows: pallor, drawn face, crouched sitting position of the body, difficulty in breathing, bad breath, weak, irregular pulse, cold body temperature, etc. A physician should be consulted immediately. While awaiting his arrival, place very hot poultices of linseed or fenugreek on the abdomen, give frequent hot drinks but only a little at a time, preferably with a spoon: tea made from cinquefoil. Even better is tea made from

cinquefoil boiled in milk with the addition of a little fennel and honey; you can also use barley water or chamomile flower tea.

4) For colic in children you can use the following. If the stools are green, combine 2 sugarspoons magnesia, 2 sugarspoons sugar, ½ egg yolk, 1 cup fennel seed tea. Mix all ingredients thoroughly. This mixture should be given every two hours. In the opposite case, give aniseed tea. Wet nurses can take the same; this will stop the child's colic and improve the quality and quantity of the milk. Or, mix 1 tablespoon sugar with 1 table-spoon olive oil; this should be taken in one dose. It is very good for adults, too.

Colic/Cramps from Hemorrhoids (Piles)

Place hot compresses of water and vinegar on the abdomen; boiled hayseed compresses are even better. Also drink 1 cup common chamomile tea. If common chamomile is not available, ordinary chamomile flowers may be used. Grated carrot can be applied to painful external swellings; this is an excellent remedy to take away the burning. It is also good to spend ten minutes a day sitting on a cold, wet, wrung out towel folded in eight. Itching and painful hemorrhoids should be washed with the following mixture: 1 teaspoon (4 grams) Hoffman's Balsam[6] dissolved in 1½ cups (350 grams) strong chamomile tea.

1) Take dried horse chestnuts with the rind and pound them to a powder and ingest a pinch of the mixture twice a day. This remedy is especially recommended if the piles itch severely, are very painful and are not bleeding.

2) Smear the piles twice a day with Dutch Drops: this causes them to shrivel up. In addition drink 2 cups of tea every day that is made from stinging nettles, white horehound, or yarrow. It is recommended to take 1 tablespoon olive oil every morning and evening. Note: Dutch Drops may be replaced by the fol-lowing excellent ointment. Boil ⅔ cup (125 grams) melted tallow with ½ cup (100 grams) olive oil for a few minutes. This is very

---

[6]Hoffman's Balsam is a mixture of eugenol oils of cinnamon, lavender, lemon, myristica (nutmeg) and thyme in ⅖ p. c. alcohol.

good ointment to use on children when they have injuries, burns, chapped hands and feet.

3) Fry spearmint very slowly in a little unsalted butter, but do not let the butter brown. Smear the piles with this mixture three times a day. Also take a daily hot hip-bath (see Part III, The Water Cure) of chamomile flowers or common figwort. Use approximately 1 cup (100 grams) for each bath.

4) Pile Powder: Mix 2½ cups (40 grams) purified flowers of sulfur[7] with 3 tablespoons (40 grams) cream of tartar and ⅓ cup (40 grams) powdered sugar; take a sugarspoonful three times a day in a little water or milk. This is an efficacious remedy.

CONGESTION OF BLOOD IN THE HEAD (CONGESTIO)

The symptoms of congestion of blood in the head are the following: the face is very red; the head heavy and drowsy, there is dizziness, ringing in the ears, strong pulsation of the veins in the neck and temples, sparkling eyes and dryness in the nose. To relieve this, try the following:

1) Every morning and evening do a cold upper body wash; every other day a half-bath, taken kneeling, for three to five seconds; hot footbaths containing a handful of salt and two handfuls of wood ash, for twelve to fourteen minutes; every week a cold compress of vinegar on the back for half an hour and the same for half an hour on the chest, but these compresses should not be applied at the same time. A wet shirt may be alternated with the compresses; on retiring, cold foot compresses are highly recommended.[8]

2) Drink 1 or 2 cups speedwell tea daily; this remedy cannot be praised highly enough as it certainly hastens recovery; the potency of this tea is astonishing. Taking 20 to 25 drops of rue tincture twice daily is also beneficial.

3) Take 15 to 25 drops of rue and valerian tincture twice a

---

[7]Flowers of sulphur are a form of sulphur crystals that are still available at some pharmacies. These are not to be confused with precipitated sulphur.
[8]See section on the Water Cure.

day—equal quantities of both mixed together. This should be taken in a spoon of cold water one hour before or one hour after meals.

4) A cup of tea made from equal quantities of speedwell and vervain taken twice daily is a powerful remedy.

5) In addition, the following water applications are highly efficacious: Every morning and evening an upper body wash; once a week a cold compress of water and vinegar on the back for three quarters of an hour and a similar compress daily on the chest; three knee waterings and walking on wet stones for five to ten minutes every day.

CONSTIPATION

To avoid this condition, one should acquire the habit of regular bowel movement at an appointed time each morning; the body will gradually become accustomed to it. I advise anyone plagued by constipation to eat tonic soup[9] every day, to eat invigorating, easily digestible food, and to walk for three minutes barefoot every day on wet stones. In addition:

1) Take 1 tablespoon of unbruised white mustard seed in water daily.

---

[9]Tonic soup is probably the soup recommended by Sebastian Kneipp, in his book entitled *My Water Cure* (1892), and called strength-giving soup. Two loaves of black bread (preferably homemade or using whole ground flour, such as used in the country in the 1800's) are cut into cubes and dried on tin plates on the hearth. The bread should be dried into very hard cubes. These can be ground up as needed into a fine powder using a mortar. Whenever you need this soup, add 2 or 3 tablespoons of the freshly ground powder to some boiling broth and use very little, or preferably no spice, and very little salt. The powder can also be added to boiling milk. The soup is ready in 2 minutes. Modern people would dry the bread in a slow oven for a few hours until the bread is very dry. You can probably grind the bread to a powder in your food processor. The broth you would use today would probably be a vegetable broth, which can be made by cooking various vegetables and straining the liquid left when the vegetables have cooked together for half an hour or so. Good vegetable broth can be made from garlic, onions, celery, carrots, etc., and large quantities can be made so you can use this soup several times a day. A large quantity of vegetable broth would probably last a week in the refrigerator. Pub.

2) Twice a day take 1 tablespoon of linseed in water, after first letting it steep in cold water.

3) Every hour take 1 tablespoon of cold water.

4) Fry an apple in butter, eat this on an empty stomach and follow it with a glass of cold water.

5) Soak sliced fresh figs in olive oil, the longer the better; take 6 half figs each day. After eight days the constipation will cease. Purgatives are very bad in such cases; they eventually cause even more constipation and spoil the stomach.

6) Fenugreek tea is also good for constipation.

7) Every morning, on an empty stomach, take a small sugar-spoonful of salt dissolved in half a glass of cold water; or take 1 to 2 sugarspoons of milk sugar powder (lactose) in half a glass of water in the morning on an empty stomach.

8) Mix 1 tablespoon finely chopped black currant leaves with 2 teaspoons licorice and an equal quantity of lemon peel; steep these ingredients in 2 cups (½ liter) boiling water for half an hour. Drink cups of this remedy throughout the day.

CONSTRICTION OF THE CHEST

Take a head vapor bath (see The Water Cure) of chamomile flowers for fifteen to twenty minutes every two days, and every day take a whole body wash. The head vapor bath should immediately be followed by a whole wash and one hour in bed. In addition take 1 tablespoon of tea made from coltsfoot, sage and angelica with a little sugar every two hours.

CONTAGIOUS DISEASES—PREVENTIVE MEASURES

Before going among people suffering from contagious diseases, scrupulous people should drink a little gin in which garlic has been steeped. It is also beneficial to keep a piece of camphor in the mouth, to sniff some camphor powder, or to chew either common wormwood, mint, angelica or orange peel.

CONVALESCENCE

Take 1 tablespoon common centaury tea every two hours and ½ sugarspoon of bone-dust twice a day. In addition, a whole body wash on one day may be alternated with an upper body wash the next day.

CONVULSIONS AND CRAMPS IN CHILDREN

Convulsions frequently occur without there being any obvious reason. The child may be cutting teeth, it may happen from shock, worms, stomach complaints, brain disease, etc. The symptoms are: the eyes are wide open and staring, the limbs are stiff, the lips are tightly closed, the mouth is motionless, the fingers shrink, the face turns blue, breathing is oppressed, sometimes the whole body stiffens, the head falls backward, the arms and feet stiffen. Sometimes the child remains in this condition for only a few minutes, and other times for hours, and it may disappear quite suddenly or consciousness may return slowly. If the convulsions return, they can be fatal for many children. When this illness occurs, one should not hesitate to call a doctor.

1) An efficacious remedy for convulsions is the following: take fresh pounded rue and place this on the child's abdomen. If no fresh rue is available, compresses of dried rue infusion should be applied. This remedy is harmless and will almost certainly help. If no rue is available at all, apply hot compresses from hayseed decoction, from hot water and vinegar, or cinquefoil.

2) Every half hour give 1 tablespoon tea made from *Viola tricolor* (heartsease) or cinquefoil. Cinquefoil boiled in milk is the best remedy for all kinds of cramps; it should be taken as hot as possible.

3) Take powdered dried common St. Johnswort; mix a knifepoint of this in porridge twice a day.

4) Mix 2 spoons olive oil, 1 sugarspoon gin, ½ eggyolk and ⅓ cup (60 grams) lemon juice. During the convulsions, a sugarspoonful should be given every ten minutes, thereafter every half hour.

CORNS

1) Every morning and evening tie pure cotton wool around the corn; after a few days it will have gone.

2) Let ivy leaves steep in vinegar or salt; apply one leaf every day.

3) Apply a compress of vinegar or beer and a piece of tar or wax four times a day.

COUGH (DRY CHEST)

Take 2 tablespoons (15 grams) milled barley and a handful each of borage, coltsfoot, lungwort and ground ivy; a little more or less can do no harm. Boil all the ingredients in 2 quarts (liters) water until half a quart (liter) has boiled away, then add 2 tablespoons (10 grams) marshmallow root; leave this to steep for a further fifteen minutes, strain through a cloth without squeezing and then add 2 tablespoons (45 grams) honey; boil for a few minutes and skim off the scum. Take a wineglass of this, lukewarm, every two hours.

COUGH (TUSSIS)

1) A simple yet very efficacious remedy is sage. Take 1 cup (30 grams) sage to 2 cups (½ liter) boiling water, strain it, add enough honey to sweeten the infusion, add 1 tablespoon vinegar and take 1 tablespoon of this remedy hot every hour or two. This is also an exceptionally good gargle for throat complaints caused by chills. This remedy dissolves a great deal of phlegm.

2) Boil ½ cup (30 grams) marshmallow root and 6 teaspoons (8 grams) licorice in 1 quart (liter) water until reduced by half, strain and add 2 tablespoons (15 grams) licorice powder. So as to dissolve the licorice powder, the mixture should be briefly boiled again. When the licorice powder has dissolved, it should be bottled, well shaken until nearly cold and then ½ ounce (15 grams) sal ammoniac (ammonium chloride) should be added. A tablespoon should be taken every two hours.

3) Mix well together: 1¼ cups (250 grams) sugar syrup (a normal glassful), 2 tablespoons olive oil. Take 2 sugarspoons of

this mixture, mix with an egg and take a sugarspoonful every half-hour.

4) Boil ½ cup (150 grams) peeled onions, cut in rings, with a scant ½ cup (120 grams) honey and ¾ cup (120 grams) white sugar for three or four hours; allow it to cool and strain through a cloth. This juice should be kept in a well-corked bottle. Take 1 tablespoon lukewarm every two hours. This is an excellent remedy for a cough.

5) Drink tea made from 1 tablespoon (2 grams) pellitory (*Parietaria officinalis*), 6 teaspoons (2 grams) horsetail, 2 teaspoons (2 grams) licorice and 5 teaspoons (2 grams) white horehound.

6) Mix 2 tablespoons thyme with 1 tablespoon aniseed and 1 tablespoon licorice. Let this steep for twenty minutes in 2 cups (½ liter) boiling water, strain through a cloth and add 1 tablespoon honey. Take one spoon every hour.

7) In the evenings, drink the juice of a lemon.

8) For a dry, old cough, boil a handful of elder leaves with ½ handful elder flowers in 2 cups (½ liter) wine and take this with a spoon throughout the day.

9) Mix linseed meal with honey to make a syrup, and take 1 to 2 sugarspoons every hour for a dry, old cough.

10) Drink a cup of comfrey and licorice tea every day for a dry old cough.

11) Boil 1 tablespoon linseed in 4 cups (1 liter) water and drink this throughout the day for dry, old coughs.

12) A daily cup of tea from the plant and roots of parsley, taken lukewarm, will dissolve phlegm from the chest and lungs and expel it. This is particularly beneficial in the case of a heavy cold. For one cup of tea, use 1 tablespoon chopped roots and herbs mixed together and let it boil for twenty minutes.

13) A daily cup of goldenrod tea is also an excellent remedy for coughs and colds.

14) A remedy worth recommending is as follows: before retiring take a glass of hot tea made from equal quantities of elder

flowers and chamomile flowers mixed together and sweetened with sugar.

15) Every day drink one or two cups of thyme tea sweetened with honey. This is an excellent remedy for a stubborn cough.

16) For stomach coughs, drink a daily cup of tea made from walnut septa.[12] Use 1 sugarspoon septa for each cup of tea.

17) Use 1 to 2 tablespoons leaves and flowers of Aaron's rod boiled in 1 cup milk. Take hot in 3 doses as a very powerful remedy for a cough. This remedy is also good for consumptives and for diarrhea suffered by consumptives.

18) For a chronic cough, catarrh, throat infections, blood spitting, coughing blood, consumption, intestinal and stomach disorders, Dr. Hufeland recommends the following treatment: Mix ⅔ cup (50 grams) linseed meal, 4 teaspoons (5 grams) powdered fennel and 4 teaspoons (5 grams) licorice powder. Let 1 tablespoon of this mixture steep for twenty minutes in 4 cups boiling water. Strain and take half a cup every two hours.

Cough Caused by an Elongated Uvula (Uva)

A stubborn cough is often treated without success and is eventually considered to be a lung complaint. It may indeed become so if the cause of the complaint is not removed. The complaint is speedily cured by a small, insignificant operation, i.e., by cutting the elongated uvula. This must naturally be done by a physician. In the case of a protracted cough, it is advisable to have the throat examined by a physician.

Cracked Lips

1) Smear with glycerine.

2) Ointment made from 1 part salicyl mixed with 9 parts vaseline brings rapid relief.

3) Melt 1 part white wax with 2 parts sweet almond oil, stirring

---

[12]Septa is the membrane in the nut that separates the nutmeats.

continually until it begins to boil. Remove from the fire and add a few drops of rose oil as perfume.

CRAMPS (HANDS, LEGS, AND FEET)
1) Bathe the limbs in hot soda water, or in a foot or hand vapor bath of chamomile flowers.

2) Cut corks into slices, thread them on a string like a rosary and tie it round the legs.

3) If a piece of camphor the size of two grains of barley is taken in the evenings, the cramp disappears (Dr. Raspail).

4) Measure 1 tablespoon (10 grams) camphorated oil, ½ teaspoon (1 gram) spike oil, ¼ cup (50 grams) turpentine, 1 cup (250 grams) gin. Mix these ingredients and rub on the legs three times a day.

5) Take 10 to 20 drops valerian tincture in water daily.

6) Tie a lamp-wick cord around the legs.

CROUP
Croup is a very dangerous childhood illness. It affects children at any season of the year, but particularly in the Spring and Autumn, with a north and east wind prevailing, and especially boys from 2 to 6 years; girls are less likely to be affected. The danger of croup lies in the fact that, as a consequence of inflammation of the larynx and the windpipe, a membrane forms which blocks the air passages; the result being that the child concerned runs the risk of suffocation. It is vital for this illness to be recognized at a sufficiently early stage since every hour brings danger and the hope of recovery consequently diminishes.

Croup always begins with mild symptoms of catarrh, the voice becomes hoarse, there is a barking, dry cough, the face is bluish and swollen. The cough sometimes resembles the crowing of a cock. The child coughs up slimy, sticky phlegm, has a high fever and the breathing is fast and oppressed. Should such symptoms appear, there is every reason to consider croup. It usually breaks out at night. The startled child becomes very restless, breathing deeply and with difficulty. Such attacks are repeated; after the first attack the child appears to be cheerful, but fevers generally follow and the intervals between the attacks become increasingly shorter. The breathing becomes faster and more oppressed; the cough has a rattling sound, and the whole chest seems to be full of phlegm. A doctor should be summoned at once. At the onset, 1 tablespoon of fenugreek tea should be given internally every hour; in addition, twice a day upper body waterings and one or two whole washes. I have seen four fine cures by means of this method. After the first upper body watering, they felt much refreshed and all danger seemed to have passed. It is also good to rub the neck with walnut oil; this dissolves the phlegm.

1) The following remedy is also highly praised: put 1 tablespoon purified flowers of sulphur in a glass of cold water. Stir well and give the small patient 1 tablespoon every hour. It is also advisable to brush a little flowers of sulphur inside the throat, using a fine brush. It is very good to make croup patients sneeze by allowing them to sniff some kind of snuff.

2) A woman in Germany recently cured her child who was given up for lost by giving him 1 sugarspoon of honey every five to ten minutes. After taking a few spoonsful, the child was much better, but later refused the honey which was then boiled in milk and given with a spoon.

3) In addition to the above mentioned waterings, Monseigneur Kneipp recommends three further water cures for children who have croup: A) The small patient takes a half-bath, then goes to bed and is wrapped in a blanket; this divides the blood and expels it since we are dealing here with blood poisoning. If the burning returns, the second half-bath should be given as long as the fever still continues. B) The patient is given a whole body watering (full watering) and then goes to bed as described above. If the patient is so weak that doubt arises as to the possibility of recovery, hot salt water should be used for the watering; the salt attacks the skin and causes irritation; after the watering the patient should return to bed. If the fever returns, the treatment may be repeated with cold water. C) The

patient should be given a compress cloth (scarf) or neckwrap: the first time hot, the second and subsequent times, cold. These compresses or wraps should be renewed every fifteen minutes.

4) Croup can also be cured by washes—for example, every fifteen minutes. These washes should be reduced as the fever subsides. Application of the washes is indeed sometimes dangerous, if not done quickly enough.

CROUP (DIPHTHERIA)
1) Mix a sugarspoon of salt with a spoon of honey; take some of this frequently throughout the day.

2) Every five minutes, give the child a sugarspoon of the following remedy until he begins to vomit: the white of an egg with sugar. Also apply a piece of flannel soaked in hot water around the neck and cover it with a dry cloth.

3) Grind sugar to a very fine powder and blow this as far as possible down the child's throat several times throughout the day.

4) Every fifteen to twenty minutes, smear the throat with a feather dipped in gin; this remedy is highly recommended for croup.

CURVATURE OF THE SPINE
Children who suffer from this evil must remain in bed for six weeks or more. The mattress should be rather hard so that the parts of the body may be brought into the correct position. It is essential to ensure regular blood circulation, excretion of diseased matter and above all nourishing food. The small patient should be given a hay shirt and a whole wash daily. The former expels all waste matter, the latter has a strengthening, dissolving effect. Instead of the whole wash, the child can also be dipped in cold water (up to the armpits) for two to three seconds and laid in bed without being dried.

The patient should be given tonic soup twice a day, a pinch of bone-dust twice a day and 1 tablespoon of milk every hour. The following tea is particularly invigorating: mix equal quantities of common centaury, white horehound and thyme; to make 1 cup of tea, allow 1 tablespoon to steep for twenty minutes in boiling water and give 1 tablespoon every two hours.

DEAFNESS

1) If the deafness is caused by hardened earwax, 5 drops sweet almond oil should be put in the ears every other day; after a few days the ears should be syringed out with warm water.

2) Allow the vapor from chamomile tea to rise into the ears (by reversing a funnel for example); the ears should also be syringed out with horsetail tea.

3) Every day, place a cold compress around the neck for half an hour and use a daily footwrap; in addition, bind a compress of sauerkraut water on the ears; syringe with horsetail tea every eight days.

4) Every day for several days put 2 drops sulfuric oil on cotton wool and place in the ears each morning before eating or drinking.

5) Every morning and evening put 5 or 6 drops houseleek sap in the ears.

DIABETES (DIABETES MELLITUS)

The most obvious signs of diabetes are acute thirst, dry mouth and throat, and excessive urination. The urine is thick and contains a large quantity of sugar. These patients generally have a large appetite; but although they eat a great deal, they become thinner by the day and feel their strength waning. If there is no appetite, the patients gradually become weaker; this is followed by a dry cough, a sign that the lungs are affected, and the patient's condition deteriorates every day. A strict diet is usually prescribed for these patients—particularly farinaceous food. Monseigneur Kneipp permitted them to eat everything. Well-toasted bread, rusks and Kneipp's tonic soup are allowed; fish, meat and eggs are advised. Egg-cake with fat bacon is usually recommended for diabetes; also a glass of good, old wine. Beer is strictly forbidden; coffee should be taken infrequently. Cold baths are of great value, cold washes and waterings also. Such patients can make a good recovery by making use of them. The following remedies are most highly recommended:

1) Boil old linseed slowly in water until it becomes slimy. Take 1 cup of this three times a day. After some time, the sugar level will have considerably decreased.

2) Every day drink 3 cups knotgrass tea, and take three or four sugarspoons of tormentil tincture in water.

3) Blueberry leaves as tea are also indicated in cases of diabetes.

4) Take 3 handsful white beans, boil slowly for three hours in 3 quarts (3 liters) water until reduced by half. Drink this throughout the day, but drink nothing else.

5) Take 4 tablespoons (30 grams) limewater throughout the day, or drink 2 cups of goldenrod tea daily.

6) Boil a handful of eucalyptus leaves, a handful of knotgrass and a handful of goldenrod in 5 cups (1½ liters) water until reduced by half. Drink half of this quantity daily.

7) Boil 1 tablespoon tormentil root with 2 tablespoons blueberry leaves and 2 tablespoons knotgrass in 8 cups (2 liters) water until reduced by half. Take 2 cups (½ liter) daily.

8) Twice a day drink a cup of tea made from equal quantities of blessed thistle (*Cnicus benedictus*) and centaury (*Centaurium erythraea*). The infusion is 1 tablespoon for an average cup of tea.

9) Let 1 tablespoon eucalyptus leaves steep for twenty minutes in 1 cup (200 grams) boiling water. Take this quantity daily in two doses. With diabetes, all cheese without exception is recommended, as well as almonds, nuts, sour plums, apples, raspberries, strawberries, hazelnuts, cream without sugar and skimmed milk.

DIARRHEA (ACUTE)

If diarrhea is caused by overloading the stomach or by a chill, the patient should keep warm, especially the feet, and eat little or nothing. Gruel is recommended. Irregular diarrhea, with or without pain, is usually a symptom of a diseased organ; such patients seldom grow old. Diarrhea should never be suddenly cured by strong, astringent remedies; the bad or diseased matter must first be evacuated. Diarrhea should not be confused with dysentery. Diarrhea is usually a small indisposition which is easy to cure. The diarrhea is often more beneficial than detrimental. If it continues too long, causing general weakness, it is advisable to stop it. You can use one of the following methods:

1) Use hot compresses of hayseed decoction, or of water and vinegar, on the abdomen for half an hour; in addition use one of the following remedies.

2) Tea from silverweed, oak bark, shepherd's purse, blackberry leaves, chamomile flowers, agrimony, plantain, wood avens, knotgrass, or acorns will help the condition.

3) Take 1 sugarspoon tincture of bilberries (blueberries) twice a day in half a cup of hot water.

4) Lime blossom enemas, 1¼ cup (100 grams) per quart (liter) of water are helpful.

5) Take 3 or 4 raw eggs per day mixed with sugar.

6) Take 3 to 6 sugarspoons tincture of tormentil in water.

7) Taking 1 tablespoon common centaury tea every hour is an invigorating, efficacious remedy.

8) To cure diarrhea with abdominal pain, and thick, red water use tea from linseed or comfrey, enemas from starch water. Mix 1 tablespoon starch with 2 cups (½ liter) hot water. Rest and diet are essential here.

9) For diarrhea due to weakness of the stomach, you could do the following: Make tea from 5 teaspoons (3 grams) each of sage, common wormwood and oak bark in 2 cups (½ liter) boiling water; take 1 tablespoon every hour. Or let 3 tablespoons (10 grams) walnut septa steep in a bottle of Bordeaux wine; take 1 tablespoon every two hours.

DIARRHEA (CHRONIC)

Every morning, midday and evening, take 3 tablespoons of tea made from oak bark and common centaury. Also three half-baths and three upper body washes per week. Or you could do the following:

1) Dissolve 2½ tablespoons (20 grams) gum arabic in a glass of hot water, add 2 tablespoons (20 grams) sugar, and drink this in one dose.

2) Drink 1 cup tea made from blessed thistle, or from purple loosestrife (*Lythrum salicaria*) every day.

3) Take dry pieces of starch throughout the day. If the diarrhea is not accompanied by pain, from the fifth day onward take ½ teaspoon (½ gram) of rhubarb daily. If there is indeed pain, take a decoction of rice, or barley water, or gum water, or sago.

4) For diarrhea in old people, give a cup of blackberry leaf tea daily.

5) For diarrhea in children, rub the abdomen every morning and evening with hot, raw linseed.

6) A potent remedy for diarrhea is as follows: mix the powder of half a nutmeg, the powder from a piece of alum the size of a pea, with an egg yolk, and swallow the mixture. This brings rapid relief.

7) Diarrhea and intestinal infections can be cured by eating 1 tablespoon (15 grams) raw onion on bread each day.

DIARRHEA (IN CONSUMPTIVES)

1) Beat the whites of 5 eggs to a froth, add ¼ cup (30 grams) sugar and 1 quart (liter) distilled orange flower water. Drink this throughout the day.

2) A highly recommended remedy for this complaint is preserved dog rosehips (*Rosa canina*).

3) The following remedy is exceptionally potent: mix an egg yolk with a spoon of sugar, continue to stir and slowly add a

spoon of French brandy and 1 tablespoon olive oil; take 1 sugarspoonful every fifteen minutes.

4) Drink 2 cups fennel seed tea a day.

5) Every fifteen minutes take 5 drops camphorated spirits on sugar.

6) Take a piece of alum the size of a pea, let this dissolve in 3 tablespoons water and then drink it in one dose. This may be repeated if necessary. This is certainly the most efficacious remedy for diarrhea.

7) Lime water with milk is also effective.

DIZZINESS/VERTIGO

1) Drink tea from blessed thistle (*Cnicus benedictus*).

2) Mix 1 tablespoon (6 grams) speedwell with 2 teaspoons (4 grams) valerian, and let it steep for twenty minutes in 2 cups (½ liter) boiling water; take 3 tablespoons four times a day.

3) Fill half of a glazed earthenware pot which holds at least 2 quarts (liters) with fresh common wormwood leaves, then continue to fill it until nearly full with fresh sage leaves. Add a good handful of bruised juniper berries and, finally, 2 quarts (liters) gin, without pressing the herbs too close together. Bind the pot and seal it with dough to make it air-tight. Leave to stand for a few months in the cellar or in the shade, then carefully press it through a cloth and store in well-corked bottles. A sugarspoonful of this should be given in an empty glass which is then filled with water so that the infusion is thoroughly mixed with the water. This should be taken in the morning on an empty stomach for two weeks; breakfast may be taken an hour later. After two weeks respite, the treatment should be resumed; one should then wait three weeks or a month and then take it again for two weeks. This strengthens the brain and promotes digestion. It is also a potent remedy for the avoidance of strokes.

DROWNING (PREVENTION)

Advice from an old soldier: if one should fall in the water, keep the head tipped back and the hands and arms under water; in this way the water cannot enter the mouth. One should breathe out as little as possible and breathe in deeply. In this way one can really not drown. Anyone who cannot swim only needs to tread water like a horse, or like a man climbing the stairs, keeping the arms under water.

DYSENTERY

This complaint occurs in two forms: it can be mild or dangerous. In the first instance, it differs little from diarrhea and should be treated in the same manner. In the second case, it is a most prevalent illness with the following symptoms: frequent bowel movement, sometimes with blood, mixed with membrane or shreds of skin, commonly called intestinal scrapings.

Dysentery is usually characterized by shivering accompanied by colic. In serious cases, a great change in the features is apparent; after a few days the patient may look very strange; the pulse is weak, difficult to find; the patient is attacked by fits of shivering and death may swiftly follow. With dysentery, remedies for stopping the diarrhea should not be used while the illness is severe; even if it becomes chronic, they may only be used if the abdominal pain has completely ceased, if the bowel movements no longer contain blood and have decreased in quantity and frequency.

Only after five or six days may an absorbent be used. During this illness the patient should follow a strict diet, take no solid food, in particular no meat or fish. The food should consist of gruel, porridge, or farinaceous soup mixed with a little milk. Milk alone would have a most detrimental effect. As soon as the diarrhea stops, the patient should gradually be given more solid food. Treatment is as follows:

1) Hot compresses can be placed on the abdomen three or four times a day. Drink comfrey tea or shepherd's purse tea; take 2 teaspoons (2 grams) powdered walnut septa in a glass of Bordeaux wine three times a day. Take 2 egg yolks, 2 tablespoons sugar and an equal quantity of Bordeaux wine and beat well

together. This mixture should be drunk in one dose. These three remedies for dysentry are all most efficacious.

2) Plantain seed boiled in milk is an excellent medicine.

3) Take the white of 3 eggs beaten to a froth, mixed with a little sugar every day.

4) Take a hot drink of plantain seed boiled in milk or a strong infusion of greater plantain (*Plantago major*) or let plantain seed steep in gin and take 1 tablespoon three times a day.

5) Fill a normal drinking glass with hot water, a sugarspoon salt, and 15 drops vinegar; take this every half hour or hour with a spoon. This is highly recommended.

6) A successful remedy—although it may seem odd to many—for remaining free from dysentery is: eat plenty of fruit and grapes, but no meat or fish.

DYSPEPSIA/INDIGESTION

The treatment of indigestion lies chiefly in tonic, bitter medicines.

1) Mix the following ingredients together:

> ½ cup (25 grams) wormwood
> 1 cup (15 grams) lemon balm
> 3 teaspoons (5 grams) rhubarb powder
> 5 tablespoons (20 grams) common St. Johnswort
> 2 tablespoons (10 grams) juniper berries
> 1½ quarts (1½ liters) white wine

Every morning and evening take 2 tablespoons with an equal quantity of orange peel syrup.

2) Take 2 to 3 sugarspoons of charcoal powder in milk.

3) Twice a day take 1 to 2 sugarspoons of unbruised white mustard seed.

4) Tea made from common centaury, gentian, angelica, white

horehound, blessed thistle, rosemary or sage, either alone or mixed, are powerful remedies for indigestion.

5) The tincture described in number 3 under Dizziness, is also a good remedy.

DYSPEPSIA (WEAK STOMACH)

Weakness of the stomach is usually caused by foul matter. The symptoms are as follows: lack of appetite, indisposition after taking food due to pressure, tension in the stomach region, the skin temperature is poor compared to that of a healthy person, the skin is pale, the pulse sluggish and weak, there is weariness after the least work, sluggish digestion, much wind, vexation, drowsiness, etc. If these symptoms lead one to believe that it is only weakness of the stomach and not inflammation, a speedy recovery may be expected by the use of the following prescription. Every week take four whole washes, three upper body washes, three hot compresses of hayseed decoction on the abdomen for one hour, to be renewed after half an hour; twice a day drink a glass of sugar and water. Take Kneipp tonic soup one or two times a day. Four times a day take 2 tablespoons of the following tea:

> 5 teaspoons (3 grams) sage
> 1 tablespoon (3 grams) common wormwood
> 1 teaspoon (1 gram) juniper berries
> ¼ cup (2 grams) mint

This should be left to steep in 2 cups (½ liter) of boiling water.

EAR INFECTIONS

Inflammation of the ears may have external causes (for example, hardened wax, insects, other foreign objects which have entered the ear, or a fall, bang or knock), but it is mostly caused by chills and draughts. In cases of ear inflammation, a doctor should always be consulted.

1) To treat earache (Otalgia), put 1 to 3 drops aniseed oil on cotton wool and place in the ear; this frequently gives immediate

relief. You can also put 2 to 3 drops arnica tincture in the ears; then place a piece of cotton wool in each one. Use 4 drops warm sweet almond oil in the ears for earache.

2) Running ears can be treated as follows: drink walnut leaf tea and syringe the ears twice a day with the same tea. Take 1 quart (liter) plantain leaf decoction, add ¼ teaspoon (1 gram) alum. Syringe the ears with this twice a day, or syringe them with horsetail tea. Each week take four whole washes, three upper body washes, one hay-shirt and one half-bath.

3) Insects in the ear can easily be treated. Let 5 to 6 drops of sweet oil, olive oil or almond oil run into the ear. The insect will rapidly leave its hiding place.

4) Ringing in the ears may be helped by the following treatments. Every other day put 5 drops sweet almond oil in the right and left ear; after a few days syringe the ears with warm water. Or, take a head vapor bath of chamomile flowers for twenty minutes.

ECZEMA

There are two kinds of Eczema—dry and wet. In order to cure the eczema, cleanliness of the body and pure fresh air should be ensured. Abstinence from stimulating food, such as coffee, tea, beer and spirits is essential. A good Kneipp cure nearly always cures eczema. The treatments are as follows:

1) Take freshly chopped roots of greater celandine (*Chelidonium majus*); allow this to steep in strong vinegar and add a little salt. Smear the eczema well with this twice a day.

2) Apply compresses of wheat bran decoction.

3) Apply compresses of clay, water and vinegar.

4) Unsalted soft cheese compresses are highly efficacious.

5) Compresses of hayseed decoction (hay residue) are also helpful.

6) Smear the eczema twice a day with Petroleum.

7) Boil 3½ tablespoons (30 grams) of elecampane root powder (*Inula helenium*) in 1 quart (liter) of water until reduced by half and then strain. Apply constant compresses of this.

8) Take 4 teaspoons (10 grams) each of burdock root, couch-grass (quack grass), juniper berry tops and long-stalked cranesbill; boil these ingredients together in 1 quart (liter) water. Take one cup in the morning on an empty stomach for 2 weeks. Make a decoction from the same herbs, but add 3 tablespoons (20 grams) of each herb to 1 quart (liter) water and smear the eczema with this every day; in the meantime no more of the decoction should be taken.

9) Every day drink 1 cup of tea made from 5 teaspoons (10 grams) dock and 1 cup (10 grams) ash leaves in 2 cups (½ liter) of water.

10) See *Deadly Nightshade*.

11) Every morning smear the eczema with egg white; after half an hour, wash it off with hot water.

12) Mix a pinch of finely ground alum and the white of an egg thoroughly, and smear the eczema with this.

13) Wash the rash with burdock root decoction.

14) Smearing the eczema with glycerine is also effective.

15) Boil plantain leaves in milk and wash the eczema with this or, better still, apply compresses of this mixture.

16) Drink a cup of goosegrass tea every day; also apply daily compresses of the decoction.

17) Carefully mix 6 teaspoons (30 grams) vaseline with 2 tablespoons (15 grams) zinc oxide and 2 tablespoons (15 grams) starch powder; rub the rash with this mixture twice a day or apply a plaster of this ointment twice a day. In the case of wet eczema, it is very good to wash it four times a day with tea made from walnut leaves with 1 tablespoon sugar to 2 cups (½ liter) water.

18) Twice a day apply the following ointment: 3 tablespoons (30 grams) fresh butter with 3 teaspoons (7 grams) flowers of sulfur.

19) Boil 2 handfuls of common mallow in 1 quart (liter) water and apply as a compress.

20) Mix cream with a little chalk powder; smear with this twice a day.

21) Mix ½ teaspoon (½ gram) flowers of zinc[10] (*Flores zinci*) with 3 tablespoons (30 grams) sweet butter and smear with this twice a day.

22) Boil walnut leaves, apply these on the rash; add some sugar to the decoction and wash with this twice a day.

23) Mix 1 cup (250 grams) rose water, 4 teaspoons (12 grams) alum, ½ ounce (15 grams) white lead, ¼ ounce (6 grams) sublimate,[11] and the white of an egg. Apply in the form of compresses and wash the eczema with it twice a day.

24) Take a fresh burdock radical leaf, remove the top skin of the leaf and place this on the eczema. This is a very simple but excellent remedy.

25) Mix 3 tablespoons (70 grams) wool fat with 3 teaspoons (15 grams) vaseline, 8 grams Peruvian balsam and 3½ teaspoons (7 grams) myrrh. Rub with this twice a day. This remedy is also good for chapped hands and feet.

EMPHYSEMA/LUNG COMPLAINTS

Those who suffer from this complaint generally have a dry cough, are very breathless and also have attacks of asthma. It is frequently confused with consumption. The symptoms are as follows: the lungs, overfilled with air, have lost so much strength that they cannot evacuate sufficient air from the air-cells; since this causes insufficient pure air to be breathed in, both the changing of the blood and the circulation are inter-

---

[10]Flowers of zinc: an early name for zinc oxide, which has a mild astringent and antiseptic action.

[11]Sublimate is the act or process of sublimation, which results in corrosive sublimate or mercuric chloride. This chemical is poisonous if taken internally, but contains antiseptic qualities for disinfection. Modern day use is in surgeon's hand soap and for sterilization of clothing and diapers. Sublimate is the manufacturing process used to produce mercuric chloride.

rupted. The heart is also more or less hindered on this account, is overfilled with blood, and therefore swells, frequently causing palpitations. Since the abdominal organs suffer from the impeded blood circulation in the heart and lungs, various intestinal illnesses may occur. The patients should avoid bad air, cold wind, especially north and east wind, dust, smoke, chills, walking, mountain climbing, heavy work.

A mild water cure can be of good service here, for example, each week take four whole washes, three upper body washes, and three short compresses of water and vinegar. Hip baths, half-baths, knee waterings and upper body waterings gradually follow. Good bowel movements should be ensured, to which end a cup of buckthorn bark tea with a sugarspoon of aniseed taken in the evenings is most efficacious. In addition, a cup of lime blossom tea with honey, or tea made from stinging nettles, ground ivy or plantain may prove helpful.

ENEMAS

1) Enemas of 1 to 2 cups (2–400 grams) cold water are useful for constipation and attacks of dizziness.

2) A salt water enema can be made as follows: use 1 tablespoon salt in 1 to 2 cups (400 grams) warm water for congestion of blood in the head, and especially for intestinal worms and maggots.

3) A softening enema is made as follows: combine 3 tablespoons (15 grams) linseed, 10 cups (125 grams) Aaron's rod leaves, and 2 cups (½ liter) boiling water. Let steep until lukewarm, strain through a cloth and add the yolk of an egg. This enema should be used in two doses.

4) A refreshing enema is made as follows: take 2 cups (400 grams) lukewarm water and add 4 to 5 tablespoons vinegar. This is highly recommended for diarrhea.

5) A purgative enema can be used for constipation. Boil ½ cup (30 grams) marshmallow root in 2 cups (½ liter) water until reduced to 1 cup (¼ liter), then strain and add 1 to 2 tablespoons (30–35 grams) honey, and 3 tablespoons (30 grams) castor oil.

EPILEPSY/FALLING SICKNESS

Those who suffer from the so-called falling sickness have cramp-like movements of the body and fall down quite unconscious with a loud cry, foaming at the mouth, the hands clenched together. They bite on their tongues and usually thrash about with the hands and legs. Biting on the tongue is a major characteristic of this illness, likewise unconsciousness and insensibility. Epilepsy is frequently an inherited disease. Those who suffer from falling sickness must refrain from excesses, spirits, wine, beer, gin, coffee, heavy food such as peas, beans, onions, garlic, heads of mammals, eel, mustard, pepper, rancid bacon, etc.

Many children are cured of this illness by Kneipp's water cure; there is little hope for adults with water treatment, although an occasional cure has taken place. As long as the memory remains good, there is always hope for a cure. The following remedies are recommended:

1) Drink a cup of mistletoe tea every day.

2) Let alder buds steep in gin and take 1 tablespoon twice a day.

3) Every day drink a cup of tea made from white bedstraw (*Galium album*).

4) Let 2 teaspoons (3 grams) of mistletoe, 3 tablespoons (3 grams) horsetail and 2 teaspoons (3 grams) valerian root steep in 2 cups (½ liter) boiling water and take 2 tablespoons four times a day.

5) Drink cinquefoil or vervain as tea.

6) Drink a daily cup of hyssop tea.

7) Take 2½ teaspoons (3 grams) angelica seed in some kind of liquid.

8) I found the following very simple remedy in a book which is 300 years old; I have often recommended it with excellent results; after taking it some patients even had no further attacks at all.

For adults, every evening take 2 tablespoons olive oil mixed with sugar; for children take 1 tablespoon. Nearly all those who take it recover quickly, and many who take it regularly recover completely. If the memory has suffered a great deal, or if the patient is a half-idiot, the remedy is no longer effective. With the oil, I also give a daily cup of mistletoe tea and additionally recommend a mild water cure. For example, each week four whole washes and three hot compresses of hayseed decoction on the abdomen for half an hour, or three cold hip-baths for fifteen seconds or three half-baths for five seconds.

•   •   •

A few cures: a young lady had fits of falling sickness every month. I recommended the oil, tea and mild water applications. Six months later, she wrote me saying that it was not helping, upon which I replied: "Keep on trying." And now—it was ten years ago—she has no more fits. A young man of 18 suddenly began to have epileptic fits in rapid succession, defying all medicine. I let him try the above mentioned remedies; he is now a soldier and has not had a recurrence.

A Father of about 40 years of age, suffering from epilepsy, was advised by me to take the oil cure with four whole washes and three half-baths per week and a daily cup of mistletoe tea. After he had taken the first spoons of oil, not the slightest sign of the illness was seen again. After having had no fits for a whole year, he came to thank me personally; but a few days later he wrote that he had had a fit that very evening. This was now some months ago and he has had nothing since. He had probably eaten or drunk something injurious.

Sufferers from this appalling complaint, I am writing this for your benefit, try the oil cure!

ERYSIPELAS

Erysipelas may be recognized by the following symptoms: shivering, great thirst, fever and lack of appetite. It is often accompanied by burning itching and light stabs of pain. The affected part becomes red, even rather purple, and swells up; the patient is not in pain but has frequent attacks of nausea and vomiting. Erysipelas usually affects the head; it begins on both sides of the nose and is accompanied by headache. You can try the following treatments:

1) In the first place, good bowel movements should be ensured and the patient should be given hot elder tea to drink. Food should be mild; in this condition the patient should definitely not eat pork or mutton and must always stay in bed. If the erysipelas develops internally, it should be brought out in the same place by the application of very hot compresses of hayseed infusion or a mustard plaster.

2) Allow a sugarspoon of finely chopped walnut septa to steep for twenty minutes in 1 cup of boiling water and use this amount daily until a cure has taken place; this is an efficacious remedy. If there is erysipelas on the arm or leg, a poultice of unsalted soft cheese should be applied (as in erysipelas on the head).

3) With erysipelas it is always good to put on a hay-shirt of hot hayseed decoction daily and to take a whole bath (with the exception of the head) three to four times a day.

4) Erysipelas can frequently be cured simply by keeping warm and drinking two or three cups of meadowsweet tea every day.

5) The following simple remedy can cure erysipelas in three days. Take a linen cloth, folded double, make an opening in it for the eyes, nose and mouth; thickly smear the cloth with fresh, unsalted soft cheese and bind it around the face like a mask; the plaster must be renewed as soon as the cheese begins to dry and this must be continued day and night. The cheese soaks up all poisons, takes away the burning and prevents swelling. This remedy never fails.

ERYSIPELAS (IN WOUNDS)

This particularly occurs in careless people, if the wound was not correctly treated at the beginning or was neglected, or the sufferer has laid himself open to a chill. Erysipelas is dangerous; if there is a sudden decline in strength, the patient should take a couple of glasses of good wine. It is also very contagious; everything with which the patient has been in contact must be disinfected. Erysipelas can be recognized by the swellings in the affected places, the redness of the skin and in particular by the blisters which look exactly like burn blisters. Erysipelas can soon turn into gangrene. (See Gangrene).

1) Experience has shown that unsalted soft cheese—applied directly on to the area very thickly—is an excellent remedy and there is then no need to be afraid of contagion.

2) Erysipelas is accompanied by severe itching. This can be counteracted by applying cold compresses of clay, water and vinegar alternately with the cheese; these clay compresses also heal the erysipelas.

3) Three times per day apply a poultice of potatoes and buttermilk, or a clay poultice. The latter should be renewed every hour.

EYE COMPLAINTS

If the eyes feel tired doing certain kinds of work, if they begin to feel painful, one should allow them to rest. Eyes deserve to be treated carefully, although generally very little thought is paid to them. If one has weak eyes, one should read as little as possible, and only with a good light; it is especially damaging to read in a railway train. Always ensure that when the eyes are exerted, the light is clear. Take one or two cold eye-baths daily by simply keeping the eyes in water for 3 to 4 seconds and opening them for a moment in the water. For inflammation of the eyes use one of these remedies:

1) Put one drop of salt water in the eyes daily.

2) Place unsalted, soft cheese on the eyes; this is one of the best remedies.

3) Let elder flowers steep in boiling milk and place the warm compresses of this over the eyes.

4) Dissolve 3 teaspoons (5 grams) zinc sulphate and ¼ cup (40 grams) sugar candy in 1 quart (liter) rainwater or pure spring water. Put two drops of this in the eyes every two hours.

5) Take 5 cups (1½ liters) rainwater or springwater; add 2 tablespoons (15½ grams) zinc sulphate and 1 tablespoon (15½ grams) kitchen salt. Apply warm compresses of this throughout the day.

6) Take 2 tablespoons fresh milk, the white of a fresh egg, and a little rosewater; beat all together until frothy and apply compresses of this over the eyes. This remedy always helps exceptionally quickly.

7) Burning eyes can be helped if you beat the white of an egg to a froth, mix with rye flour and apply over the eyes.

8) Or, take ½ cup (50 grams or half an average drinking glass) of rainwater, 1 spoon sugar and ¼ teaspoon (1 gram) zinc sulphate, beat an egg white to a froth, mix all together and place compresses of this over the eyes to relieve burning in the eyes.

9) Sniffing galangal powder is advisable with all eye complaints.

10) With eye complaints it is beneficial to have the ears syringed and to take hot footbaths.

11) If you get lime in the eyes, place as much sugar in pure water as the water will dissolve, dip the eyes in this and ensure that the water goes well into the eyes. This is the best remedy to avoid harmful consequences. Cod liver oil or olive oil may also be dripped into the eyes. Rapeseed is also good.

12) For bleary eyes, apply compresses of an infusion of greater plantain leaves, adding a little rosewater. Before retiring, smear the rims of the eye with a little unsalted butter.

13) For an eye rupture, take fresh bramble (blackberry) leaves, pound well to a pulp, and place over the eye. Dried bramble leaves can also be steeped in boiling water and applied in the form of compresses, or a mixture of egg white with a little saffron can be placed over the eyes.

14) Eye powder for weak eyes can be made by combining:

⅔ cup (30 grams) eyebright
4 teaspoons (7 grams) fennel seed
1 teaspoon (1⅓ grams) ordinary loaf sugar
1 tablespoon (15 grams) white sugar candy

Pound all the ingredients together to a powder and mix very carefully. In the evening before retiring, take 1 teaspoon (3 grams) in a little wine. This should be continued for some time.

15) To treat eye fistula, wash the eyes four times a day with tea made from oak bark.

16) To treat spots on the eye, take equal quantities of saltpeter and sugar candy, pound to a very fine powder and blow through a paper tube or straw into the eyes. Or, you could put a little dandelion sap in the eyes three times a day.

17) For inflammation of the eyelids, apply unsalted, soft cheese. Or, smear a very little of the following mixture on the closed eyelids: 3 teaspoons (15 grams) vaseline and 3 teaspoons (2½ grams) flowers of zinc. Mix very carefully.

18) For red, running eyes, wash the eyes with cinquefoil tea and sniff powdered galangal root. You can also wash the eyes with tea made from common wormwood mixed with a little aloe.

19) Four times a day, put a few drops of houseleek sap in the eyes, or apply as compresses to relieve red, running eyes.

20) Take fresh bruised betony leaves; place a pellet of them in each nostril and repeat several times to relieve running eyes.

21) Erysipelas in the eyes can be treated as follows: Apply compresses of rose leaves and elder flowers boiled in milk. Or, mix rose leaves, elder flowers and wheat bran together; place in one or two fine linen bags; warm them and place on the eyes.

22) To treat skins on the eyes (dark sight), take ¼ cup (60 grams) greater celandine sap and 2 teaspoons (15 grams) honey; boil together, skim and put one drop in the eyes four to six times daily.

23) Painful ulcerated eyes can be treated as follows: mix together 3 tablespoons (30 grams) sweet butter, 3 tablespoons (30 grams) lily oil, beat the white of an egg to a froth, stir well together and apply as compresses. Or, soak a piece of white bread in hot milk, place betwee two fine linen cloths, and apply on the affected area.

24) Swollen eyelids can be treated as follows: apply compresses of elder flowers. If accompanied by a burning sensation, and if the eyelids are red, boil the elder flowers in milk and apply as compresses.

FAINTING (SYNCOPE)

Poor functioning of the heart is frequently the cause of fainting. It is often also of nervous origin and occurs not infrequently in hysterical people. In such cases there is nothing to fear. If it is really caused by the heart, a doctor should be consulted at once.

For swift recovery, take 20 to 24 drops gentian tincture in a glass of cold water, or drink a cup of tea made from common centaury. The best and simplest remedy is a lump of sugar.

FAT LUMPS (NEOPLASMATA)

Mix an egg yolk with an equal quantity of lard, rub the fat lumps with this twice a day and cover with a piece of cotton wool.

FEVER

Fever is not an illness in itself, but a symptom of illness and usually the forerunner of a serious illness. If a person is shivering or feels first very cold and later hot; if the pulse is fast, (for example 100 beats per minute), if the breathing is faster than usual (20 times per minute), there is fever. If the thermometer registers 99.5°F (37.5°C) and more, there is fever; 101.3°F (38.5°C) is still a mild fever, 102.2°F (39°C) is moderate fever; if it goes higher, it is critical. The highest temperature is 108°F (42.5°C), but then there is seldom any hope of a cure left. Fever is generally accompanied by dry tongue, thirst, headache, sweating, lack of appetite, general weakness, and dark or cloudy urine with sediment. Fever is always higher in the evening. In the case of feverish illness, there should always be sufficient fresh air, but care should be taken that the patient is not in a draft; the patient should also not have too many heavy covers.

1) For feverish patients: a whole wash with cold water every two hours is recommended; as the fevers subsides, so the number of washes should be decreased. For the thirst, cool, but not too cold, drinks should be given with a spoon. Do not force the patient to eat too much; strong people can easily go without

food for three to four days, but cooling drinks should always be provided. With weak patients, ensure that they partake of a little fortifying food; for example: clear soup with a beaten egg, taken with a spoon (clear soup alone does not provide nourishment). Fowl, pigeon, chicken, and gradually a little veal, may also be served in addition to milk and thin Kneipp tonic soup.

2) Remedies to lower the temperature: use tea made from common centaury, white willow, celery, arnica, alder, chamomile flowers, wild chicory, gentian, or wood avens root.

3) Quartan cold fever is a type of malaria and occurs every fourth day. Use parsley juice as an excellent remedy. This juice can be obtained by cutting a good handful of parsley (with the stalks) close to the root, pound it fine, add 4 tablespoons (30 grams) water and then squeeze. Take ⅓ cup (90 grams) one or two hours before the attack of fever. Or you can mix 3 tablespoons each rose water, rainwater and French brandy. The patient should take this one or two hours before the onset of the fever and stay in bed for five hours. During this time the patient should drink nothing, howver thirsty he or she may be, and should be well covered so as to sweat. If the fever does not subside, the treatment should be repeated until the fever disappears.

4) For quartan cold fever, one can also let 1 tablespoon white horehound steep in 4 to 5 tablespoons (30–40 grams) gin for twenty-four hours. Take 1 tablespoon every half hour until this quantity has been used up. Or, one can boil ¾ cup (31 grams) fresh holly leaves (*Ilex aquifolium*) in 2 cups (½ liter) water. The patient should take an ordinary drinking glassful before the onset of the fever. Another remedy is to drink a cup of heartsease tea an hour before the onset of the fever.

5) For tertian fever, drink tea made from cross-leaved heath (*Erica tetralix*) sweetened with sugar. In the case of protracted fever, common centaury tea is one of the best remedies. Common wormwood tea and fumitory tea are also both highly efficacious.

6) For fever in general, take 20 drops of gentian tincture twice a day. Or, boil together 3 tablespoons (15 grams) valerian root,

1 cup (90 grams) licorice, and ⅛ cup (20 grams) skinned raisins in 1 quart (liter) water and drink a wineglassful twice a day.

7) Vervain, taken as tea, drives away the fever.

8) The following remedy is very effective against fever: take 1 ounce (30 grams) devil's-bit scabious root and 1½ cups (30 grams) of the dried herb Robert, boil in 1 quart (liter) water until reduced by half and drink this quantity in three doses, a third each time. The fever generally subsides after the second dose and the remedy can be used for all kinds of fever.

9) For fever in general, take 10 to 15 drops of quassia tincture in a spoon of water three times a day.

10) For intermittent fever, drink tea made from decoction of tormentil.

11) For putrid fever (Septicemia) the characteristic symptoms are: teeth and tongue coated with white mucus, bad breath, evil-smelling sweat, general weakening of the senses and contraction of the muscles. Mix the following:

> 1½ cups (150 grams) rye dough
> 3 ounces (90 grams) black soap
> 1½ cups (30 grams) white or dead-nettle
> ½ ounce (15 grams) gun powder

Pound the gunpowder with the dead-nettles and mix well with the other ingredients. Make this into four plasters on linen and place a plaster under each foot and around each wrist. Leave these plasters on for twenty-four hours. Before removing them, place a cloth dipped in vinegar around the nose, to avoid danger from the putrid smell, and bury the plasters in the garden.

FISHSKIN DISEASE (ICHTHYOSIS)
This complaint is congenital, usually inherited from parents or grandparents. The skin of those affected is dry due to the absence of natural oil; it is rough and covered with thick or thin scales, so that it very much resembles a fish or snakeskin. Sometimes the whole body is affected, with the exception of

the joints. Some sufferers are tormented by unbearable itching which makes life a burden, all the more so since the complaint is considered incurable. I treated a number of patients for months without success. After having treated the last person for four months also without success, I let him wash twice a day with a rather strong decoction of walnut leaves, and two weeks later the itching and scales had gone, the skin was quite normal and the patient was naturally overjoyed. Anyone suffering from this complaint should try this simple remedy.

FISTULAS IN GENERAL
If the limbs can be bathed, hot baths of chemically pure soda are highly recommended; four baths should be taken daily, each lasting ten to fifteen minutes. A good handful of soda should be dissolved in each quart (liter) of boiling water. If the limb cannot be bathed, a hot soda compress should be applied four times a day for one-half hour. In addition, take 2 cups of tea made from sanicle with honey, or 1 to 2 cups of tea made from goldenrod, yarrow, or herb Robert daily. These teas work as well, if not better, than the external remedies; one should therefore not hesitate to use them together. A gentleman suffering from a fistula under his foot had tried all possible remedies but was cured in a month by the above prescription. A girl with a fistula on one arm recovered by means of the same remedies in three months, yet another in six months. So if one has patience and follows the cure to the letter, the reward for one's pains will be a complete cure.

FISTULA IN THE RECTUM
1) Take enemas made from oak bark infusion (cold) alternating with cold enemas of horsetail infusion.

2) Fresh yarrow leaves can be crushed to a pulp, mixed with half as much beef suet, and used as an excellent remedy for fistulas.

FLATULENCE

1) Take half-baths, back waterings, upper body washes, cold water compresses on the abdomen. See also Monseigneur Kneipp's juniper berry cure on page 292.

2) Drink thyme, or common chamomile, or mint, or lemon balm, or fennel, coriander, caraway or aniseed tea.

3) In the case of children, the abdomen should be rubbed with the following mixture: 1 tablespoon (10 grams) water and 5 drops oil of cloves.

FOOT PROBLEMS

1) Cold feet usually occur in anemic people and in patients with stomach disorders; it is also caused by poor blood circulation. The feet should be hardened by treading water, washing the feet with cold water before retiring, applying cold water and vinegar compresses, walking barefoot as much as possible, walking in wet grass in the summer, by knee waterings, etc.

2) Every morning and evening wash the feet with 1 part spirits of ammonia and 2 parts cold water; this opens the pores and warms cold feet.

3) Take 1 tablespoon mustard seed, ⅓ cup rye flour, mix this to a paste with vinegar, place between two linen cloths which should be large enough to cover the soles of the feet. If this is done for ten days, the feet usually stay warm.

4) Take a hot footbath (five minutes is sufficient) every evening before retiring for several days; dry the feet and rub them with 5 to 10 drops turpentine to alleviate cold feet.

5) Swollen feet can sometimes be caused by a kidney complaint. If the swelling is of a rheumatic or gouty nature, see Rheumatism (page 140). For swollen feet in general, the following recommendations have been found useful: compresses of clay, water and vinegar, also hardening and strengthening the body by means of a mild water cure, washes, compresses, knee waterings, half-baths; and, if the condition of the patient permits, powerful waterings. Swollen feet are usually a sign that the body is ill, especially if the feet are swollen in the mornings upon rising.

FOOTBATHS

1) If blood is rising to the head, footbaths serve the useful purpose of drawing it away or of drawing blood away from the chest. They are often used for inflammation of the eyes, headaches or toothaches. One should always ensure that the footbaths are not too hot; lukewarm is best. Put ¾ to 1 cup (100 to 125 grams) mustard flour in a bucket of hot water and stir well; the feet should be kept in it for ten minutes.

2) Take 2 handfuls wood-ash and 1 handful salt, place in a bucket of hot water. Put the feet in it for ten minutes and then rinse them with cold water.

FRECKLES FROM THE SUN

1) Take ¼ cup (60 grams) rosewater, add 1 teaspoon (4 grams) borax; wash the face with this every morning and evening.

2) Wash the freckles with parsley water.

3) Take ⅓ cup (90 grams) lard, 4 teaspoons (15 grams) borax powder, 2 teaspoons (5 grams) mint oil and mix together. Rub on freckles twice a day for five minutes.

4) Pound fresh roots of Solomon's seal and rub the freckles with it twice a day.

5) Make a strong infusion of common centaury and wash the freckles with it four times a day.

FRESH WOUNDS/INJURIES

1) With fresh wounds, one should first take care to bandage the wound so that it is not exposed to the air. It is highly recommended to place the wounded or injured limb immediately in cold water. Then wash the wound thoroughly with cold water to which arnica tincture has been added. When the wound is quite clean, dip cotton wool in half water, half arnica tincture and place on the wound or injured limb. When the cotton wool begins to dry, do not remove it but tip a little water and arnica over it. In this way the largest wounds often heal in three days. This also staunches bleeding wounds immediately.

2) Apply a lanolin plaster twice a day.

FRIGHT

Immediately after the fright, one should drink a good quantity of hot boiled milk or, if it is not available, a fairly large quantity of sugar and water.

FROSTBITE

To avoid frostbite, rub the limbs with spirit of camphor and take 2 drops spirit of camphor on sugar three or four times a day.

FROZEN LIMBS

1) Take 3 handsful fresh rose leaves and 2½ cups (500 grams) olive oil and boil together for a few minutes in a double-boiler. Leave to cool and pour, with the leaves, into a bottle or glass with a wide neck; tie down well with a piece of paper or blotter and prick a few holes in the paper with a pin. Leave this to steep in the sun for a couple of months. In the Autumn take fresh turnips, mince or scrape them, pound them a little so as to be able to extract the sap all the better, and squeeze well through a cloth so that about ¾ cup (250 grams) of sap remains. Place the olive oil and rose leaves on the fire (double-boiler), leave to boil a while, then add the turnip sap and let all the ingredients boil together for fifteen minutes, stirring continually. Remove from the fire and leave to cool a little. Keep stirring, and add 9 ounces (250 grams) red lead and return to the fire, still stirring and let it boil until brown. When it has cooled a little, add, while continuing to stir, 3 tablespoons (45 grams) camphor, 3 spoonsful olive oil and 1 tablespoon (15 grams) Peruvian balsam. When everything is thoroughly mixed together, the ointment should be poured into boxes or pots which should be sealed after a few days. This is an excellent ointment for frozen limbs.

2) Take hot baths from potato peelings.

3) If the frozen limbs have not cracked, they should be washed with salt water or alum water.

4) Mix 3 teaspoons (8 grams) of spirits of turpentine with 1 teaspoon (1 gram) camphor, and use as an ointment.

5) Arnica tincture with an equal quantity of water is excellent; also if the frozen limb is cracked.

6) Mix 1 part salicyl with 9 parts vaseline, and use as ointment.

7) Marigold ointment is excellent for chapped hands or feet, also for burns.

8) Rub two or three times per day with tincture of southern-wood (*Artemisia abrotanum*).

9) Dissolve 2¼ cups (500 grams) alum in 4 quarts (4 liters) hot water; bathe the hands or feet in this for fifteen minutes every evening.

10) Hot oatstraw baths rapidly cure chapped hands and feet.

GALLSTONES (CHOLELITHIASIS)

Gallstones are stonelike formations in the gall bladder or gall ducts. The patient has a feeling of external pressure and obstruction in the area of the upper abdomen and the stomach, pains in the right side, and a tendency to vomit bitter matter. After a few days, the skin turns yellow and gallstones are found in the feces. Use one of the following treatments:

1) In the morning on an empty stomach, take 1 cup (200 grams) of pure olive oil, lie on the right side for half an hour with the hip higher than the shoulder; this causes the oil to run into the gall bladder. Any gallstones that may be present will come to light in the first bowel movement. At least a hundred people to whom I have given this advice have been cured.

I would also recommend squeezing 2 or 3 lemons and drinking the juice in a little water and a cup of tea made from common St. Johnswort over some period of time. The lemon juice takes away the pain and dissolves the gallstones. A tablespoon of castor oil should be taken the evening before.

2) For a blocked gall bladder, drink parsley tea.

3) Let box leaves (*Buxux sempervirens*) steep in gin and take a couple of tablespoons throughout the day for a blocked gall bladder.

4) Drink fenugreek tea for gall and mucus.

5) For gall and mucus you can also take a pinch of Carlsbad salts[13] with a little water every morning on an empty stomach. Follow an hour later with 2 cups of common St. Johnswort tea. This remedy is worthy of recommendation.

6) Every eight days, take 3 tablespoons (25 grams) of the tincture given for bilious vomiting, in the morning on an empty stomach. Those who suffer from gallstones should refrain from fatty food, spices and spirits. I would recommend plenty of vegetables and fruit and a daily cup of tea made from knotgrass or common St. Johnswort or common centaury.

GANGRENE

Gangrene is the extinction of life in the tissues of a part of the body and requires careful, energetic treatment. With this illness, a doctor cannot be called quickly enough. Gangrene may occur externally or internally. Internal gangrene may be caused by dropsy, scurvy, putrid fever, consumption, or heart disease. External gangrene may be caused by internal injury, by neglected or badly treated wounds, or severe infections of the latter, etc. It can be recognized by a lack of feeling, a deathly pallor and cadaverous smell. If gangrene is caused by great old age, or from some other internal cause, there is no hope of a cure. Use the following treatments:

1) Poultices of white bread and milk, sprinkled with powdered walnut septa are a very good remedy for external gangrene; 1 teaspoon (1 gram) of this powder should also be taken in wine three times a day.

2) If the gangrene is dry, apply constant compresses of camphorated oil.

3) Take ½ teaspoon (1 gram) cinchona powder every three hours for several days.

---

[13]Carlsbad salts: also known as Carlsbader salts, is a mixture of the more important chemical salts naturally present in several of the well-known mineral springs in Europe.

4) Drink 2 cups walnut septa tea every day.

5) Let 1¾ cup (200 grams) of oak bark boil in 5 quarts (5 liters) of rainwater until reduced to 1 quart (liter); strain through a cloth; apply this fresh compress every half hour by using a clean cloth each time. On the second day the complaint will have improved and a fresh compress should be applied every hour until a cure takes place. Cinchona powder and walnut septa tea can also be taken.

6) Another excellent remedy is as follows: apply constant compresses of a decoction made from teasel leaves; it helps even more if fresh leaves are applied. Above all, one should not forget the use of internal remedies, especially tea made from walnut septa.

7) Dissolve a handful of sea salt in 1½ quarts (1½ liters) hot water, then add a handful of common wormwood (*Artemisia absinthium*), leave to boil for fifteen minutes and apply compresses of this mixture.

GASTRITIS (INFLAMMATION OF THE STOMACH)
With inflammation of the stomach, the membrane, or the internal skin of the stomach, is inflamed. The best and easiest way to distinguish between stomach cramps and inflammation of the stomach is to press on the stomach. If the pain increases, becoming sharp and biting, it is inflammation of the stomach; if the pain lessens, it is stomach cramp. These illnesses are frequently confused. True inflammation of the stomach occurs rarely. In such a case, soothing remedies must be applied, such as hot poultices or compresses on the stomach and abdomen; cold washes; drink tea made from marshmallow or linseed. Mild food should be taken: mild kinds of meat, farinaceous foods, especially tonic soup which is very mild and easily digestible.

GASTRITIS (MUCOUS STOMACH)
A mucous stomach is frequently caused by too little exercise, a sedentary life, food that is too fatty and indigestible. It is also caused by worms, damp, unhealthy houses, and is found in people with weak constitutions. The usual symptoms are: lack

of warmth; thirst and hunger; a nauseous sweet taste with much slimy saliva in the mouth, especially in the mornings; the tongue is coated white; after eating there is pressure and a bloated feeling; slimy stools; frequent constipation; blue rings around the eyes; pallor; lassitude, constant inclination to sleep, etc. Chronic gastritis is, in fact, quite simply caused by a weak stomach. The following tea is excellent for a mucous stomach; it dissolves the mucus, strengthens the stomach, and is both a diuretic and a depurative.

> 2 tablespoons (4 grams) wild chicory
> 3 teaspoons (3 grams) angelica
> 1 tablespoon (3 grams) rosemary
> 4 teaspoons (2 grams) blessed thistle
> 2 teaspoons (2 grams) calamus
> 1½ teaspoons (3 grams) fennel seed
> 4 teaspoons (2 grams) buckbean
> 4 teaspoons (3 grams) meadowsweet

Leave to boil for fifteen minutes in 2 cups (½ liter) of water. Take 2 tablespoons four times per day before meals. It is advisable to eat a dry rusk after meals.

GOUT (RHEUMATISM)

Remedies to dissolve and expel gout are as follows: Apply compresses of hayseed, or even better, pour boiling water over hayseed, squeeze it out and apply hot on the gouty parts. Also use compresses and baths from oatstraw, clay compresses, washes, waterings, etc. The following teas are excellent in cases of chronic gout:

1) 1 teaspoon (1 gram) juniper berries, 2 tablespoons (5 grams) rosemary, 3 teaspoons (3 grams) licorice. Boil together in 2 cups (½ liter) water and take one to two cups daily.

2) 4 teaspoons (3 grams) thyme, 2 tablespoons (3 grams) heather, 3 tablespoons (3 grams) chamomile flowers. Let steep for twenty minutes in 2 cups (½ liter) boiling water. Drink one cup twice a day.

3) Each day drink three cups agrimony tea, and before retiring drink one cup of elder flower tea.

4) Drink a daily cup of tea made from buckbean and an equal quantity of lime blossom.

5) Let inner rind of elder wood steep in gin and take 2 to 3 tablespoons of this per day.

6) Every morning and evening, while in bed, rub the affected parts with the following mixture: 8 parts olive oil and 1 part juniper berry oil.

7) Rub twice a day with the following mixture from Raspail:

    3 tablespoons (30 grams) spirits of ammonia
    3 tablespoons (15 grams) alcohol
    3 tablespoons (30 grams) camphor
    1 quart (liter) rainwater
    1 cup (250 grams) coarse salt

8) Take lemon juice for ten days. Begin with the juice of one lemon and increase to five each day, then decrease each day to one again. This is an excellent remedy that can be repeated if it does not immediately bring about a full recovery.

9) A honey plaster applied to the painful area relieves the pain.

10) Take hot baths or use compresses of chemically pure soda.

Those who suffer from gout must eat little protein (meat, eggs, peas, beans, etc.). Beer and alcoholic drinks are forbidden. Good bowel movements are essential. Honey and fruit are very good, especially apples and stewed fruit. Pork is permitted.

GOUT (ARTHRITIS CHRONICA)

To treat chronic gout, twice a day, take a cup of tea made from a mixture of equal quantities of chamomile flowers, thyme and common heath (*Erica vulgaris*). Let a tablespoon of this herbal mixture steep in 1 cup boiling water and drink one or two cups daily.

GOUT WITH SWELLINGS (ARTHRITIS DEFORMANS)

1) The following simple plaster, applied once a day, dissolves the lumps and makes them disapper. Take burgundy tar[14] (*Piceus navalis*), liberally smear it on a linen cloth, sprinkle with a thin layer of flowers of sulphur and apply on the swellings. Also take a sugarspoon of white mustard seed every morning, midday and evening.

2) A flannel cloth, dipped in rosemary tea, wrung out and applied, then covered with dry linen and woolen cloths, left throughout the night, should cure the swellings after repeated treatment.

3) Boil 1 tablespoon fresh ash leaves with an equal quantity of finely chopped young ash twigs in 2 cups water. Take 1 cup daily with a spoon.

GOUT (GALLOPING)

This is usually cured by the application of one or two goose-wraps (see p. 410) of oat straw decoction for an hour to an hour and a half. I have experienced this twice. Drink one or two cups of tea made from juniper berries, rosemary and licorice. Or, boil a handful of buckbeans for a few minutes in 1 quart (liter) water and drink two cups daily. The latter tea is an excellent remedy for gout and rheumatics.

GREEN SICKNESS (CHLOROSIS)

This illness is peculiar to young girls and arises from anemia, a too watery quality of the blood, growing too quickly, food of poor quality, impure or damp air, severe illnesses, too much sitting and sleeping, etc. It begins with lack of strength, palpitations, difficulty in breathing and depression. The principle characteristics are: a yellowish-white color, with bluish rims to the eyes and pale bluish looking lips, white swollen gums, unpleasant breath, decreased menstruation or its absence, indigestion, lack of appetite, and, in particular, melancholy.

---

[14]Burgundy tar is probably made from the Norwegian spruce.

1) Green Sickness can be permanently cured by water applications (see Water Cures, p. 401), good food and a healthy way of life. Every morning and evening an upper body wash with cold water and a little vinegar, a hot compress applied for half an hour on the abdomen every two days, and daily knee waterings are most efficacious. This treatment should be continued for fourteen days or three weeks. Then three times a week an upper body watering, with four knee waterings, two thigh waterings, two hot compresses of hayseed decoction, or water and vinegar on the abdomen for half an hour. This should be done for two weeks. Following this, every week: two half-baths (three seconds); three waterings on the upper part of the body and two compresses for half an hour on the abdomen. In addition, each morning 1 tablespoon of milk boiled with fennel and tonic bread are easily digested and are healthy invigorating food for those suffering from Green Sickness. Also tea from bitter herbs such as white horehound, common centaury, thyme, angelica, etc.

2) Tincture of tormentil: a sugarspoonful taken in water twice a day; a piece of bread dipped in wine, taken every hour, is highly recommended. Sufferers from Green Sickness who live in cities should repair to the country.

3) The following mixture is an excellent invigorating remedy: mix an egg yolk with 1 sugarspoon brown sugar and 1 sugarspoon brandy; take this at ten o'clock in the morning and at four o'clock in the afternoon.

4) Mix 1 sugarspoon of pure iron filings (from the chemist) with 1 tablespoon powdered cinnamon, 1 tablespoon powdered eggshell and 1 tablespoon powdered sugar; take a pinch of this mixture every morning and evening.

5) A glass of goat's milk with a little honey, every morning and evening, is very efficacious.

6) Drink daily 1 cup milk in which 1 tablespoon dead-nettle and a pinch of cinnamon have been slowly simmered for fifteen minutes.

7) A nun used the following remedy for years with optimal results: Take 2 small nutmegs and finely grate them, 3 sticks

good double cinnamon, a handful angelica, a handful lovage, 12 cents (a pinch) of saffron, a handful of rue, a handful of common wormwood and a good pinch of nightshade (*Solanum nigrum*). Put everything in a glazed earthenware pot, add 3 quarts (liters) pure white wine, close the pot tight and place a quantity of bread dough around the earthenware lid; leave it to boil over a gentle fire for three hours. Before use, make a small hole in the dough and seal this with a cork; keep the medicine in the same pot in which it was cooked. (To facilitate opening, use a pot with a lip that can be sealed with dough before boiling; the position can be noted and the opening made there.) Dose: A liqueur-glassful, lukewarm, three times a day, the first glass in the morning on an empty stomach, the two subsequent glasses one hour before meals. If the medicine is finished and a cure has not yet been satisfactorily achieved, it may be repeated once or, at the most, twice more.

HAIR-LOSS, SCURF, DANDRUFF (SEBORRHEA SICCA)

1) Let a quantity of nettles steep in vinegar for six days, then filter them and add 10 percent glycerine.

2) Take a quantity of finely chopped burdock roots, steep ten days in 5 parts of 75 percent alcohol; rub the scalp with this two or three times a week.

3) Let a quantity of hop flowers draw in 5 parts of 70 percent alcohol for six days and rub the scalp with this twice a week.

4) Let ½ cup (60 grams) *Cortex chinae* (cinchona) steep for two days in 1 quart (liter) of gin, then strain. Dissolve 1 cup (250 grams) salt in 1 quart (liter) boiling water. Add 2 tablespoons (20 grams) medicinal soap. When this soap has dissolved, add 1 cup (200 grams) Eau de Cologne with the *Cortex chinae* (cinchona) infusion. Rub the scalp well with this every day. It will encourage the hair to grow and the scurf or dandruff will disappear.

5) A good remedy to prevent hair from falling out is to wash the head twice a week with salt water.

6) To remove hair (depilatory): mix 1 teaspoon (2 grams) alcohol, ½ teaspoon (75 centigrams) iodine, 1½ ounces (35 grams) collodion,[15] 1 teaspoon (1½ grams) extract of turpentine, and 1 teaspoon (2 grams) castor oil. A layer of this should be smeared on the part which is hairy; this should be done for several days.

HAYFEVER

Spray the inside of the nose twice a day with 2 cups (½ liter) lukewarm horsetail tea and drink a daily cup of the same tea. In addition, sniff a little galangal powder four times a day. I have cured many people with this remedy.

HEADACHE

Headaches are usually merely the result of some kind of illness or indisposition. If the headache is caused by a stomach complaint, the pain is felt in the forehead. If the headache is caused by congestion of blood in the head, the pain lies more toward the back of the head. If the pain is felt above one eye on one side, it is generally a nervous headache (migraine). Rheumatic headaches do not appear in any fixed position but move from one place to the other.

1) A remedy recommended for a severe headache, with a coated tongue and lack of appetite, caused by the stomach, is a cup of tea made from sage, common wormwood and juniper berries. Put a hot compress made from hayseed decoction on the abdomen for one hour; it should be renewed after half an hour.

2) Lay a fresh cabbage leaf on the forehead, and renew it every now and then.

---

[15]Collodion is a solution of gun cotton in ether, which forms a colorless, gummy liquid that dries rapidly, and is used in surgery for coating wounds, burns, etc. *Tr.*

3) Mix clay with water and vinegar and apply in the form of compresses on the forehead; it should be renewed every fifteen to twenty minutes.

4) Take 5 drops spike oil (lavender oil) twice a day on sugar.

5) Nervous headache (migraine) is cured by drinking a daily cup of strong tea made from speedwell (*Veronica officinalis*) over a long period of time. In addition take 4 whole washes, 2 half-baths and 2 hot vinegar and water compresses on the abdomen for half an hour per week.

6) A remedy for migraine is to sniff lukewarm ground ivy tea into the nose.

7) Should the headache be caused by congestion of blood in the head, the best remedy is to drink a cup of speedwell tea twice a day; this is most efficacious in drawing the blood away from the head.

8) A headache which had lasted for years was cured with the white of 3 eggs mixed with a little saffron, smeared on a linen cloth and bound around the forehead.

9) Take 2 teaspoons of powdered vervain with an equal quantity of powdered common wormwood, the white of 3 eggs and 1 spoon of flour; mix all the ingredients well and apply around the neck.

10) For headaches with severe burning on the forehead, sniff a little camphor powder, or sniff a little wine vinegar up through the nostrils. Also drink lemon water.

11) For headaches caused by a chill, thick phlegm, etc., without burning—sniff galangal powder.

12) Rub a few drops of aniseed oil on the forehead.

13) Bind freshly crushed mint on the forehead. This sometimes gives immediate relief.

14) Pour boiling water on a quantity of vervain, pound it all together and place on the forehead. In addition, drink 1 cup of tea made from 1 tablespoon of vervain steeped for twenty minutes in 1 cup of boiling water.

HEAD COLDS (INFLAMMATION OF THE NASAL MEMBRANE)

Little attention is usually paid to this complaint and it is also usually of little significance, but can have serious consequences if the cerebral cavity, for example, is affected.

1) Take ¼ cup (25 grams) powdered sugar, 3 tablespoons (25 grams) alum powder, 2 tablespoons (25 grams) camphor powder, and mix these ingredients together carefully. This powder should be sniffed at the onset of the cold; it is most efficacious.

2) A chronic head cold is cured by sniffing a strong infusion of bramble leaves (blackberry) every half an hour.

3) Sniff a little cod liver oil into the nose two or three times a day.

4) Rub the neck with camphorated spirits every morning and evening.

5) Inhale chamomile vapor.

6) Snuff for head colds: take 1¼ cup (125 grams) finely powdered alum, ⅔ cup (125 grams) starch powder, 1 cup (125 grams) powdered sugar, 1 cup (125 grams) camphor powder, and grind this mixture until it is very fine and sniff it throughout the day.

7) Sniff powdered salt. This is both a simple and an efficacious remedy, but should be used at the onset of the cold.

HEAD INJURIES

To treat swellings on the head caused by a fall or push, or for bruises caused by hitting your head, do one of the following:

1) Apply parsley pounded with vinegar. If the skin is grazed, add some water.

2) Apply compresses of diluted tincture of arnica. (The arnica should be diluted by adding a ⅓ or ½ part water. This is a homeopathic remedy.)

3) Apply a poultice of clay, water and vinegar, mixed with a

little arnica tincture, or apply freshly bruised common St. Johns-wort or common daisy or wallflower or Solomon's seal.

HEADLICE AND OTHER INSECTS ON THE BODY

Every evening before retiring, rub the head and affected places with the following mixture: 3 tablespoons (30 grams) lavender oil and 2 tablespoon (15 grams) sweet almond oil. A piece of blotting paper should be dipped in this mixture and used to rub it in; in the morning all the vermin will be dead.

HEART CRAMP (ANGINA PECTORIS)

1) According to Professor Martin, the best remedy is tincture of arnica. Mix 7 drops with ⅓ cup (100 grams) water. Take 1 sugarspoonful every five to ten minutes.

2) Mix 5 teaspoons (5 grams) cinquefoil, 2 teaspoons (2 grams) rue, 3 teaspoons (2 grams) lemon balm, ⅓ cup (3 grams) watermint and 2 teaspoons (3 grams) valerian root. Boil in 1 quart (liter) milk. Take this remedy hot throughout the day. It is essential to ensure regular bowel movements.

HEART DISEASE (VITIUM CORDIS)

Heart complaints can only be diagnosed by a physician. The symptoms of heart complaints, such as palpitations, painful dis-tressed feelings, pressure, constriction, breathlessness, etc., also occur in those who suffer from nerves. The heart can be per-fectly healthy and still be affected by severe palpitations; this often occurs in nervous patients, particularly hysterical people, or in those who suffer from Basedow's Illness. Heart patients must avoid excitement, excessive worries or troubles, deep depression, climbing stairs and walking. Extreme cold is also injurious; they should abstain from spirits and smoking; wine may only be taken in water (diluted) or in small quantities; hot food, coffee and tea are forbidden. Good bowel movements are necessary and the patient should take daily walks in the fresh air.

In the case of heart complaints, poultices made from clay, water, and vinegar, and placed over the heart region, have been found very useful; likewise upper body and whole washes, plus hot compresses made from water and vinegar (or hayseed decoction) on the abdomen for half an hour seem to help. If the palpitations are severe, compresses of camphorated spirits placed over the heart region are the most effective; they usually help after only a few minutes. A cold clay poultice may also bring great relief.

A recommended remedy is: drink 2 glasses of rosemary wine every day and take 5 drops of false hellebore tincture in a spoon of water three times a day. Or take 8-10 drops of tincture of *Flor. acaciae* in a spoonful of water three times a day.

For swollen legs and feet, which often accompany heart complaints, clay poultices around the legs are highly recommended. The clay compresses may be replaced by a poultice made from boiled leek: this is also most efficacious.

If there is numbness in the heart and hands (or in general) with heart complaints, a hot sage armbath (five minutes) is recommended daily. Great weakness of the heart may be controlled by taking 30 drops of equal quantities of tormentil and cinquefoil tincture in a spoon of cold water three times a day.

HEART (FATTY DEGENERATION, DEGENERATION ADIPOSE CORDIS)

Those who suffer from this complaint should avoid excessive tension or any kind of excitement. Their food should be easily digestible—little fat, no flour, no sugar or spirits, no tea or coffee. A little wine diluted with water is the best drink. Plenty of walking in the fresh air is beneficial.

1) Drink 4 cups (1 liter) of raw buttermilk daily. In addition take 5 drops arnica tincture in a spoon of cold water three times a day.

2) A daily dose, 2 cups (½ liter) Vichy water is very good.

3) Two wineglasses of rosemary wine daily is a well-known efficacious remedy. Let two good handfuls of bruised rosemary steep for twenty-four hours in a bottle of Mosel or Rhine wine.

4) Drinking a glass of hot water every morning on an empty

stomach has been a highly recommended remedy in recent times.

5) By using the following prescription, I discovered that the complaint swiftly improved. Every week take 4 whole washes, 3 short compresses made of water and vinegar (hot or cold according to choice), and 3 half-baths of five seconds. Three times a day take 5 drops of false hellebore tincture. Drink 2 glasses rosemary wine, and eat 1 cup (150 grams) dried meat and a few eggs.

Hematuria (Blood in the Urine)
The remedy for this is tea made from comfrey with common St. Johnswort, from horsetail and shepherd's purse, or yarrow, thyme, agrimony and shepherd's purse, or plantain and bearberry. Two people who suffered from hematuria for years were cured after a few weeks by drinking 1 cup thyme tea (*Thymus serpyllum*) every day with honey. Or try the following:

1) Take 15 Dutch Drops (see index) with a spoon of milk every other day.

2) Thyme tea is a very efficacious remedy.

3) Two sufferers from hematuria were cured in three days by drinking 1 to 2 cups of goldenrod tea every day. (It makes no difference if the blood is coming from the kidneys or the bladder). Goldenrod cannot be recommended highly enough for bladder and kidney disorders and several other complaints besides. See Goldenrod.

Hemorrhoids (Piles)
Hemorrhoids are generally swellings of the veins around the edge of the rectum, which appear in the form of small, painful, internal or external lumps. When these swellings remain small, they cause little trouble; but if they become larger and more numerous, they can cause considerable pain and annoyance. Special characteristics are: an itching, burning sensation around

the anus; stabbing pain and often pressure in the rectum; pain in the tailbone (coccyx) extending into the spine and neck; a feeling of anxiety; abdominal swelling which is usually due to trapped wind; indigestion; sluggish, irregular bowel movements; often diarrhea alternating with constipation, etc.

People who suffer from hemorrhoids should be on guard against all passions, particularly fornication, anger and depression. They should abstain from stimulating or sharp food, from celery, peas and beans; from heavy food, strong drinks, coffee, vinegar, etc. They should avoid soft beds, should not sleep too long or sit on hard chairs, and they need moderate exercise. An effective treatment is to drink a cup of yarrow tea daily.

If hemorrhoids bleed extensively and no infection arises, they are often beneficial to the health since they purify the blood; it is then dangerous to stop them.

If the hemorrhoids become inflamed, they cause great pain; bowel movements are very painful, sometimes impossible. In this case one should apply softening enemas—linseed, for example. A hot hip vapor bath of chamomile flowers or yarrow can also be taken twice daily. (See the Water Cure, Part III.) If the hemorrhoids bleed too heavily and thus weaken the patient, it is advisable to drink yarrow tea (2-3 cups per day) or calamus root tea.

A successful remedy for very swollen internal piles is to swallow 2 tablespoons olive oil daily.

HERNIA (RUPTURES)

1) Place grated comfrey on the rupture and then the truss; as soon as the comfrey is dry, the poultice should be renewed. This is a very simple but excellent remedy.

2) Monseigneur Kneipp cured a rupture by rubbing in fat from a fox and applying a pitch plaster on top.

3) Ruptures in children may be healed by rubbing the place twice a day with Peruvian balsam and giving a hot bath of oatstraw decoction every day.

4) Take 2 pounds (1 kilo) of fat from a male swine (pork fat, or lard), 6 cups (300 grams) comfrey, 4 ounces (100 grams)

Marchantia polymorpha,[16] 2½ cups (100 grams) *Vinca minor* and a handful of earthworms. Cook all these ingredients gently in a double boiler until the plants are really soft; press well through a cloth and store in an earthenware pot. A mustardspoon of this should be applied on the rupture every two days on a small piece of pig's bladder. This cures ruptures in children very quickly.[17]

HICCUPS

1) If hiccups occur during a severe illness, it is generally *not* a favorable sign; in such a case, a doctor should be consulted. The common hiccup can easily be stopped by drinking a glass of cold water with a spoon or by holding the breath as long as possible.

2) Hiccups can also be stopped by putting a pinch of very fine salt at the back of the throat on the uvula.

3) Marjoram tea is also good for hiccups.

4) Take a sugarspoon of strong vinegar with sugar.

HOARSENESS (RAUCITAS)

1) The best remedy, especially at the onset of the condition, is to place cold compresses around the neck for one to one and a half hours; but these compresses must be renewed every ten to thirty minutes if one does not wish to aggravate the illness.

2) Hot footbaths of potash and salt are recommended. One hot footbath is sometimes sufficient.

3) Drink tea made from hedge mustard (*Erysimum officinale*); a few cups are sufficient to bring about a cure.

4) An excellent remedy for chronic hoarseness is the following: Boil in a well-sealed pot until reduced by half: 8 cups (2 liters) water with a handful of haricot beans, ½ cup (94 grams) figs,

---

[16]*Marchantia polymorpha* is also known as brook liverwort; however, we were unable to locate any of this.

[17]We do not recommend people using earthworms and pig's bladder as remedies, but have included this recipe for its historical and folk recipe value.

and ½ cups (94 grams) raisins. Strain, and add 2 tablespoons olive oil, ⅓ cup (100 grams) French brandy and ⅓ cup (94 grams) honey. Mix well, bottle, and take 1 tablespoon every two hours.

5) Boil finely grated parsnips in 2 cups (½ liter) milk, strain through a cloth, add a little sugar and drink this throughout the day.

6) Take 4 to 5 teaspoons (2 to 3 grams) sage, let this boil with 1 cup (200 grams) milk, strain through a cloth and add a good tablespoon of sugar. Take before retiring.

7) Drink licorice tea.

8) Gargle with fenugreek or agrimony tea. A cup of tea from both of the above may be taken daily.

9) Pour boiling water over a quantity of vervain, soak for a few minutes and mash it together; apply this to the neck as hot as possible. This will cure even the most acute hoarseness. In addition drink a cup of vervain tea.

HOUSEMAID'S KNEE (BURSITIS PRAEPATELLARIS)
Boil leeks to a pulp which should be applied thickly on the swelling three times a day. (See also Swollen Knees.)

HYDROTHORAX (WATER ON THE CHEST)
Hydrothorax is frequently difficult to recognize. The symptoms are as follows: difficulty breathing, a feeling of constriction, unexplainable anxiety, a dry cough, breathlessness, palpitations, hoarse, weak voice, lack of sleep or restless sleep, red or bluish cheeks, neck stretched forward, watery swelling of the eyelids, swollen hands and feet, etc. This illness must be treated by a qualified physician. Do not postpone this long. You can also do the following:

1) Let a handful of rosemary steep for forty-eight hours in a bottle of Rhine wine (or white rather sweet wine), shake the bottle well occasionally and drink 2 wineglasses of this daily.

2) Take 1 or 2 cups white horehound tea, or rosemary wine. Both are recommended.

3) In addition: alternate half and whole washes. Soft cheese applied as a plaster on the chest and renewed when dry has an excellent effect.

HYPOCHONDRIA

People affected by this illness are deplorable; they are an annoyance to both themselves and others, and in general little sympathy is given them. Medicine is of very little or no help at all.

The Kneipp water cure gives every hope of recovery if the patient has forebearance and does not expect to be cured in six weeks as is usually the case. Water applications are particularly beneficial and these patients should occupy themselves during the day with gardening.

HYSTERIA

Hysteria is an illness of the brain; it appears at any age from ten to sixty. Moments of deep emotion, great distress, disappointment, tension, pampering, etc., are followed by this illness. It is especially peculiar to women. They have palpitations, nervous cramps, constriction of the throat, breathing becomes difficult, the chest tightens spasmodically; the patient has the feeling as though a bullet has been released low down in the abdomen and slowly rises to the throat where it causes a kind of suffocation that impedes breathing. This is followed by convulsions very similar to epileptic fits. The patient sometimes laughs and weeps at one and the same time, or screams, hits and bites the people around him or her. When in bed, the patient sometimes forcefully rips the sheets and blankets to shreds. Such severe attacks may last from a half-hour to two hours. The patient subsequently feels very tired and falls asleep. Many such people are cured by water applications.

First week: upper body washes with hot compresses on the abdomen.

Second week: four whole washes, three upper body washes, three hot compresses made from hayseed decoction for half an hour on the abdomen.

Third week: four whole washes, three knee waterings, one cold compress made from water and vinegar on the back for half an hour. Then one cold compress on the chest for half an hour.

Fourth week: four upper body washes, three half-baths, two compresses as in the third week.

In addition, the patient should take waterings of the upper body, back, thigh, depending on his or her condition. The patient should drink one or two cups of tea made from lemon balm and mint every day. In the evenings, the patient's abdomen should be rubbed with camphorated oil. Balsam tea (*Balsamita suaveolens*)[18] is also good. If hysterical patients have a headache, a cold clay compress should be placed on the forehead.

IMPURE BLOOD

Every week take four whole washes, three short compresses of hayseed decoction for one hour, and three hip-baths for fifteen seconds or three half-baths for five seconds. In addition, take 1 cup depurative[19] tea daily, as detailed later in this book (see p. 375).

INDIGESTION

Drink lemon water; if this does not help, drink sufficient lukewarm water to cause vomiting; or strong tea made from chamomile flowers. The following day, remain on a diet. Or, mix a sugarspoon of salt in half a glass cold water and drink it.

INFANTILE PARALYSIS (POLIO)

Paralysis may occur in children due to sudden illness caused by an infection of the brain or spinal cord. The cause and course is as follows: usually the child quite suddenly becomes restless at night and begins to toss and moan. A high fever,

---

[18]We are not certain if the author was referring to sweet balm, lemon balm or *Impatiens balsamina,* garden balsam.

[19]Depurative means to remove impurities.

accompanied by severe cramps causes the little one much suffering; this cramp-fever usually subsides after one or two days, but can sometimes last longer. It is followed by paralysis in one or more limbs. Sometime after the fever has subsided, most of the paralysis also disappears, so that only an arm or leg remains paralyzed; it is generally the left leg. Some time later, this limb becomes emaciated and backward in its development, sometimes becoming shorter than the other. The following remedies may be applied with good results: every day a hay-shirt and a whole wash, or twice a day a hot compress of hayseed decoction around the paralyzed limb with a whole wash. Instead of this, the child may also be dipped in cold water up to the armpits. The following is highly recommended: four times per day use a hot compress of chemically pure soda water with one whole wash daily.

INFECTION (CONTAGION)
Boil leeks to a pulp, apply hot three times a day and drink two cups of the decoction every day.

INFLAMMATION OF THE CEREBRAL MEMBRANE (MENINGITIS)
This complaint must be immediately verified by a physician; it may occur because of a fall, bang, push, from walking bareheaded in the burning sun, from extreme cold, becoming soaked, drinking too much spirits, etc. At the onset of meningitis, the patient has high fever, sleeplessness, severe headache, fast pulse, ringing in the ears and vomiting; this is soon followed by unconsciousness, hypersomnia and paralysis, and death a few days later. Occasionally there is a lucky case where recovery takes place, but very seldom; if the meningitis becomes a chronic condition, the patient is generally dull or insane.

At the onset of this illness, it is good to apply a cold poultice of clay, water, and vinegar on the neck. Renew it as soon as it begins to dry; it is also good to alternate this with a clay poultice on the back. If the feet are cold, dip hot cloths in a solution of water and vinegar, wring out well, and wrap these around the feet until they are warm. To combat the headache, a clay poultice should be applied on the forehead and renewed as soon as it becomes warm. The most advisable internal remedy is to give cold water with a spoon. The physician should be consulted as soon as possible.

INFLAMMATION OF THE HIP JOINT (COXITIS)

This complaint frequently occurs in scrofulous[20] children and is generally tubercular. It can be caused by a fall, bang, push or injury. The first symptoms of the illness are: limping and pain in the knee, although there is nothing to see and a mistake is possible. Sooner or later the hip joint becomes painful and completely stiff, so that the child puts his weight on the one healthy leg and touches the ground with the toes of the affected leg, just as though it is shorter, which is not the case. Those who suffer from this complaint should stay in bed and apply a hot compress of soda water (chemically pure) on the hip four times a day for half an hour; for the rest of the day a poultice of clay, water and vinegar should be applied and renewed as soon as it begins to dry; at night a poultice of fenugreek. In addition, take a pinch of bone-dust twice a day, and 1 cup goldenrod tea daily.

• • •

A child of 14 had suffered for three months from inflammation of the hip joint and all remedies had been tried without any sign of recovery. I advised that the child should be washed all over daily with cold water and that poultices of clay, water and vinegar should be constantly applied to the hip. After three weeks, the child had completely recovered and now, ten years later, is still healthy and well.

A young lady from Antwerp lay for a year in bed with this complaint. She could only move her leg with the greatest pain; I wrote and advised a daily whole wash and a soda compress four times a day, applied as hot as possible; she should drink a cup of tea made from thyme, white horehound, and common centaury daily, and take half a sugarspoon of bone-dust twice a day. After strictly following my advice, the lady was cured.

A 15 year old child, on whom they were preparing to operate, recovered in three months by means of washes, soda

---

[20]Scrofulous means a swollen condition of the glands, usually of the throat.

compresses and a poultice of fenugreek at night. I could quote still more examples, but time and space are dear. It is far better to try the cure oneself when the occasion necessitates it.

INFLAMMATION OF NERVES (NEURITIS)

Neuritis can have many causes; for example, poison which has been taken, not sleeping at night, nicotine and alcohol, dangerous contagious diseases, gout and rheumatism, syphilis, diabetes, injured limbs, a fall or bang, etc. Neuritis can cause severe pain, sometimes at the least movement; it frequently begins with fever and affects several nerves, such as in the hands, arms, and legs. Dangerous paralysis can also occur with muscular tuberculosis. I should like to quote the following example:

A German gentleman came to me with a very swollen, very painful blue hand. I asked him the cause and what remedies had been applied, and he answered, "My doctor said that it is neuritis, that he knew of no remedy and that I should go to a certain specialist in Aachen. This I did. The specialist in Aachen called it 'Nervenentzündung,' but could not help me. The same day I consulted two other doctors and received the same answer—Inflammation of a nerve, no remedy."

Following this tale, I prescribed bathing the hand twice a day in hot chemically pure soda water and the rest of the day applying a poultice of clay, water and vinegar, which had to be renewed as soon as it became dry, and at night a poultice of fenugreek. After two weeks he was to show me the hand again. He kept his word and what he showed me was a fully recovered hand—swelling, pain, blue color, powerlessness and immovability of the fingers—all had gone and the gentleman was as happy as his advisor.

I was able to cure a second case of neuritis by bathing the arm a whole day in soda water and applying a poultice of fenugreek at night. On the second day I prescribed bathing four times in soda water and the rest of the time fenugreek; on the third day a poultice of potatoes and buttermilk was to be renewed three times. Ten days later it had also completely recovered.

INFLUENZA

Influenza is a severe cold which has frequently visited us in the last few years and is not to be trifled with. The symptoms are: severe headache, general weakness, tiredness, sometimes nose-bleeds, lack of appetite, intermittent fever, pain in the knees, cough, etc.

The best remedy for a quick recovery is to take whole washes every hour, until the sweat breaks out, then continue with a whole wash every three hours, and so on gradually decreasing. Should burning or fever reappear, a whole wash should immediately be given. Drink one to two cups elder flower and chamomile flower tea. Also give 1 tablespoon of tea made from sage, common wormwood and juniper berries every two hours.

An excellent remedy for influenza is the following: mix 2 tablespoons olive oil with 1 tablespoon French brandy, 3 fresh egg yolks and ⅓ cup (100 grams) honey. Take a sugarspoon of this mixture every fifteen minutes; the patient should stay in bed and apply the washing treatment as above.

INGROWN NAILS

1) First apply a poultice of fenugreek to soften the skin, then cut out the nail and place a little lint underneath. In future cut the nail for quite some time more in the middle than at the sides; in this way, the nail will assume a different shape and will no longer grow into the flesh.

2) Take one or two hot footbaths from chemically pure soda water every day for about twenty minutes (1 handful soda to 4 cups (1 liter) boiling water).

INSECT BITES (PREVENTATIVE)

Mix 1 tablespoon (10 grams) tincture of *Pyrethrum roseum* with ⅓ cup (100 grams) water; rub the face with this. Pyrethrum powder kills flies, crickets, ants, and other insects; it should be scattered in places where insects collect.

INSOMNIA

Insomnia is usually caused by some kind of illness; those who suffer from nerves are the most inconvenienced by this. If the insomnia is caused by an illness, it is the latter which should be fought. If one wishes to sleep well by using one of the following remedies, it is essential to avoid stressful business, especially in the evenings, and to remain as quiet as possible.

1) Those who suffer from nerves are recommended to take a cup of yarrow tea before retiring. In addition, the bed should be so placed, if possible, that the head is pointing north and the feet south, then the patient will sleep much more peacefully.

2) Rub the abdomen with cold water two to four minutes every evening, or place a cold compress around the feet or on the neck.

3) If insomnia is caused by congestion of blood in the head, take a cup of speedwell tea in the evenings.

4) Take 3 drops onion tincture in a spoon of water three times a day.

5) Every morning, midday, and evening crunch a piece of camphor the size of a grain of wheat and swallow with a little wild chicory tea; or put this quantity of camphor in a glass of sugar and water, add 3 drops sulfuric ether. Drink this in one dose before retiring and it will be followed by the most pleasant sleep (Raspail).

6) An excellent remedy for insomnia is to take 1 or 2 raw onions in the evening.

INTESTINAL BLEEDING

Every day take 2 cups sanicle tea with honey.

INTESTINAL CATARRH (ENTERITIS CATARRHALIS)

There is rarely fever with intestinal catarrh; but there is always diarrhea alternating with constipation, and tough, jelly-like, slimy feces. The release of wind and bowel movement always bring relief, while the constipation tires and depresses the patient. The abdomen is tense and there is a feeling of pressure, particularly following meals; the patient has heartburn, nausea, and is spiritless and weak. Hot compresses should be laid on the abdomen and the patient should be given upper body washes; after a few days a whole wash may be given. Every hour he or she should be given 1 tablespoon hot tea made from sage, common wormwood and fennel, or tea made from common centaury, sage, and juniper berries.

If the diarrhea lasts too long or is too severe, the patient should be given 1 to 2 sugarspoons of tincture of bilberries (blueberries) in hot water every two hours. The strictest diet should be observed here: thick soups made from gruel, oats, sago or rice; a little red wine is also permitted; meat dishes, black bread, vegetables, and fruit should be avoided.

Intestinal Inflammation (Enteritis)

The symptoms of enteritis are burning pain in the region of the navel or lower, external pressure; every movement increases the pain which, at the onset, is only felt in one place but rapidly extends and frequently affects the whole abdomen. The pain becomes worse, eventually unbearable; the abdomen is sometimes very swollen and sometimes depressed. There may be considerable oppression, nausea, even severe vomiting; such symptoms take away almost all hope. It goes without saying that in such a case one should not hesitate to consult a qualified doctor. Water and vinegar washes are recommended. Every half hour a hot compress of water and vinegar should be placed on the abdomen; each week one half-bath and two hip-baths should be given.

If the patient has cold feet, they should be well rubbed with water and vinegar and then wrapped in a dry linen cloth and a woolen blanket. With this illness, no purgatives should be given, as every movement or shock of the body increases the pain and aggravates the inflammation. Take 1 tablespoon hot tea made from common wormwood, sage, and fennel every two hours; also take 8 to 10 drops wormwood tincture in lukewarm water twice a day.

A highly efficacious remedy for enteritis is as follows: boil 1 tablespoon linseed in a quart (liter) of water for fifteen minutes and take 1 tablespoon, hot, every hour.

ITCHING (PRURITUS)

For itching on the lower part of the body, wash the area twice with tea made from sage or goldenrod. Or boil chervil in milk and wash the affected area with this. A good ointment against itching, even when deep-rooted, is as follows: mix 2 tablespoons (30 grams) lard with 1 tablespoon (15 grams) wood tar. Smear the areas with this twice a day.

JAUNDICE

Yellow colored skin and eyes are symptoms of jaundice. This is caused by gall mixing with the blood. If the liver is healthy, jaundice is not a serious matter. The following remedies can be used with good results:

1) Drink tea made from soapwort, agrimony, woodruff, or white horehound.

2) Vervain steeped in wine is very good.

3) Every week use two or three short compresses at night, a whole wash, and 3 tablespoons of common wormwood tea three times a day.

4) Mix 2 egg yolks and 1 teaspoon (1 gram) dried saffron with 2 cups (½ liter) French brandy. Take 1 tablespoon three times a day after meals. Recovery takes place after a few days.

5) I have found the following remedies to be the best for chronic jaundice: Boil 6 tablespoons crushed hempseed in 1 quart (liter) of milk; take this quantity every day. Or, let a handful of elder skins (*Sambucus ebulus*) steep for thirty-six hours in a bottle of white wine and take three wineglasses of this remedy daily. Or, drink walnut blossom tea as a highly efficacious remedy for chronic jaundice.

6) The following remedies must be used over a long period of time. (If the urine becomes cloudy and thick with a profusion

of sediment, it is a sign that the illness is nearly cured.) Take fresh elder roots, scrape them down to the hard wood, squeeze them out, and take 4 to 6 tablespoons. This brings about a very swift recovery, sometimes in one day. Or you can combine a small tablespoon of rhubarb and 3 egg yolks in 2 cups (½ liter) Bordeaux wine and take 1 tablespoon of this every hour.

7) A remedy for the severe itching that often accompanies jaundice is to apply a short compress of hayseed infusion every other day for one hour.

KIDNEYS (BLEEDING)
If the blood comes from the kidneys, it is mixed with the urine; if it comes from the bladder, urination is followed by clear, red blood.

1) By drinking two cups of goldenrod tea daily, two patients were cured from passing blood in three days when their urine was completely clear again.

2) Dutch Drops, 15 every other day taken with milk, are sometimes very beneficial.

KIDNEYS (ULCERATION)
1) Drink tea made from plantain (the seed is also good), or comfrey tea.

2) Tea from sanicle mixed with licorice and mint is highly recommended for ulcerated kidneys.

3) Tea from ground ivy, and especially a mixture of goldenrod and sanicle with the addition of a little honey is recommended. It is best to take 1 cup of these teas daily. In addition, take a daily hay compress around the loins for one hour.

KIDNEY STONES
1) Mix ½ cup (100 grams) old walnut oil and ½ cup (100 grams) sweet almond oil. Take 2 to 3 sugarspoons per day. Also drink tea made from licorice and oats decoction.

2) Tea made from thyme and common St. Johnswort is also good.

3) With kidney complaints, it is also good to drink a large quantity of buttermilk.

4) Boil a handful of rosehips with the pips (the pips are the most powerful part) for three-quarters of an hour in 5 cups (1-½ liters) water. Take 2 cups daily. Milk and sugar may be added to improve the taste; it is then a very pleasant drink.

5) If there is much pain, a hot compress of horsetail or oatstraw decoction can also be applied. Linseed tea is also recommended.

6) Dutch Drops are also effective in the case of kidney stones.

7) Tincture of mistletoe (*Viscum album*) is prepared by letting a handful of mistletoe leaves steep in a liter of gin. Take a liqueur-glassful every morning and evening. This is an excellent remedy for kidney stones.

8) Take ⅔ cup (30 grams) goldenrod, boil in a bottle of white wine for fifteen minutes and drink 2 wineglasses per day; this will destroy and expel the kidney stones. In addition, it is advisable to drink 1 cup linseed decoction tea every day.

9) The seed from ash trees (*Fraxinus exelsior*) steeped in gin, is a most efficacious remedy, but one should begin very carefully with small amounts. Use 6 to 8 tablespoons of seed per bottle of gin. First take 1 tablespoon a day and increase to 2 to 4 tablespoons. This remedy expels the water most powerfully.

KNEES (SWOLLEN)

1) Apply compresses of clay, water and vinegar.

2) Apply compresses of rue or horsetail.

3) Boil ¼ cup (32 grams) powdered oak bark in 4 cups (1 liter) water until reduced by half, then add: 3½ teaspoons (8 grams) alum powder. Apply in the form of compresses.

4) Boil equal quantities of walnut leaves and elder bark in

water, add a little Spanish soap[21] and some gin. Apply as compresses.

5) The following tincture is an excellent remedy for swollen and bruised knees:

> 2 cups (50 grams) arnica flowers
> 2 tablespoons (10 grams) cloves
> 5 teaspoon (10 grams) cinnamon
> ¼ cup (15 grams) balsam flowers
> 3 tablespoons (10 grams) St. Johnswort flowers
> 1 quart (liter) 75% alcohol

Leave this to steep for ten to fifteen days and then strain. Use this tincture diluted with an equal quantity of water; it should be applied as a compress.

6) For internal bruising, 1 sugarspoonful of the above mixture should be put in a glass of sugar and water and given to the patient three times a day.

7) If there is inflammation, see Bone Diseases.

8) If there is no inflammation, apply a poultice of lard boiled with an equal quantity of green soap three times a day; this remedy is particularly effective if water has collected on the knee. It is also effective in the case of so-called housemaid's knee. The latter is a spongy swelling which is mostly caused by too much kneeling, and I brought about numerous cures by using the above mentioned lard and soap poultices. This may be used without the slightest fear and continued until the knee has fully recovered. A nun had to apply them constantly for about five months before the swelling completely disappeared. In other patients treated by me, it took three months, for some people two or three weeks. The older the swelling, the longer the treatment.

9) For other knee swellings, hot compresses of chemically pure soda (a good handful to each quart of water) are very effective; the more compresses each day, the better.

10) Apply fresh scrapings of bryony root.

---

[21]Castile soap.

LEGS (SWOLLEN)

1) Boil leeks to a pulp, apply this three times and also drink a cup of the decoction. A nun who had had a swollen leg for months was cured by this remedy in one day.

2) Boil potatoes without salt, mash them very fine and mix them with unboiled buttermilk to make a thick poultice. Apply this thickly on the leg and renew it as soon as it begins to dry. This is also an excellent remedy for old sores.

3) Legs swollen by weakness, anemia and dropsy can be cured by cold compresses of water, vinegar and clay; to be renewed as soon as it begins to dry.

4) Buttermilk compresses are also effective.

LIVER COMPLAINTS (HEPATITIS)

1) Apply hot hayseed compresses and take cold washes.

2) The following kinds of tea are highly recommended for liver complaints: white horehound, agrimony, vervain, common St. Johnswort, and greater celandine. The latter is most efficacious but poisonous. It should be used in wine: 1⅓ cups (20 grams) of the fresh plant to 1 bottle white wine; take 1 tablespoon four times a day.

3) One of the best remedies is to rub the liver area with olive oil, especially if the liver complaint is caused by obstructed gall. This oil should be rubbed in hot.

4) Combine the following: ¼ cup (5 grams) horsetail, 2 tablespoons (5 grams) common wormwood, 1 teaspoon (1 gram) juniper berries, 3 tablespoons (6 grams) agrimony, 4 teaspoons (3 grams) vervain and 2 tablespoons (3 grams) wild chicory. Leave to steep for twenty minutes in 2 cups (½ liter) boiling water and take 2 tablespoons every two hours.

5) For inflammation of the liver (hepatitis), the symptoms are a swelling of the liver, pain when the liver area is pressed, little fever, green vomit, restless sleep, melancholy disposition, itching all over the body, hard, sticky stools. Those who are weak should take a whole wash daily and a hot compress of hayseed

on the liver area. Those who are stronger can take a short hayseed compress every other day and a half-bath alternating with a whole wash. At the onset of the inflammation, it is advisable to take compresses made from hot water and vinegar.

6) Let ⅔ cup (10 grams) of the herb or root of greater celandine steep in 4 cups (1 liter) of water. Take this quantity, with a spoon, over a period of twenty-four hours.

7) Four times a day, take 2 tablespoons tea made from sage, common wormwood, horsetail and juniper berries. Those who suffer from liver complaints should abstain from spirits and eat only a little meat. The best diet in this case is: in the mornings milk, bread and eggs; in the middle of the day, fatless soup, a little meat, vegetables, farinaceous foods and fruit; in the evenings, vegetables and no meat.

8) Carrot juice is an excellent medicine: take a normal glassful every morning on an empty stomach.

9) The following kinds of tea are recommended: rosemary or gentian, fumitory or soapwort, the roots of couch grass or wild chicory. Fresh herring is excellent.

10) For a blocked liver or gall bladder, drink tea made from common centaury or angelica. For a blocked liver only, drink tea made from rosemary, vervain, valerian, or mint.

LIVER SPOTS (CHLOASMA)
The brown, so-called liver spots have nothing in common with the liver; these brown-yellow spots appear especially on the neck, chest and arms, sometimes so numerous that the latter are almost completely covered. They are quite harmless, although sometimes unpleasant on account of the itching. Before using one of the following remedies, scrub the patches hard with a brush and green soap.

1) Let ¼ cup (30 grams) American white hellebore (*Veratum viride*) steep in 1 cup (240 grams) alcohol for ten days. (This tincture should not be filtered.) Rub the spots with this three times a day.

2) Mix 1 part nutmeg flower oil with 10 parts cod liver oil; rub in every evening and tie a cloth around it.

3) Moisten the spots with a solution of ½ teaspoon (2 grams) borax in 4 tablespoons (32 grams) rosewater.

4) Wash the affected area with parsley water.

LOSS OF STRENGTH

About fifteen years ago, a gentleman came to me and said, "I have with me a patient who, according to a doctor treating him, has at the most three months to live. He is losing four pounds every week." The patient looked very sorrowful, discontent and thin; his eyes were deep and cavernous in their sockets, and his whole body was just like a skeleton. The aforementioned doctor had declared that there was nothing organically wrong and the patient only complained of backache and loss of strength.

I began by encouraging the patient, assuring him that everything would turn out well and urging him to follow my instructions strictly. Every day in the first week he was given an upper body wash, a hot hay compress on the abdomen, tonic soup and bone-dust, and every two hours 1 tablespoon tea made from angelica, common centaury, sage, common wormwood and juniper berries. During the second week he was given four whole washes, three knee waterings, three hay compresses on the abdomen, and three cold hip-baths for five seconds. In the third week he was given three upper body washes, three knee waterings, three half-baths for five seconds and three compresses. During the fourth week he had the same application, plus walking for ten minutes in wet grass and three minutes of treading water.

And after the fourth week? The gentleman was healthier than he had ever been before; the backache had long since vanished, he had gained twenty pounds and I have heard that since his stay here he has enjoyed constant good health.

A young lady was so anemic and so weak that she could hardly stand on her legs. She had no appetite at all; in three weeks she had taken nothing more than a little chocolate. My prescription for her was: every day a lukewarm compress of hayseed decoction on the abdomen, a daily upper body wash

with lukewarm water and vinegar, and every two hours 1 tablespoon common centaury and white horehound tea with
sugar. In addition, twice a day she took a knife-point of bone-
dust with water and milk, and every hour 1 tablespoon milk.
On the second day, she already ate a little thin tonic soup; on
the third day, she really enjoyed the tonic soup and took a piece
of bread with a little egg yolk. Her appetite gradually improved,
she regained her strength, and after two weeks she was able to
sit at the communal table. The doctor who had previously been
treating her paid her a visit and accidentally met her at the
door. The young lady, delighted to see her doctor, gave him a
friendly greeting, but he failed to recognize her and asked if
he could speak to the young lady, and although she assured
him that it was she, he could and would not believe it because
she looked so fresh and strong.

The same performance occurred here twice: a father came
to visit his daughter whom he had not seen for two months; he
would never have recognized her if she had not made herself
known. I could quote more examples of weak patients making
a full recovery, but time and space render it impossible.

LUMBAGO (PAIN IN THE LOINS)

1) Every hour place a hot compress of hayseed decoction, or
hot water and vinegar on the back.

2) Mix together ½ teaspoon (1 gram) spirits of ammonia and
3 teaspoons (8 grams) olive oil. Smear the back with this mixture
twice a day.

3) Mix 1 tablespoon (10 grams) spike oil, 1 tablespoon (10
grams) cod liver oil, and 1 tablespoon (10 grams) opodeloc.[22]
Rub the back with this three times a day.

4) Rub the back with arnica tincture.

5) Rub with rue tincture three times a day. Also take 10 to 15
drops of this tincture twice a day in a spoon of water, one hour
before or after meals.

---

[22]Opodeloc is also known as camphorated soap liniment or white castile soap,
which is made from potassium hydroxide (KOH) and olive oil.

6) Three times a day take 20 to 30 drops of the following mixture on sugar: 3 parts ether with 1 part spirits of turpentine.

7) Place a piece of gutta percha paper in the painful area until the pain subsides.

LUPUS

1) Apply compresses of the following remedies: ⅓ cup (6 grams) arnica flowers, 6 teaspoons (6 grams) rue, 4 tablespoons (6 grams) plantain, 4 tablespoons (6 grams) horsetail, and ¼ cup (6 grams) chamomile flowers. Let steep for twenty minutes in 2 cups (½ liter) boiling water.

2) The application of finely pounded chickweed is an efficacious remedy for lupus.

3) Mix 1 part Peruvian balsam with 6 parts sweet butter. Smear on cotton wool and place over the lupus sores.

4) Smear with cod liver oil two to four times a day.

5) Boil 4 teaspoons (10 grams) oak bark and 1 tablespoon (10 grams) tormentil root in 2 cups (½ liter) water for fifteen minutes, then add ½ cup (10 grams) horsetail and let boil for a few minutes. Strain through a cloth and add 3 tablespoons honey. Let boil again for a further two minutes and pour into a bottle. Smear the lupus sores with this four times a day.

6) Use compresses of clay, water and vinegar. A little arnica tincture may be added; these compresses have a beneficial effect on lupus sores.

7) Especially at the onset of lupus, head vapor baths are useful: one or two head vapor baths are sufficient to dissolve foul matter in the head. It should not be forgotten that the remedies must be frequently changed: even if a remedy is found to be most effective, it is never for long. If a different remedy is then used for a few days, one is quite free to choose the previous one and start all over again. Two or three different remedies can be used on the same day, or another remedy can be used at night. If the lupus sores are burning, apply unsalted soft

cheese, or whey in which elder flowers have been boiled, in the form of compresses.

8) Place grated carrots on the lupus sores; this is excellent.

9) Boil a handful of walnut leaves in 1 quart (liter) water for fifteen minutes, strain through a cloth, add ¼ cup (30 grams) sugar, and apply continually as compresses.

10) Wash the sores four times a day with sweetened walnut leaf tea; also drink 1 cup of the same tea every day and take 1 tablespoon cod liver oil daily. Every two weeks use a mild purgative, such as St. Germain.

11) Soda water compresses are highly recommended.

MAGGOTS OR THREADWORMS (OXYURIS VERMICULARIS)

Maggots are white, ⅛ inch (½ centimeter) long, the thickness of a thread. They are generally found in the rectum of weak children, but sometimes occur in adults, too. They sometimes appear externally, particularly at night and cause severe itching. Children who have maggots are pale, their eyes deeply sunken in the head; the eyeballs are large, there are blue shadows under the eyes and the patients persistently pick their noses. These children generally have a coated tongue, little appetite; they prefer to eat farinaceous food and potatoes; they frequently wet the bed in their sleep; their sleep is restless, they grind their teeth and wake with a fright while sleeping. A large number of these worms are often found in the stools.

1) See Salt Water Enema.

2) Boil garlic in milk, give 4 to 6 tablespoons every morning and evening. Give enemas of the same decoction; this is best before going to bed.

3) An enema made from walnut leaves is also very effective.

4) Give quassia wood enemas every evening. This should be prepared as follows: boil 4 tablespoons (30 grams) quassia wood in 1 quart (liter) water. After the enema, smear the anus with cod liver oil. If there are worms in the vagina, it should also be syringed out.

5) Instead of the last remedy, enemas of fresh rue decoction can be used.

6) Thoroughly boil 2 teaspoons (3½ grams) lemon pips in 2 cups (½ liter) milk; give teacups of this throughout the day. The first cup should be taken half an hour before breakfast; the last before retiring.

MALARIA (MARSH FEVER)

This is an illness which rarely occurs in our marshy regions but is very wide-spread in hot southern countries. The causes of this illness give rise to disagreement: it is thought to be caused by a small insect that nestles in the blood and is then passed on by the bite of a mosquito which has sucked the blood of a malaria patient.

Malaria is usually characterized by intermittent fever. The patient has a feeling of paralysis, there is no desire to work and the appetite is much diminished. Each time there is an attack of fever, the spleen swells up to a greater or lesser extent. Sometimes the fever occurs daily, at other times every three or four days.

1) Treatment: every day, one or two whole washes; each week, three short compresses of hayseed decoction for one hour. Every day 1 to 2 cups tea made from goldenrod, or 1 cup tea made from heath spotted orchis, juniper, calamus, blue lilac leaves, or tormentil root.

MASTITIS (BREASTS SWOLLEN THROUGH CHILL, THICKENING OF THE MILK, ETC.)

1) Fry some old butter and pour it, while it is still hot, into cold water; remove it from the water and add as much French brandy as the butter will absorb. Smear this thickly on cotton wool and apply it to the swollen breasts three times a day. This mixture does not spoil.

2) Mix 3 parts olive oil with 2 part rosemary; smear this over the breasts with a feather four times a day.

MEASLES

Measles is a contagious childhood illness. It usually affects children age 2 to 10 years. Symptoms are: numerous red spots on the skin, similar to flea bites; after three days they disappear, leaving numerous pink-colored flakes of skin. Before the outbreak of measles, there is generally a little fever, also a head cold; the children complain of headache and pain in the limbs; the eyes are red and running and cannot bear the light. Sometimes patients have severe headache, diarrhea, vomit bile, have a bleeding nose and a barking cough. The measles first break out on the face, temples, and both sides of the nose; then the neck, chest, legs, and last of all the feet. If the red spots are pressed with a finger, they disappear, becoming white and when the pressure is released, become red again. The treatment is very simple. The child should be given nothing to eat; tea should be provided made from palliative herbs such as lime tea, Aaron's rod flowers, coltsfoot, or licorice. One should always ensure sufficient warmth. This illness takes a favorable course by the patient simply being kept warm and taking the kinds of tea mentioned above. While there is fever, a whole wash should be given every hour or two, and a daily hay-shirt for an hour and a half.

MELANCHOLY

Each week four whole washes, three half-baths and two short compresses, or instead of short compresses a back watering and upper body watering should be given. Every day the patient should take a cup of tea made from speedwell, valerian, pennyroyal, or agrimony.

MENORRHAGIA (EXCESSIVE MENSTRUAL BLEEDING)

The patient should go to bed, supported by a pillow underneath the legs but the head lying low; cold compresses of water and vinegar should be placed on the abdomen and 2 cups of tea made from mistletoe, shepherd's purse and horsetail should be taken daily. You can treat as follows:

1) The following remedy is one of the most potent for this menstrual condition, particularly in the menopausal years: let ⅛ cup (30 grams) of finely powdered alum steep in a bottle of Bordeaux wine for twenty-four hours. The patient should take a sugarspoonful of this every ten minutes. After two or three hours, the flood of bleeding should diminish; then 1 sugarspoon should then be taken every fifteen minutes. If it continues to decrease, 1 sugarspoon may be taken every half hour. Heavy bleeding is generally followed by leukorrhoea, in which case the patient should remain in bed for three or four days and continue with the medicine. During this time, the patient should not take hot food, or coffee or strong alcoholic drinks; a little wine is allowed.

2) A remedy that has often helped where nothing else was successful is the following: grind a quantity of best sealing wax with an equal amount of alum to a powder and give 1 teaspoon (2 grams) of this in a glass of Bordeaux wine three times a day.

3) Take 1 sugarspoon of powdered walnut blossom three times a day in Bordeaux wine. This is a very efficacious remedy.

4) Likewise, powdered walnut septa, but only ½ sugarspoon should be taken in Bordeaux wine three times a day.

5) Comfrey tea, or a daily cup of yarrow or lady's mantle tea or 2 cups blackberry leaf tea daily, or 1 cup agrimony tea with 1½ teaspoons honey; the last two are most efficacious.

• • •

All these different remedies have been mentioned as some ingredients may not always be easily at hand. They are all excellent as I have helped hundreds of people by means of them.

MENSTRUAL DISORDERS

1) For weakness drink white horehound tea.

2) Let 4 tablespoons (3 grams) common centaury, 4 teaspoons (3 grams) thyme and 7 teaspoons (3 grams) white horehound steep in 2 cups (½ liter) boiling water. Take 2 tablespoons four times a day.

3) For menstruation delayed because of shock or cold take a

hayseed hip vapor bath for twenty minutes two or three times per week. In addition drink 1 to 2 cups of yarrow tea daily.

4) For late menstruation, drink tea made from buckbean or long-stalked cranesbill.

5) For late menstruation, take a knife-point of eggshell powder twice a day, or 4 to 5 drops of spike oil twice a day on sugar.

6) Drink tea made from lemon balm, catmint, marjoram, or angelica for late menstruation.

7) Let 6 tablespoons bruised hempseed steep for ten days in 1 quart (liter) gin, and take 2 to 4 tablespoons daily. Or take 3 whole washes of water and vinegar every week. Also take three hot compresses of hayseed decoction on the abdomen for an hour, to be renewed after half an hour when menstruation is late. Also drink the tea mentioned above when using the washes.

8) To stimulate menstruation, drink tea made from calamus or thyme.

9) For excessively heavy menstruation, drink rue tea, 2 to 4 teaspoons (2 to 5 grams) per 2 cups (½ liter) boiling water. Or take 4 to 6 sugarspoons of tormentil tincture in cold water daily, or drink horsetail tea, or tea made from shepherd's purse or snakeroot. You can also drink tea made from knotgrass or wild strawberry leaves.

10) There is no better remedy for cramps, pain and heavy uterine bleeding than a few days in bed. If this fails to help, the patient should take one or two hot hip-baths (probably 100 to 111°F for fifteen minutes in a warm room. Immediately after the bath, she should go to bed with a hot compress—as hot as possible—on the abdomen for half an hour up to an hour. Between periods, the patient should take three cold hip-baths for four seconds each week; this is best done at night straight out of bed and then immediately back to bed without drying. Excess water may be quickly rubbed off.

MENTAL CONFUSION

Several people suffering from this have been cured by mild water applications. By regulating the blood circulation and treating the patient with gentleness and patience, one can successfully combat this complaint. I usually advise giving a daily whole wash, three hot short compresses of hayseed decoction or three cold water and vinegar compresses per week, gradually introducing—in accordance with the patient's degree of improvement—knee waterings and upper body waterings, plus walking for fifteen minutes in wet grass or ten minutes on wet stones every day. Every day drink 2 cups tea made from speedwell (*Veronica officinalis*) and twice a day take 25 drops rue and valerian tincture, equal quantitites of each mixed in a spoon of cold water one hour before or one hour after meals. This remedy should naturally be applied at the onset of the illness.

MIGRAINE (HEMICRANIA)

Migraine, also known as bilious headache, is nothing other than a nervous headache that appears to be caused by the stomach and abdomen, while there is a total lack of appetite and the patients have a real aversion to eating. It is generally accompanied by vomiting, irregular bowel movement and such unbearable headache that the sufferers are forced to stay in bed.

1) A refreshing remedy is to rub the head with menthol or lavender water, mixed with eau de cologne and rosemary.

2) A further recommended remedy is to drink a strong cup of *Veronica officinalis* (speedwell) daily for several weeks and to take each week four whole washes, three hot compresses of hayseed decoction on the abdomen for half an hour and three cold hip-baths for ten to fifteen seconds.

3) Sniffing ground ivy tea through the nose makes the headache subside, sometimes after a few minutes.

4) Others are helped by cutting a lemon into slices, leaving it to steep in a cup of boiling water and then drinking it in one dose.

5) A good remedy for migraine is to take 5 drops spike oil daily on a lump of sugar.

6) Drink a daily cup of vervain tea.

MILK RASH (CRUSTA LACTEA)

This complaint chiefly occurs in children and scrofulous persons. The rash first appears on the cheeks, making the skin red, followed by blisters which are filled with a yellowish-white fluid. The blisters burst open and form crusts. Crusta Lactea does not only affect the face, but also the head, and sometimes spreads over the chest, back, abdomen, and nearly over the whole body. Although this complaint sometimes stubbornly resists medicines, it can just as well be cured by simple remedies. I have cured many children in a short period of time by means of the following home remedies:

1) Apply alternating compresses of the following: bran decoction, heartsease, walnut leaves, unsalted soft cheese, or compresses of clay, water and vinegar, or horsetail, on the rash for two or three days. If the whole body or part of it is covered with a rash, take, in addition, a whole wash and a hay shirt every two days. Every day give 2 to 4 teaspoons (1 to 2 grams) dried heartsease boiled in 2 cups (½ liter) milk or water.

2) Give 4 drops tincture of greater burdock roots (*Lappa major*) mixed with a half glass water, daily in three doses.

3) Boil walnut leaves; apply them as a poultice until the crusts have softened and loosened; then wash the skin frequently with the decoction. Throughout the day give the child several spoons of milk in which a couple of walnut leaves have been boiled.

MOTHER'S MILK (INCREASE/IMPROVE)

⅓ cup (45 grams) English magnesia[23]
5 teaspoons (6 grams) orange peel powder
5 teaspoons (6 grams) fennel powder
2 tablespoons (12 grams) powdered sugar

Mix well together and divide into 18 equal portions; the nursing mother should take 1 portion daily.

2) Eat a bowl of pea soup every day.

3) Take a sugarspoon of fennel seed, a spoon of elder flowers

[23]We assume English magnesia is a brand name for a certain type of milk of magnesia.

and a spoon of chervil; let steep 20 minutes in 1 cup (¼ liter) water and drink 1 cup daily with a spoon.

Mother's Milk (Involuntary Leakage)

In nursing mother's, if there is an involuntary leakage of milk, drink sage tea. If a burning rash appears on the breasts, apply a poultice of unsalted, soft cheese.

Mother's Milk (To Dry)

To dry up mother's milk or milk that had hardened in the breast, take a quantity of fresh alder leaves, put them over the fire until they begin to sweat and become moist. Place them immediately on the breasts; the blockage will soon disappear and the milk likewise. Or, take 4 handsful fresh, chopped parsley, add white breadcrumbs, boil together in a little sweet milk and place this poultice on the breasts, or put bruised parsley under the arms.

Mumps (Inflammation of the Parotid Glands)

These glands are situated close to the ears; inflammation occurs in children and young people, generally in Spring and Autumn when the weather is cold and damp. It is contagious, so that sometimes a whole school and even a whole village may be affected. The symptoms begin with a poor appetite, restless sleep, a low fever and headache; the tongue is coated, the breath bad and foul; sometimes there is offensively smelling diarrhea and vomiting. The parotid glands swell up and stretch from the eyelids right down to the neck so that the earlobe is pushed upward. Sometimes the swelling is painful, other times not; opening the mouth, chewing and swallowing is difficult; the face is swollen and misshapen, the head stiff. This illness usually runs a favorable course as children rarely ever die from it. The treatment is very simple: fluid food only should be given—milk, tonic soup, or some other soup. Dry, warm bran should be applied in small cushions, or the swollen glands should be smeared with warm oil and covered with cotton wool. Should the swelling form an abcess or suppurate, fenugreek poultices should be applied; or it should be opened by a doctor, otherwise there could be inflammation of the testicles in men after the swelling has subsided.

MUSCULAR RHEUMATISM (MYOPATHIA RHEUMATICA)

This is not so dangerous as articular rheumatism. It is seldom accompanied by fever. The symptoms are pain in the muscles, especially in the upper part of the trunk, which increases when touched or with movement. It is sometimes accompanied by articular rheumatism, but usually occurs alone. The principal remedies may be found under Gout and Articular Rheumatism. It usually speedily disappears if one of the rubbing remedies is applied. With all rheumatic complaints, it is particularly important to make good use of the following kinds of tea which have a dissolving, expelling action.

1) Take 1 tablespoon (7½ grams) sassafras, boil in 2 cups (½ liter) water and take ½ cup twice a day.

2) Every day drink 1 cup of burdock root tea, or use stinging nettles mixed with licorice, or hyssop, or cowslip (*Primula officinalis*).

NASAL CATARRH (CORYZA)

1) Apply a mustard plaster between the shoulder blades for fifteen to twenty minutes and put hot compresses of French brandy on the forehead. Poke bruised sage into the nostrils.

2) Mix ½ teaspoon (4 grams) wood tar, 1 teaspoon (1 gram) camphor and 2 teaspoons (7 grams) ether and sniff it throughout the day.[24]

NAVEL RUPTURE

This usually cures itself if the rupture is held in place by a bandage. Take a piece of wax, roll it into a ball, wrap it in cotton

---

[24]Publisher's Note: We don't recommend this recipe! Included as a curiosity only.

wool and place on the navel which has been pressed inward; cover with a cross of sticking plaster and finally another large piece of plaster on top so that it cannot move. Renew after two to three weeks; the rupture will have healed after four or five weeks.

NERVE PAIN (NEURALGIA)

Neuralgia is an affliction of the nerves that can affect all parts of the body, and can only be diagnosed by a doctor, as it is sometimes difficult to recognize. The face is particularly affected by neuralgia. With facial pain, the teeth are also frequently affected. The eyes are not excluded from this complaint although such cases occur infrequently. If neuralgia affects the ears, the pain is felt deep in the ear and it is almost unbearable. Neuralgia in general is a terrible pain wherever it may be seated. The best and surest remedy for this complaint is the cold water cure which has cured hundreds. It is difficult to give any one prescription without first seeing the patient.

1) Those who suffer from neuralgia should always ensure good bowel movements, strictly abstaining from coffee, tea, beer, and spirits. Cold washes and cold compresses of clay, water, and vinegar are always useful for neuralgia.

2) Dried elder flowers placed between muslin on the painful area relieves the pain; the pain may also be relieved by painting with one part camphor and three parts ether.

3) Neuralgia usually immediately subsides after the application of hot compresses followed immediately by pouring cold water over the compress. Repetition of this several times will bring about a full recovery; or dip a piece of flannel in turpentine, wring it out and apply for ten to twenty minutes on the painful area and so make a speedy recovery. Application of fresh, bruised herb Robert is also a very good remedy for neuralgia.

NETTLERASH (URTICARIA)

Nettlerash frequently occurs after the consumption of overheating food, such as fish, smoked or salted meat, mussels, etc.

The body is covered with spots as though one has been in contact with stinging nettles; it is accompanied by severe itching. The best remedy is a mild purgative, hay-shirts, water and vinegar washes and tea made from lemon balm and mint. Every day take whole washes with water and vinegar as well as a hay-shirt for one and a half hours. Drink 2 cups mint and lemon balm tea daily.

NEURASTHENIA (FATIGUE)

Those who suffer from neurasthenia can be recognized by their anemia, pallor, cold hands and feet, irritability, sleeplessness, weak pulse, headaches, etc. Such patients should have complete rest and a mild water cure, spending some time in a healthy country spot or taking a course of fresh air treatment. The principal water applications are: washes, compresses on the back and chest, knee waterings, half-baths, upper body and back waterings.

1) The following remedies are highly recommended for nerve patients in general: Equal quantities of valerian tincture and orange peel. Take 10 to 15 drops in water twice a day.

2) Valerian tea or valerian tincture.

3) Tea from motherwort (*Leonurus cardiaca*).

4) The use of celery has been of great service to many nerve patients. Taking celery daily is highly recommended, but those who suffer from piles should not eat it as it could cause them much harm.

5) The following kinds of tea will be of use to nerve patients: lemon balm, valerian, mint, pennyroyal, cinquefoil, rue, rosemary, cowslip, lavender, lady's bedstraw, common St. Johnswort, balsam, long-stalked cranesbill, woodruff.

NEURASTHENIA (WEAKNESS OF THE NERVES)

This complaint encompasses a complex of different symptoms of illness that appear as the result of the entire nervous symptom. It should not therefore be confused with neuralgia or nerve pain, which simply arise from an irregular functioning of the nerves in any one particular part of the body. Neurasthenia affects the whole body. The sufferer is oppressed by acute despondency; severe irritability, coupled with restlessness, weak pulse, sleeplessness, facial pallor, cold hands and feet, headache, etc. Sometimes, nevertheless, only one or other part of the body is particularly, even visibly, affected by this weakness. This is why the symptoms of neurasthenia are so very varied. The normal development of the illness is as follows: there is a permanent state of excitability, followed by a condition of weakness that is the main characteristic of this illness. Since this complaint is rather difficult to treat, and since in our age, particularly, very many people have a tendency to neurasthenia, there is a special obligation to avoid it by taking the rest and relaxation demanded by nature at the requisite moment, by avoiding excesses and dissipation, by ensuring good nourishment and bowel movement. If more thought were given to these matters, how many people would now be leading useful lives instead of being a burden to society. Such patients should have complete rest and a mild water cure and stay for a lengthy period in a healthy country spot or take a fresh air cure.

The principal water applications are as follows: washes; compresses on the back and chest; knee waterings; half-baths; upper body, back and full waterings. It is not advisable to use one's own judgement in applying these treatments; it must be decided by the condition of the patient. Kneipp repeatedly warned against excessive applications and always said, "The milder, the better!" This should especially be borne in mind with nerve patients.

The following kinds of tea are useful: lemon balm, valerian, mint, pennyroyal, cinquefoil, rue, rosemary, cowslip, lavender, bedstraw, common St. Johnswort, balsam, long-stalked cranesbill, woodruff, gentian, juniper berries, white mustard seed, wallflower, sage, and ground pine. A highly recommended remedy is to take 20 to 25 drops valerian tincture and rue tincture, in equal proportions, twice a day in 1 tablespoon water, one hour before or one hour after meals.

NIGHTMARES

Each week take one or two salt-shirts for 1½ hours, four whole washes and three upper body washes. In addition, before retiring, take a sugarspoon of magnesia in cold water, or eat 1 to 2 sugarspoons of aniseed before retiring.

NIPPLES (INJURED)

1) Smear with lily oil.

2) Smear with fresh butter mixed with white wine.

3) Smear with gum arabic dissolved in rosewater.

4) Rub frequently with houseleek.

5) Rub the nipples with rosewater mixed with an equal quantity of French brandy.

6) Lip pomade is a good remedy for injured nipples.

7) Rosewater in which quince seeds have been dissolved is a very efficacious remedy. These seeds can be dissolved by boiling the ingredients together.

NIPPLES (PAINFUL)

Smear the nipples with a little lily oil, or fresh butter, or gum arabic dissolved in rosewater. Or wipe them frequently with fresh houseleek sap, or mix rosewater with an equal quantity of French cognac or apply scrapings of fresh comfrey.

NOSE COMPLAINTS

1) For a red nose, take 2 teaspoons (5 grams) borax, mix well with 4 tablespoons (35 grams) rainwater, and moisten the nose with this three times a day.

2) For loss of smell, rub several leaves of catmint or sage between the fingers daily and strongly inhale the fragrance through the nose.

3) For ulceration of the nose, smear it with glycerine. Or, melt ¼ cups (50 grams) lard, add 5 teaspoons (6 grams) camphor;

allow it to cool and then add 1 teaspoon (6 grams) Peruvian balsam. Rub this in three times a day.

4) For a blocked nose, spray the nose every day with salt water or horsetail tea.

5) To cure nose catarrh (chronic) mix together 6 tablespoons (60 grams) water, 15 drops tincture of arnica, 10 drops tincture of tormentil. Sniff this up the nose four times a day. Or, another excellent remedy for both nasal catarrh and head congestion is as follows: Sniff a little galangal powder up the nose four times a day, or use a little very finely ground horse chestnut powder. Inhale lukewarm horsetail tea through the nose two or three times a day, keeping the mouth open so that it may run out again.

6) Polyps in the nose can be treated by carefully mixing together ⅛ teaspoon (70 centigrams) alum powder, ½ teaspoon (70 centigrams) flowers of zinc (*Oxydum zincicum puris*), and 1 teaspoon (2 grams) ordinary snuff. Sniff a little of this four to six times a day. Or wintergreen sap, smeared inside the nose, makes polyps and bad air disappear. Polypody root, ground to a fine powder, mixed with honey, smeared inside the nose, eats away the polyps. Another remedy is as follows: twice a day, spray the inside of the nose with horsetail tea.

7) Stink Nose (Ozena), is an unpleasant complaint that may sometimes be cured by using one of the following remedies over a long period of time. Internally, take tea made from burdock root or yarrow; four times a day sniff an infusion of bramble leaves (blackberry) or horsetail through the nostrils; in addition sniff a little galangal powder twice a day. Chamomile vapor introduced into the nose through an upturned funnel is also worthy of recommendation; likewise tying a cloth dipped in hot French brandy around the forehead each day.

8) To get rid of an object in the nose, the empty nostril should be held closed and one should blow very hard into the mouth by pressing one's mouth firmly against that of the other. The pressure of air which comes out through the nose forces out the object. This is usually a problem only with small children.

9) To treat inflammation of the nasal membrane see also Cold

in the Head. Smear wintergreen sap inside the nose, or sniff the sap gently into the nostrils; this also drives out the bad air. The polypody root remedy mentioned earlier can also be used here. Or, spray the nose three or four times per day with luke-warm horsetail tea.

10) For a blocked nose, sniff a little galangal powder or pow-dered horse chestnut four times a day. In addition spray the nose with tea made from horsetail or bedstraw twice a day.

NOSEBLEEDS

The causes of nosebleeds can be very varied and the bleeding itself is sometimes dangerous. If the cause of the nosebleed is not *external,* for example from a blow, knock or fall on the nose, it is frequently caused by congestion of blood in the head. In such people, including children, it is generally preceded by a headache which usually subsides after the nosebleed. Nose-bleeds usually stop on their own accord and generally take the form of dripping, but it may also happen that the blood streams from the nostrils for a long period, so that sometimes the best of remedies are applied in vain. In such a case, one should not fail to consult a doctor. Should the bleeding be too profuse, one should attempt to arrest it by means of one of the remedies given below. If nosebleeds occur frequently, it is the result of some kind of disorder of the mucous membrane in the nasal cavity which could possibly cause anemia.

1) The best home remedy is shepherd's purse (*Bursa-pastoris*); a strong, cold infusion of this should be sniffed up the nose and one should drink one or two cups of tea made from this herb. If the herb is freshly picked, so much the better.

2) Sniff vinegar through the nose, or salt water, or horsetail tea. The latter is most efficacious.

3) Pound fresh leaves of lady's bedstraw (*Galium verum*) or goosegrass (*Galium aparine*) and place a pellet of this in the nose.

4) A cold pebble, placed under the tongue, sometimes quickly stops the bleeding; also keeping both hands and feet in hot water.

5) Dip a little cotton wool in water and then in alum powder and place this in the nostrils.

6) Raising both arms in the air also stops nosebleeds.

7) Place a cold compress on the neck and forehead. In the case of a persistent nosebleed, cold compresses can also be placed on the abdomen.

8) The best remedy for a persistent nosebleed is to tip 1 to 3 buckets of cold water over the upper part of the body. I experienced this in two instances where nothing which had been applied had been of any avail; the water immediately helped.

9) If the nosebleed occurs neither too frequently nor too profusely, it can do no harm; on the contrary, it alleviates the head, giving a more pleasant feeling.

OBESITY

Those who suffer from obesity must refrain from too many farinacous foods, potatoes and vegetables; drink as little as possible; eat lean meat, dried meat and eggs, drink 3 glasses of Bordeaux wine daily and take plenty of exercise; gardening is highly recommended. Each week take two short compresses, two half-baths, two back waterings and two full waterings. Drink a cup of hawthorn blossom tea daily.

More about diet: no oily food, no butter, sugar or carrots; no food or spirits prepared with sugar. The diet should be rich in nitrogen and contain protein—for example, egg whites, meat, cheese, non-oily fish, moderate quantities of spinach and other vegetables such as asparagus, various kinds of cabbage without potatoes, salads, etc. It is advisable to drink a glass of hot water every morning on an empty stomach and a glass of rosemary wine twice a day. Every day eat 1 cup (50 grams) raw or dried meat and the whites of 2 or 3 eggs. In addition, each week take four whole washes, three half-baths, three short compresses of water and vinegar, and water or hayseed decoction; two back and two full waterings. In addition to the hawthorn blossom tea, take 5 drops adonis tincture three times a day in a glass of cold water. If these recommendations are strictly followed, 2 to 5 pounds (1 to 2 kilos) weight can almost certainly be lost each week.

OVERHEATING WITH CHILL
Suck the juice from a lemon.

OVERLOADING THE STOMACH
An emetic or purgative is usually the best remedy. Sugar and water is sufficient to cure a simple case of an overloaded stomach; one glass of well-sugared water should be taken. Overloading the stomach is usually the cause of a disordered stomach. One should always avoid overloading it.

PAIN
For pain caused by lifting, or for internal pain, take a liqueur-glass of cod liver oil, immediately followed by a small glass of French brandy.

PAIN IN THE SIDE
1) If this pain is felt in the chest region and is accompanied by fever, burning and coughing, one is dealing with pleurisy or pneumonia. If there is no fever or coughing, hot compresses of hayseed decoction or hot water and vinegar should be placed around the loins. In addition, drink knotgrass or valerian tea, or take 20 drops gentian tincture in water twice a day.

2) If the pain in the side is caused by wind, which often happens, take 5 drops of spike oil on sugar twice a day.

3) Drink goldenrod tea.

4) Chronic pain in the side is treated with the following remedy: 6 spoons linseed meal or rye flour, 3 spoons honey, and 6 spoons lard should be melted over the fire; mix thoroughly and apply a plaster of this embrocation three times a day.

5) For pain in the side, apply a piece of gutta percha paper until the pain has subsided. Also drink a cup of goldenrod tea.

PALPITATIONS (PALPITATIO CORDIS)

Palpitations are a troublesome, annoying complaint, although little danger is involved. Hysterical people are frequently tormented by palpitations at night, causing them great distress. Treatments are:

1) A good remedy is: before retiring drink a glass of cold water and take a cold upper body wash, or use a cold compress on the abdomen for half an hour. The latter is particularly efficacious.

2) Mix tincture of valerian with an equal quantity of rue: take 20 to 25 drops twice a day in a spoon of water one hour before meals.

3) Let the following mixture steep for twenty minutes in 2 cups (½ liter) boiling water and take 3 tablespoons three times a day:

> 3 teaspoons (2 grams) lemon balm
> 2 teaspoons (2 grams) rue
> 2 tablespoons (1 gram) arnica
> 2 teaspoons (3 grams) great burnet root
> 1 tablespoon (1 gram) borage

4) Lemon water is highly recommended for palpitations.

5) Woodruff tea strengthens the heart.

6) Take 5 drops of false hellebore tincture three times a day in a spoon of water.

PERITONITIS

Peritonitis is a dangerous, much feared, and very painful illness which is occasionally caused in healthy people by chills, but usually by bruising or injury of the abdominal organs, such as the stomach, intestines, liver, spleen, etc. There is usually inflammation which gradually effects the peritoneum.

If an abcess bursts in the abdominal cavity, a chronic stomach ulcer for example, peritonitis generally occurs. A tear in the stomach or intestines, or some other accident, can also cause peritonitis. It generally begins with fever and severe pain in the abdomen on which the patient cannot bear the slightest pressure. The abdomen swells, there is acute thirst, accompanied by nausea, frequent vomiting of green matter and stubborn constipation. Death generally follows after a few days. If the inflammation takes a turn for the better, the fever lessens and the vomiting stops, the abdominal pain and swelling decrease and the bowel movement becomes normal. The patient should still be handled with the greatest care as recovery takes quite some time. It is unnecessary to mention that one should strictly adhere to the physician's instructions.

1) At the onset of the inflammation, while awaiting the doctor, cold compresses should be constantly applied to the abdomen and renewed as soon as they become warm, sometimes every five or ten minutes. Every hour the patient should be given 1 spoon of cold water, or still better, 1 spoon of milk whey. If during the cure the illness takes a favorable turn, a strict diet must be adhered to: very light, digestible but nourishing food: bouillon with an egg, milk, good old wine (taken with a spoon) and soft eggs.

2) Tubercular peritonitis is incurable. Since the patient cannot usually bear a double-folded compress on account of the pain, one simply applies an unfolded linen cloth, dipped in cold water. The colder the water the better. If the patient cannot bear the compress or if the fever continues, a cloth folded three to six times, dipped in cold water and well wrung out, should be placed on the back. This is more bearable and can remain in place for three quarters to one hour. If these cold compresses cannot be borne by the patient either, hot compresses of hayseed decoction should be placed on the back.

3) Instead of cold compresses on the abdomen, soft cheese is even better; it is light and is the best for taking away the pain. This remedy may be used without the slightest danger, but this poultice must be renewed every hour at first. Also good is 1 to 2 spoons of olive oil taken daily, upper body washes, and two cups of blackberry leaf tea daily.

According to Kneipp, "If a person complains of internal pain and has nausea or is vomiting, there is no doubt that an infection may be expected."

PHLEBITIS/INFLAMMATION OF THE VEINS

Inflammation of a vein is generally the consequence of bruises, injuries from a blow, push or fall, or following an operation due to ulceration of the tissues. The bacteria causing this inflammation invade the blood, which consequently changes into pus and becomes fluid, and in doing so can cause further inflammation. The patient is generally in considerable pain and frequently feverish; the skin is very red, swollen and painful; the veins are hard, filled with thick blood. Such cases should be handled with the greatest care; the affected limb must be kept raised, and the patient should stay quietly in bed. If the greatest care is not used, there may be dire consequences. With the following home remedy, which I can highly recommend, I have cured two such cases where, according to the physician, there was very little hope left.

I boiled a quantity of potatoes without salt, mashed them and mixed them with enough unboiled buttermilk to make a not too stiff poultice. I applied the mixture three to four times a day directly on to the leg and renewed it as soon as it began to dry. When the pain and swelling had ceased (after approxiately one month), I sprinkled a piece of flannel cloth with pure chalk-powder and wrapped it around the leg. The patient could now leave her bed and do her housework; there was subsequently not the least sign of any further occurrence of the inflammation. I have had the greatest success with this remedy in cases of inflammation, tumors, erysipelas and old sores, and I cannot recommend this simple home remedy highly enough.

A poultice of leek applied three times a day is also very efficacious.

PHLEGM

1) Boil ⅛ cup (15 grams) finely chopped elecampane root in 5 cups (1½ liters) water until reduced to 1 quart (liter); then add a good tablespoon hyssop, a spoon of ground ivy, and 3 tablespoons (50 grams) honey. Boil all the ingredients for a few seconds, skim and remove from the fire. One or two cups should be taken daily with a spoon. It is highly recommended for asthma; it dissolves phlegm with ease, purifies the lungs and is also good for gravel, kidney and bladder complaints.

2) To cure phlegm in old people use honey-water. Boil 4 cups (1 liter) water, add 3 tablespoons (50 grams) honey, thoroughly skim twice and strain through a cloth. This should be drunk as required throughout the day. It is an excellent phlegm-solvent for old men and also a good remedy for lung and internal ulceration.

PHLEGM ON THE CHEST

1) Apply a cold compress of water and vinegar on the chest for half an hour every day; in addition a whole wash every two days and an upper body wash every morning.

2) Take 1 cup (60 grams) of marshmallow, 2 cups (60 grams) wild chicory, 2 cups (60 grams) coltsfoot and 1 cup (60 grams) common St. Johnswort flowers. Mix well together; take 2 cups (60 grams) of the mixture and let it boil for half an hour in 2 cups (½ liter) water, then add 3 tablespoons (15 grams) licorice, allow to steep for twenty minutes, strain through a cloth and drink 3 or 4 cups every day.

PIMPLES ON THE FACE

Smear the face twice a day with lard and sprinkle it with haricot bean powder. See also Acne.

PINS, MONEY OR SOME OTHER OBJECT
THAT HAS BEEN SWALLOWED

The best remedy is to eat boiled potatoes finely mashed with butter. No drink should be taken. One can also eat thick bread soup. Taking oil is also recommended, or use a mild purgative.

PLEURISY

This illness can only be diagnosed by a physician and occurs quite commonly. The patient complains of stabbing pains in the chest, aggravated by breathing and coughing; has a dry cough and is always feverish. The left side of the chest is generally affected; there is seldom an infection on both sides. The causes are very varied, usually from colds, contusions, a fall or blow on the chest, etc. Pleurisy may occur several times in some lung diseases and may be a complication of scarlet fever and acute articular rheumatism.

The pleura is the double membrane around the lungs; if the inflammation of the pleura is of a more or less serious nature, a watery fluid is produced which may turn into pus. A physician can drain off this fluid by means of a small, insignificant operation which is necessary because the more the fluid gathers there, the more the heart and lungs suffer from the pressure.

At the onset of this illness, serious cases can sometimes be avoided by the patient remaining, above all, quietly in bed, applying a hot, short compress of hayseed decoction daily for one hour, ensuring a good bowel movement by drinking 1 cup buckthorn bark tea steeped with 1 sugarspoon aniseed every day. In addition, every two hours take 1 tablespoon tea made from equal quantitites of goldenrod, yarrow and common wormwood; 1 tablespoon of this mixture should be allowed to steep for two or three minutes in 1 cup boiling water. Or, take 2 cups of blackberry leaf tea daily. If the fever is only modeate, the diet should consist of milk, soup, tonic soup, soft eggs, white bread and a little lean meat.

PNEUMONIA

Pneumonia is usually caused by cold, dry weather, or by catching a chill while sweating. It begins with severe shivering which rapidly changes into high fever. This is followed by: pain in the chest, breathlessness, cough, sometimes blood-tinged sputum, oppression, anxiety, restlessness, palpitations, congestion of blood in the head; the pulse is fast, the small amount of urine is red, the skin is dry and hot; the hands and feet are generally cold. It is one of the most dangerous illnesses; so it is of utmost importance to fetch a doctor.

1) If the hands and feet are cold, one should first take care to apply hot compresses of water and vinegar around them, so as to draw the blood to them. If the patient is hot, a cold compress of water and vinegar should be laid on the abdomen; if, on the

contrary, the patient is cold, the compress should be applied hot.

A large poultice of soft cheese mixed with whey and milk to make a soft ointment should be placed on the chest. This cheese poultice is very efficacious: the pain, fever, oppression, and breathlessness rapidly disappear. When the cheese begins to dry (this should not happen quickly if it has been applied thickly enough), a fresh plaster should be applied, and renewed as necessary.

When the fever has subsided, no more compresses or cheese poultices should be applied, and the patient should be given a whole wash every hour or two, as necessary, until he or she begins to sweat. This generally occurs after the second or third wash and can be regarded as a favorable sign. The washes should then be continued every two or three hours, for example, until the burning and fever have completely subsided. If the pain and burning return, a cheese poultice or plaster should again be applied. Internally, give the patient a table-spoon of olive oil every morning and evening; this is excellent.

When the danger has passed, the patient should be given an upper body wash and a whole wash every day; later on, one day an upper body wash and the next day a whole wash. The medicine to be given to the patient is very simple: water must not be too cold and is to be given with a spoon only. Apart from water, the patient can also be given raspberry juice in water; strictly no wine to be given. At the onset, patients should only take milk or porridge, or thin tonic soup. When the fever has fully subsided, chicken, pigeon, or beef soup may be served. With pneumonia, one should always ensure fresh air.

2) Several patients have recovered from pneumonia by drinking tea made from hazel catkins; this is particularly advisable at the onset of the illness; 1 cup is generally enough to cause sufficient sweating.

3) Take 2 tablespoons powdered vervain, the whites of 6 eggs beaten until stiff, 3 tablespoons rye flour, and a wineglass of gin. Mix thoroughly until the consistency of a paste, place be-tween layers of muslin and apply on the painful side for sixteen hours. If the poultice becomes too dry meanwhile, it should be refreshed with a little gin. This poultice dissolves the thickened

fluid which has been sweated from the blood vessels, filling the small pockets and causing the air to be driven out of the affected part of the lung so that the lung can no longer breathe. It sweats it out and wonderously relieves the pain. This remedy is also recommended for all kinds of pain in the side. The affected area should be covered with a cloth to absorb blood and moisture. If the pain has not fully subsided (a rare occurrence) it may be repeated. A plaster of cheese may also be placed on the chest and 1 tablespoon olive oil taken every morning and evening. This harmless remedy is most highly recommended. Instead of olive oil, 3 tablespoons (30-60 grams) of sweet almond oil may be taken daily in three doses.

4) Boil a handful each of the leaves of borage, common alkanet and wild chicory in 6 cups (1½ liters) water until reduced to 4 cups (1 liter). Strain through a cloth and add 2 tablespoons (30 grams) marshmallow syrup or 2 tablespoons (30 grams) honey. Take 3 tablespoons every three hours.

5) Pneumonia is cured the quickest by the following simple remedy, even in cases where all other remedies have failed; after twenty-four hours, all danger has passed. Beat a fresh egg well, then beat 1 tablespoon olive oil into it and when this is thoroughly mixed, add 1 tablespoon rye flour. Beat hard and finally add 2 tablespoons chopped brown-rayed knapweed (*Centaurea jacea*) flowers. Beat again for some time until everything is thoroughly mixed. Make a small bag of embroidery canvas, fill with the mixture and leave for twenty-four hours uninterruptedly over the heart. In order to keep it in place, two tapes should be sewn to the top of the bag and tied round the patient's neck. Every morning and evening the patient should be given a spoonful of olive oil. I have used this remedy on a number of patients, and after the bag had been lying there for ten hours, they all, without exception, felt much better, and the fever and pain had subsided.

PODAGRA (GOUT IN THE FEET)

1) Eat a clove of garlic daily.

2) Twice a day take a sugarspoon of unbruised white mustard seed.

3) Apply compresses of violet leaves boiled in vinegar, and also drink licorice tea. Cold washes and half-baths are also recommended.

4) Apply fresh scrapings of bryony root or a honey plaster.

5) Every day drink 1 cup of tea made from buckbean, hop, common centaury, daisy, or dwarf elder root.

6) Dissolve ⅓ cup (16 grams) potash in 4 quarts (4 liters) hot water; take a hot foot bath in this solution daily for twelve minutes. After the bath, dry the feet well, wrap in cotton wool and go to bed.

POISONING

If the following symptoms appear in a healthy person, poisoning may be suspected: stomachache, desire to vomit, colic, dry mouth, acute thirst, constriction of the throat, diarrhea or excessive bowel movements, cold sweats, weak pulse, bulging eyes, etc.

1) While awaiting the doctor, one should try to extract the poison from the stomach by giving an emetic.

2) If an emetic is not available, give the patient a great deal of chamomile tea to drink, or a sufficiently large quantity of warm water to cause vomiting. If a doctor cannot come in time, beat 5 eggs in 1 quart (liter) water and give this to the patient.

3) I have seen a person who had consumed a large quantity of softened match heads cured by constantly drinking large amounts of milk.

4) The best is to take immediately 1 tablespoon charcoal powder. This can also be used for poisoning from mussels. In the case of mussel poisoning, it is also advisable to drink 4 cups (1 liter) cold water mixed with 1 cup (¼ liter) vinegar.

PROLAPSE OF THE RECTUM

Drink 1 to 2 cups *Sirea ulmaria* (meadowsweet) tea every day and apply one of the following four remedies:

1) Apply hot compresses of lady's mantle decoction[25] (*Alchemilla vulgaris*).

2) Mix violin resin powder (gum arabic) with an equal quantity of powdered gum and spread this on the rectum.

3) Dip a pure woolen cloth in olive oil, wring it out and allow it to burn. Spread the powder which is left on the rectum.

4) Boil ¼ cup (30 grams) powdered oak bark in ½ cup (⅛ liter) water; continually apply hot compresses of this mixture.

PURGATIVES (PURGANTIO)
If these are taken often, they are very injurious to the health and therefore very inadvisable. For example, severe burns may occur when a purgative is recommended.

1) Tartar is used as a purgative. The quantity is 2 to 3 tablespoons (15 to 30 grams) in some kind of liquid.

2) Castor oil is a mild purgative. The quantity to be used is 2 tablespoons to ⅓ cup (20 to 60 grams); it can be taken in milk, coffee, beef tea, or other liquid. Castor oil can still be taken in cases of inflammation.

3) No more than 3 to 5 tablespoons (10 to 15 grams) of senna leaves should be given.

4) The tea called St. Germain is one of the best purgatives, second only to castor oil; but should, nevertheless, only be taken in cases of dire necessity. See also Constipation.

5) Take 1 tablespoon cold water every hour as a most efficacious remedy.

6) Take 2 teaspoons of buckthorn bark and a sugarspoon of

---

[25] Decoction is a "tea" or extract made by pouring cold water over the herb and allowing the mixture to simmer. This method is used primarily for hard materials, such as roots and barks. Decoctions are usually made in quantities of 1 oz. to 1 pint. It is best to start with 1½ pints of water and simmer until you are left with a pint. Once cool the decoction is strained and taken in varying herbal doses. A decoction should be prepared fresh daily.

aniseed; leave to steep for half an hour in a cup of boiling water and taken 1 to 2 cups per day.

PURPURA OR WERLHOFF DISEASE (PURPURA SIMPLEX)

A famous German physician, Werlhoff, was the first to describe this illness. It begins with indigestion, languor, depression, poor urination and general weakness, immediately followed by the appearance of small blood flecks all over the body, particularly on the legs.

The patient should remain in bed, take light food—milk foods are the best—and totally abstain from beer, wine, coffee and tea. For the first few days the patient should be given one or two upper body washes and a hot compress of hayseed decoction on the lower part of the body for half an hour. After a couple of days, a whole wash should be given, and a hot compress on the lower part of the body. From the very onset of the illness up until the radical cure, the patient should be given 1 tablespoon common centaury herb every two hours to stimulate the appetite and to gain strength, and every day 1 cup of goldenrod tea, taken with a spoon.

This treatment radically cured two German boys whose physicians had given up hope. My advice was sought at the very last minute. There is no need to be afraid of using this gentle water treatment, if such a case should occur. I should add here that the herbs played the major role.

PYROSIS (HEARTBURN)

Acid stomach may be recognized by heartburn, uncomfortable and lengthy digestion of food, a sour smell on the breath, burning in the stomach. The gums, lips and face are pale. Those who suffer from nerves especially suffer from this complaint, too, and generally complain of an upset stomach, heartburn, stomach cramps, etc., after eating fatty food, vegetables, or drinking wine or beer.

1) The simplest and best medicine for this disorder is tea made from common centaury with fennel. It is best to take this tea with a spoon; for example 2 tablespoons every two hours. In

addition, take hot compresses on the abdomen, each week one or two hot footbaths containing 2 handfuls of wood ash and 1 handful salt, for twelve to fourteen minutes. Every day take a whole wash one hour before rising. Tonic soup is one of the best foods.

2) The following tea is also highly recommended for an acid stomach: ½ cup (15 grams) white horehound and 3 tablespoons (10 grams) licorice. Allow these ingredients to steep for twenty minutes in 2 cups (½ liter) boiling water and take 1 tablespoon every hour.

3) Take a glass of sugar and water in the morning on an empty stomach.

4) Take 1 tablespoon charcoal powder every day in milk in two doses.

5) Take 5 to 6 drops of fennel oil twice a day on sugar.

6) Take magnesia or chalk powder, 2 teaspoons twice a day.

7) Before and after every midday meal take ½ to 1½ teaspoons (5 to 10 grams) glycerine with a little water; or mix ¾ cup (20 grams) white horehound with 3 tablespoons (12 grams) licorice; let steep for twenty minutes in 1 cup (¼ liter) boiling water, then strain and take 1 tablespoon every hour.

REDNESS OF THE FACE OR RED FLECKS

1) Mix houseleek sap with an equal quantity of alcohol. Smear the flecks or redness with this two or three times a day. It usually clears up entirely within a short time.

2) Moistening the patches with crushed chickweed before retiring is also good.

3) Wash the face several times a day with the following infusion: let 2½ cups (50 grams) of plant anemone (wind flowers) steep for twenty-four hours in 2 cups (½ liter) cold water.

RENAL COLIC
(INFLAMMATION OF THE KIDNEYS/NEPHRITIS)

The kidneys lie to the right and left of the spine. Inflammation of the kidneys causes severe pain in that area; urination is difficult and the patient is shivering and feverish. The feverishness increases the thirst, feet and eyelids swell, the patient's strength diminishes and there is little appetite. If the kidney inflammation is severe, there is renal colic, abdominal swelling, nausea, vomiting, constipation, the urine is very dark, mixed with blood, later with pus and only comes in drops. Inflammation of the kidneys is usually accompanied by high fever. This fever should be fought as far as possible with whole washes or short compresses. When the fever has passed, the patient should be given two to three whole washes daily.

1) Internally, give tea from knotgrass, oatstraw, plantain, rosemary, or rosehips. The following herbal mixture is most efficacious:

> ¼ cup (3 grams) knotgrass
> 2 teaspoons (1 gram) common wormwood
> 2½ teaspoons (1 gram) sage
> 2 tablespoons (1 gram) common centaury
> 2 teaspoons (3 grams) rosehips
> 2 teaspoons (2 grams) dwarf elder root

Boil for half an hour in 3 cups (¾ liter) water and take 1 tablespoon every hour.

2) Kidney patients should stay in bed and abstain from meat, salt, spices, wine, coffee, tea and spirits. Their nourishment should consist of farinaceous and milk foods, a couple of lightly boiled eggs are permitted, likewise a little white meat (for example, poultry, chicken, pigeon, and veal). Many people are cured by this diet and the following applications. Every day take a whole wash with cold water; every other day a hot compress of hayseed decoction around the loins and the abdomen for one hour; it is often advisable to apply the compress daily. In addition, drink one or two cups goldenrod tea daily and if

possible every day drink 1 quart (liter) raw buttermilk. (Note: kidney patients should never lie on their backs; it increases the pain.)

RHEUMATISM (RHEUMATISMUS ARTICULORUM ACUTUS)

Rheumatism is always caused by a chill, especially by a draught, by catching cold after sweating, by getting wet, by living in a damp house, etc. It is divided into articular rheumatism and muscular rheumatism. It is called articular rheumatism if the joints are affected by pain and fluid; muscular rheumatism if it is the muscles which are affected. Articular rheumatism generally begins with some degree of fever, stiffness and discomfort in the whole body. The pain is felt in one or more joints, knees, elbows, etc. It gradually increases and may even become unbearable; the affected areas are generally more or less swollen. Sometimes it changes place, moving from one joint to another; it may affect only one joint, or, on the other hand, several. These changes usually occur at night. Such changes constitute a danger, even a fatal one, should they strike the heart or brain. If a patient is affected by severe rheumatism, with burning and fever, coupled with a rapid pulse, do not hesitate to call a physician. If the rheumatism is chronic, dissolvent drinks and diaphoretics (producing perspiration) should be taken over a long period. The treatment of acute rheumatism (*rheumatismus acutus*) should be palliative and antifebrile. The following home remedies are recommended for rheumatic complaints:

1) In the first instance, whole washes with cold water, every hour, are highly recommended; this should be gradually followed by cold waterings of short duration after which the patient should immediately retire to bed. One should begin with knee waterings. The area where the complaint is seated should naturally be watered the most. If only a few small areas are affected, hot compresses of oat straw decoction may be applied.

2) The following remedy is highly praised for external use for pain in the joints and all rheumatic pain: Mix ¼ cup (50 grams) camphor with ¼ cup (50 grams) spirit of turpentine and rub the painful areas with this three or four times a day near a hot

stove or in bed; the pain will soon disappear along with the illness.

3) Melt together:

   3 teaspoons (7 grams) yellow wax
   1 teaspoon (7 grams) burgundy tar
   3 teaspoons (7 grams) Venetian turpentine
   1 tablespoon (20 grams) black tar

When all the ingredients have thoroughly melted, smear the mixture on glazed paper while still hot and place on the painful area until the paper drops off of its own accord.

4) Mix 2 teaspoons (5 grams) petroleum with 1 tablespoon (15 grams) glycerine and rub the painful area with this two to four times a day.

5) Fill a bag with dry fresh birch leaves and lie inside it in bed. This causes the patient to sweat heavily and the rheumatic pains to subside.

6) Vapor baths of fragrant herbs such as mint, lemon balm, yarrow, chamomile, and thyme are also recommended.

7) Let a handful of finely chopped garlic steep in a bottle of gin; take a glassful before retiring; this remedy is frequently used in England.

8) Eating quantities of gooseberries is excellent for those who suffer from rheumatism.

9) Dip a piece of flannel in hot rosemary tea, place this around the limbs at night and cover with gutta percha paper.

RHEUMATISM
(RHEUMATISMUS ARTICULORUM CHRONICUS)
1) Mix together equal quantities of bruised juniper berries, rosemary and licorice; take 1 tablespoon of this mixture and let steep for twenty minutes in 2 cups boiling water. Use this quantity daily.

2) In the evening, before retiring, rub the painful limb thoroughly with a flannel cloth dipped in hot vinegar in order to take away the pain. Also before retiring, drink a hot diaphoretic tea (for example, elder or chamomile tea, or, even better, equal quantities of both mixed).

3) Another good remedy is the following tincture with which the limbs should be rubbed every morning and evening. Put 6 tablespoons (60 grams) medicinal soap, ⅔ cup (30 grams) potash and 1 tablespoon fresh yeast into a bottle of French brandy. Tie down the bottle with a piece of parchment and prick a few holes in it; the bottle should not be corked.

RICKETS (RACHITIS)

This illness is frequently encountered in both children and adults. If scrofula attacks the legs, rickets occurs. The symptoms are: an enlarged head, an old appearance, a bloated abdomen, the body becomes thin, the appetite is good, bowel movements sluggish, the bones are swollen at the joints, especially the hand joints, legs and feet but seldom the arms later become bent; the spine also becomes more or less bent; there is often malformation of the whole body, including the hips, causing a waddling gait. This illness sometimes disappears with the development and growth of the body.

The main treatment is hardening the body by means of water; for example, washes, half-baths, waterings, hot shirts from oatstraw decoction, etc.

The best and most efficacious food for this illness is the Kneipp tonic soup, groats, and bone-dust. Meat should be eaten as little as possible. Rubbing the back every day with gin is also very good, but tincture of chicory root is even better. Tea made from walnut leaves is highly recommended. Soup from calves feet, which should be boiled, is excellent for children. Boiled buttermilk is still one of the best remedies for rickets.

ROUNDWORMS (ASCARIS LUMBRICOIDES)

Signs that there are worms present are as follows: itching in the nostrils, distention of the eyeballs, dark shadows under the eyes, frequent change of color, sour breath, sometimes ravenous hunger and other times lack of appetite, abdominal pain, a dry cough, intermittent diarrhea, the urine is sometimes milky.

1) The best remedy for roundworms is santonin powder, but this must be prescribed by a doctor.

2) Tea made from valerian, rue, common wormwood, common centaury, speedwell, walnut leaves, chamomile flowers, or tansy are all remedies that kill worms.

3) An old, effective remedy for roundworms is the following: slice one or two onions, cover with cold water, leave overnight to steep and drink in the morning on an empty stomach.

4) In the evening take a piece of asafetida the size of a pea in a cachet. This will drive the worms from their deepest hiding places (Raspail).

5) Taking a pinch of powdered savory expels worms in children.

St. Vitus' Dance (Chorea)
This nervous disease may be cured by giving the patient two or three hot hay-shirts or shirts dipped in hot water and vinegar each week, wrapping him in a dry sheet and a woolen blanket and letting him lie in bed for 1½ hours. On the days when no shirt is worn, the patient should be given a cold whole wash. Instead of the whole washes, half-baths may also be given, with an upper body wash. This is particularly advisable if the patient does not recover quickly. Also drink 1-2 teaspoons (1-2 grams) sanicle powder four times a day in some kind of liquid.

Scabies
1) Boil 7 ounces (200 grams) burnt lime[26] and 12 cups (200 grams) flowers of sulphur in 1 quart (liter) water, stirring continually. When it has thoroughly boiled, remove from the fire, leave to cool, then pour into well-corked bottles. Before using the remedy, the patient should take a hot bath, dry well and

---

[26] Burnt lime must be the same as quicklime.

then sponge the body with the decoction. The patient should then be wrapped in a sheet and laid in bed. If necessary, the treatment may be repeated, but recovery will swiftly follow.

2) Mix 2 tablespoons (30 grams) lard with 1 tablespoon (15 grams) ship's tar; rub this in every morning and evening. This is particularly efficacious in the case of old scabies.

3) The simplest and most effective remedy to cure scabies quickly is to rub the whole body with petroleum. The following day, wash well with hot water and soap. Rubbing once is usually sufficient.

4) An equally good remedy is to rub the body with alcohol.

5) Boil ⅛ cup (15 grams) elecampane root in 2 cups (½ liter) water; steep for half an hour, then strain. Wash the whole body with this twice a day.

6) Rub the joints and itching areas with Peruvian balsam.

7) Mix ⅓ cup (50 grams) styrax[27] with 1 tablespoon (10 grams) olive oil. Rub the whole body with this every morning and evening.

8) The ulceration caused by old scabies can be cured by applying the following ointment: carefully mix ½ teaspoon (1 gram) flowers of zinc with 2 tablespoons (25 grams) sweet butter.

9) The best and most careful treatment for scabies is as follows: hot baths of hayseed, and especially yarrow. A daily cold wash should be taken with the hot baths. A salt or hay shirt is also recommended. I have given these remedies because experience has taught me that most people cannot possibly stop taking hot baths and frequently cannot help themselves, even with the best will in the world.

SCALINESS, DANDRUFF, SCURF ON THE HEAD (SEBORRHEA)

1) Let a handful of hop flowers steep in 2 cups (½ liter) of 70% alcohol for six days and rub the head with this every two days

---

[27] Styrax is storax, a liquid balsam obtained from the wood and inner bark of *Liquidamber Orientalis*.

for the first two weeks; afterward, once a week is sufficient.

2) Cut two onions into small pieces, steep for ten days in French brandy in the sun or near a fire, and rub the head with this. It clears up scurf and also encourages healthy growth of the hair.

3) Mix 2 tablespoons (30 grams) glycerine, 3 tablespoons (30 grams) alcohol, and 3 tablespoons (30 grams) rainwater. Rub the head with this mixture in the evenings, after first warming the liquid.

4) Rub the head every morning with egg whites, leave it on for half an hour and then wash the head with lukewarm water.

5) Boil a good handful of Panama bark in 3 cups (¾ liter) water. Wash the head with this once a week and rinse well with cold water.

6) Let a handful of blue cornflowers steep for twenty minutes in 2 cups (½ liter) boiling water; if the head is washed with this every day, the dandruff will soon clear up.

SCARLET FEVER (SCARLETINA)

Scarlet fever has much in common with measles, but is considerably more dangerous. Children, in particular, are affected by this disease, but it also occurs in adults and is then far more dangerous than in children. It is sometimes said that if the scarlet fever disappears, the disease is cured. If it returns, the disease is usually fatal. Dropsy, hypersomnia, and inflammation of the lungs generally occurs. It is always advisable to have this disease treated by a doctor. Symptoms are pain in the throat, occasionally a cough, which nearly always immediately follows the rash; the rash is scarlet, just like raspberries. The redness (scarlet) of the mouth and throat is a *certain* sign of scarlet fever. There are few illnesses where the symptoms are so changeable or which run such a capricious course. Scarlet fever sometimes begins with high fever, rapid pulse, severe headache, thirst, swelling in the neck and exhaustion in the limbs. The symptoms are worse in the evenings.

Monseigneur Kneipp used the following applications to cure scarlet fever. First, soak a shirt in very cold salt water, wring it out thoroughly and pull over the patient; then wrap the patient in a sheet and a woolen blanket in which he or she must lie for an hour; remove the wet shirt and change it for a dry one. If the patient feels worse again after two or three hours, provide another cold, wet shirt, without salt in the water, and repeat as often as necessary. The salt shirt should only be used once.

Instead of using wet shirts, one can also give a whole wash with cold salt water. If the fever is high, particularly at the onset of the illness, it is sometimes good to give the wash every half an hour, but then only with water without salt. One should ensure that the wash does not last longer than half a minute, and that the body is not dried off. After the wash, the patient should be carefully covered, but this should not be exaggerated; never give too many heavy bed-covers; extra covers can be placed over the feet.

The best method of quenching the thirst is to give cold water with a spoon; the patient has no appetite, and even if he or she were to have some appetite, the patient should not be given any food. If an appetite is felt after a few applications, the patient should be given frequent small amounts of liquid food; for example, very thin tonic soup. See also Measles to compare both illnesses.

SCIATICA

Sciatica is really a nerve pain. It is caused by gout, rheumatism, chills, etc. At first, pain is felt in the thigh, later in the knees, feet and calves. It sometimes moves from one foot to the other and from one limb to the other. Occasionally the pain is so bad that the sufferer trembles if anyone comes near. Relief can only be found in cold waterings. Do the following treatments:

1) The affected limb should be watered until the pain subsides and should then be wrapped in a coarse linen cloth and the patient put to bed. If the pain returns, the watering should be repeated.

2) Cold compresses made from water and vinegar on the back are also recommended; in addition, alternate back and upper body waterings.

3) Take one or two thigh waterings daily. Immediately after the watering, the leg should be wrapped in a woolen blanket and the patient put to bed.

4) Rub the hip twice a day with the following mixture: ½ teaspoon (5 grams) ship's tar (*Piceus liquida*) mixed with ⅓ cup (100 grams) 75% alcohol.

SCROFULA

The principal symptom of scrofula is swelling of the glands. These generally appear in the neck, under the chin, in the groin and later over the whole body. Many scrofulous people also have an eye infection that is not easy to cure. In addition they have running ears, inflammation of the nose, head-rash, various kinds of skin rashes, swellings, caries, etc. A mild water cure is particularly recommended for these patients; they should take as much exercise as possible in the fresh air and eat invigorating, easily digestible food. They should refrain from potatoes, black bread, pork, and should not eat too many vegetables; acorn coffee is excellent.

1) For the swollen glands: take white horehound leaves, pound them to a powder and mix with chicken fat. Apply this in the form of a poultice to the swollen glands.

2) Or, crush fresh rue and place this on the swollen glands.

3) Apply fresh coltsfoot leaves to the swollen glands.

4) It is also good to smear swollen glands with cod liver oil.

5) If the swollen glands are infected, boil white beans in buttermilk; when they are thoroughly cooked, mix them with a little medicinal soap and butter. Apply this mixture hot three times a day.

6) Mix 1 sugarspoon ship's tar (wood tar) with 1 tablespoon lard (pork fat). Rub or smear the swellings with this in the evenings. This remedy cured an old gentleman in three days; the swelling had been taken for cancer and an operation had been decided on.

7) For scrofulous sores, beat the white of an egg to a froth, add 1 tablespoon rapeseed oil and sufficient chalk powder to make a soft ointment. Smear this thickly on cotton wool, place on the sores and renew as soon as it begins to dry.

8) Mix 1 teaspoon (5 grams) Peruvian balsam with 3 tablespoons (30 grams) sweet butter and apply this to the scrofulous sores on cotton wool.

9) Acorn coffee is an excellent remedy for all glandular illness.

10) Every day, drink three cups of walnut leaf tea with a little milk. This is certainly one of the best remedies for glandular illness.

11) Combine 2 cups (½ liter) milk with a small handful of chopped parsley; place on the stove until it begins to boil; then gradually add sufficient tartar for the milk to begin to curdle. Remove from the stove and steep for another fifteen minutes. Strain through a cloth and add 1 tablespoon magnesia, 1 tablespoon sulphur (purified) and 2 tablespoons sugar. Take this throughout the day, 3 to 4 tablespoons at a time, so that the entire decoction is used in two days. Before using this mixture, it should be shaken well. This dose is for adults; children should take half and infants less, according to age. When taking this remedy, the patient should keep warm and quite definitely abstain from taking any spicy, stimulating food or drink. If there is internal burning, or inflammation in the swollen glands, this should first be drawn out.

12) The following remedy is exceptionally good; it cannot be praised highly enough for both children and adults. Mix together:

   1¾ cups (300 grams) fennel water
   1½ tablespoons (30 grams) honey
   1 teaspoon (7 grams) Venetian turpentine[28]

---

[28] Venetian turpentine: also known as Venice turpentine or Larch turpentine. It has the power to increase perspiration and may also be used as a diuretic.

Note: the honey and the Venetian turpentine should be thoroughly beaten. Also note that Venetian turpentine is not the usual fluid turpentine: this turpentine is a thick as syrup.

Children 6 years old should take a good sugarspoonful of this mixture every two hours; if younger, they should naturally have less: if older, more, up to one tablespoonful. In addition, place lint dipped in this mixture on the sores and renew as soon as it becomes dry.

13) Stewed watercress or chicory is also recommended, likewise chervil soup.

14) Boil ½ cup (125 grams) quassia wood in 2 quarts (2 liters) water in an earthenware pot until reduced by half. Adults should take 1 tablespoon every morning at 10:00 A.M., but never on an empty stomach.

15) Apply hot compresses of bran water, hayseed, blue cornflowers, clay, water and vinegar, or poultices of unsalted soft cheese, or smear with glycerine.

16) Mix 1 cup (250 grams) decoction of plantain leaves, ¼ teaspoon (1⅓ grams) lime chloride and apply as a compress.

17) Boil a handful of heartsease in 1 quart (liter) milk; apply constant compresses and drink a cup of this milk daily.

18) It is always excellent to drink fig decoction.

SCURVY

1) Smear the mouth and gums several times a day with a mixture of equal quantities of cream and houseleek sap, or rinse the mouth frequently with tea made from bramble leaves (blackberry leaves) and a little alum.

2) An efficacious remedy is as follows: take 1 ounce (30 grams) finely chopped fresh horseradish root and 2 tablespoons (10 grams) pyrethrum.[29] Boil in 5 cups (1½ liters) of water until reduced to a quart (liter); then take leaves from scurvy grass,

---

[29] Pyrethrum is Spanish chamomile; in medicine the root is used. This may be another name for pellitory.

brooklime (*Veronica beccaburga*) buckbean, watercress—a half handful of each—pound together and add to the decoction; remove from the fire, tightly close the pot and leave to cool; squeeze it out gently and add 1½ tablespoons honey. Take a wineglassful three times a day.

3) To make a scurvy gargle: take a handful each of bramble leaves (blackberry leaves) and agrimony; boil in 1 quart (liter) water until reduced by half; then add a handful of scurvy grass. Remove from the fire, leave to stand for a few minutes, squeeze it out and then add 2 tablespoons (30 grams) of rose honey. Gargle with this several times a day and also drink 2 cups sanicle and honey tea daily.

SEMINAL DISCHARGE AT NIGHT (POLLUTIO NOCTURNA)

Before retiring, drink a glass of sugar and water, chamomile tea, or tea made from wild strawberry leaves. In the evening, take light food, no coffee, tea, or chocolate.

SHINGLES

The characteristics of this complaint are: a very red blistery rash, causing burning pain and running halfway round the body like a belt. It generally appears more on the right side than on the left and never right round the body. As the first blisters subside, fresh ones appear; they cover the chest or abdomen. This rash generally lasts for 8 to 14 days, but after it has disappeared and the skin is once more its normal color, it can sometimes still be felt for months. Although this complaint is annoying, it is not dangerous.

1) Whole washes and hay-shirts cure it quickly. Unsalted, soft cheese should also be placed on the rash daily; this draws out all the poisonous matter and is miraculous in making the pain subside. Ointments should never be used here.

2) Apply poultices of fenugreek.

3) Wet a piece of soda and rub it over the rash every now and then, or apply compresses of chicory (*Cichorium intybus*), and wash the area with the decoction.

SHRINKING TENDONS

1) Combine ¼ cup (60 grams) tincture of myrrh and ½ cup (60 grams) aloe. Rub this on the numb or constricted tendons every morning and evening. Always rub in an upward direction.

2) For painful tendons, boil freshly squeezed sap from black nightshade with an equal quantity of olive oil and smear it on the tendons.

SLEEPING SICKNESS

This is a condition which is chiefly characterized by lengthy sleeping and is possibly connected with influenza. Rub the spine and limbs with spike oil. Give a whole wash and a hot compress on the abdomen daily.

SMALLPOX

Smallpox is a contagious disease. The first symptoms are fever and severe pain in back and loins, nausea. This is followed by red spots, which soon become hard, pointed pustules and subsequently suppurating ulcers. One should ensure plenty of fresh air; if possible a window should be kept open day and night; but where such dangerous diseases as this are concerned, I always recommend a doctor to be consulted.

1) Although this is a serious disease, it is easily cured by giving a quick whole wash every hour; these washes should not last longer than one minute.

2) A lady from Verviers recovered from smallpox in nine days by wearing two cold wet shirts daily; she kept each wet shirt on for 1½ hours. She also applied cold compresses on her face, day and night. No sign of a scar on her face could be traced after this treatment.

3) Stew some leeks, add linseed meal to make a poultice; if this poultice is placed on the buttocks, abdomen and legs, the pocks will appear there.

Sores (Old, Purulent)

1) Apply fresh, pounded yarrow leaves or compresses of the decoction of the dried herb.

2) Boil potatoes without salt, mash them and mix to a poultice with raw buttermilk; apply this very thickly directly on the bare sores. There are few known remedies which heal old sores as surely and swiftly as this simple, cheap remedy. If one wishes to heal a very large sore within a few days, this remedy should be tried, but the patient must stay in bed and abstain from anything stimulating, such as beer, coffee, or pork. Even if there is burning in the sore, it will disappear in a day if this simple remedy is used. If there are fleshy excrescences in the sores, they must first be removed; if not, a sore cannot possibly heal. It can be cured by sprinkling it with powdered walnut septa or finely powdered alum.

3) Place unsalted soft cheese fairly thickly on the sores. This has almost the same effect, although preference should be given to the previous remedy. Both of these remedies should be renewed as soon as they begin to dry.

4) Grated raw potatoes laid thickly on old sores is also an excellent remedy.

5) Mix white bread, soaked in warm water, with a little saffron and place on the sores.

6) Fenugreek applied as a poultice is also most efficacious.

7) Chamomile flower compresses are another well-known, old remedy for sores; these are particularly palliative if the sore is painful.

8) Sprinkle the sore with charcoal powder, especially if the sore is very wet. This dries and heals.

9) Mix 2 teaspoons (5 grams) powdered myrrh, dissolved in a little alcohol, with 3 tablespoons (15 grams) charcoal powder and 1½ cups (300 grams) lard, and apply a plaster of this mixture twice a day. This is also good for sores that itch and sweat.

10) For burning in the sore, apply rice boiled in water; or apply

a poultice of elder flowers prepared with white bread and water. With sores, it is important to ensure good bowel movements. It is also advisable to take a daily cup of depurative tea, as described in this book, from the decoction of burdock root or yarrow tea.

11) The following remedy for old sores is most efficacious: boil a quantity of carrots in milk, mix to a paste and apply directly on the bare sores.

12) For sores that itch and sweat, take 3 tablespoons (30 grams) sweet butter, mix carefully with 1 teaspoon (2 grams) flowers of zinc, smear on lint or cotton wool and apply on the sore once a day.

13) Leaves and flowers of marigold, cooked with lard, give a good healing ointment which will keep for some time and should be used on sores that itch or sweat.

14) Fry fresh butter until it is completely brown, then pour it into cold water and leave for twenty-four hours; then remove it and squeeze well in a cloth to extract all the water. This butter has a strong power to heal both fresh and old sores. It should be thinly smeared on linen and then placed on the sores.

15) Sores with fleshy excrescences can be helped as follows: take clay which has been well burnt from an oven, mix it with half wine (white) and half apple vinegar to a thick paste; place this poultice on the sore with fleshy excrescences. Or, pound raw onions, mix with olive oil and place on the fleshy excrescences. Or sprinkle with sugar or burnt alum.

SPIDERS OR OTHER INSECTS IN THE EARS

It not infrequently happens that insects enter the ear and cause the most dreadful sensation by their movements. People try to remove them by using all kinds of pins or instruments, but this can be dangerous. Insects cannot bear oil. One should therefore quite simply put a few drops of olive oil, rapeseed oil or camphorated oil into the ear. The insect immediately tries to leave its prison. As soon as it is visible, it can be removed with some kind of instrument.

SPINAL DISEASES

These are generally difficult to diagnose and even more difficult to cure. They may be congenital or may occur later; the former occur seldom and are incurable. They bring paralysis of the legs, reproductive organs, bladder and rectum and the sufferers may sometimes be completely paralyzed. This disease particularly occurs in men aged 30 to 45 and frequently as a result of an irregular lifestyle or syphilis, also from injuries, a blow or a knock, which may also cause caries of the spinal marrow; it may additionally be brought about by inflammation, or as a consequence of a contagious disease such as typhoid or chills. Good results may occasionally be obtained at the onset of the illness through taking light, easily digestible, invigorating food—especially milk—through moderate exercise in the fresh air, through mild water applications and depurative tea.

Recommendations: cold washes, cold compresses made from water and vinegar used alternately on the chest and back. Rub the back twice a day with spike oil or a tincture of wild chicory root; in addition drink a daily cup of tea made from one of the following herbs: common centaury, stinging nettle, horsetail, common wormwood, rosemary, goldenrod.

SPLEEN (SWOLLEN)

1) Apply hot compresses of hayseed, or water and vinegar, or chamomile flowers; in addition, take four whole washes and two half-baths weekly. If the spleen is severely swollen, it would be advisable to apply hot compresses twice a day.

2) Take ⅔ to 1 cup (10 to 15 grams) greater celandine herb, let steep in 4 cups (1 liter) boiling water; take with a spoon and use this quantity in twenty-four hours.

3) See Vervain.

4) Drink tea made from common centaury, calamus, scurvy grass, rosemary, mint, watermint, or peppermint.

5) Smear the swollen area with rue oil.

6) For a hard, blocked spleen, boil ivy in vinegar and place on the area. In addition, drink angelica or parsley tea.

7) For a hardened spleen, apply a poultice of fenugreek mixed with a little saltpeter and vinegar.

SPRAIN (DISTORTIO)

1) Take the white of 1 egg, beat it to a froth, then add 5 tablespoons soot from a chimney; smear this mixture on a cloth and bind it around the sprained limb. It will soon recover.

2) Boil a quantity of vervain in vinegar and apply as compresses. A sprain is quickly healed in this way.

3) If a hand or foot has been sprained, the simplest and best remedy is to plunge the sprained limb in cold water immediately and keep it there for several hours; this water should be renewed frequently; or apply constant cold compresses. Compresses of cold water, clay and vinegar are even more efficacious. When the sprained limb has been removed from the water or when the compresses have been completed, the limb can be rubbed with camphorated spirits or arnica.

4) Compresses of rapeseed oil are also most highly recommended. If a limb has been sprained, do not hesitate: *immediately* apply one of the given remedies. If the limb becomes inflamed, it does not heal so easily and may indeed be dangerous. Many people have suffered greatly through such negligence.

5) Take 4 tablespoons (32 grams) alum powder, ¼ cup (60 grams) gin and the whites of 2 eggs. Beat well together until thoroughly mixed; spread on a linen cloth and tie it round the sprained limb. Renew it once or twice a day. This treatment will bring about a speedy recovery.

6) Take a handful of common wormwood, 2 eggs with the shells, 4 tablespoons (30 grams) gin (French brandy is even better) and 1 tablespoon ox-gall; mix well together, smear on a linen cloth and place on the sprained limb twice a day.

7) Combine 1 tablespoon (10 grams) camphorated oil, ½ teaspoon (1 gram) spike oil, ¼ cup (50 grams) turpentine and 1½ cups (350 grams) gin. Rub the sprained limb with this three times per day. This remedy is also good for cramps in the legs.

8) Combine 2 tablespoons (15 grams) camphorated spirits, ½

ounce (15 grams) opodeloc (camphorated soap liniment) and 2 teaspoons (5 grams) juniper oil. Rub with this three times a day.

STIFFNESS IN OLD AGE
To avoid this as far as possible, drink 2 cups (½ liter) buttermilk every day.

STINGS
1) Put the limb in raw cold buttermilk, or, if none is available, in sour milk, or in hot soda water. At night apply a poultice of fenugreek.

2) Poultices of unsalted, soft cheese, or potatoes and buttermilk (see also section on Sores).

3) Take a fresh egg, beat it well, add a mustard spoon of salt and a little sweet almond oil. Thoroughly mix in a china mortar, smear on linen and apply; renew as soon as it begins to dry. If the bites are large, it should be renewed very frequently.

STOMACH CATARRH (CATTARRHUS GASTRICUS)
Chronic gastric catarrh is very difficult to cure. A strict diet and a thorough cold water cure are the best remedies to be rid of it. The following treatment is recommended: every week use one short compress for 1 hour; take two or three half-baths, two back waterings, after first taking cold washes so as to become used to the water and hardened by it. In addition, drink angelica tea.

Catarrhus gastricus may also be known as a stomach chill. This condition is caused by cold drinks. Drink tea made from rosemary or herb Robert.

STOMACH CRAMPS
Stomach cramps are strong contractions of the stomach and back, sometimes accompanied by oppression. These contractions seldom last more than a day, they generally subside after

a few hours, but on very rare occasions may last a few days. In the case of chronic inflammation of the stomach, however, the pain is constant, but without either oppression or fainting. One should take care to distinguish between these two complaints. Those who suffer from nerves are particularly subject to stomach cramps. A cup of hot milk boiled with 1 tablespoon cinquefoil, and hot compresses of hayseed decoction on the abdomen may be highly recommended. Take 3 to 4 drops peppermint oil on sugar twice a day. Also footbaths with wood ash and salt, tea made from chamomile flowers, mint, valerian, or yarrow are also effective. Generally speaking, what is good for stomach pain is also good for stomach cramps. One can also drink tea made from common chamomile.

STOMACH (FOUL, BAD STOMACH)

With a foul stomach, there is no appetite at all; there is a feeling of obstruction and torment in the stomach; there is great thirst, a desire for acidic or sour drinks; stabbing pain, the tongue has a yellow or white coating; filthy, stinking belching; a bitter taste in the mouth, nausea, a tendency to vomit; severe headache, especially in the forehead; a feeling of oppression in the heart region and tiredness in all the limbs; there is also some degree of fever, the urine is very cloudy and dark; the stools are dark in color, with a very bad smell. This complaint can most easily be cured by the use of a mild purgative and by eating a very small amount of food. The best cure is to eat nothing for a day. The following remedy is a little strange but it works: boil a handful of wheat bran in 2 cups (½ liter) water; take this on an empty stomach and take nothing else for five hours. If the appetite returns (which is usually the case) only a small amount of food should be eaten, the best on the first day being tonic soup or bread soup cooked with half water and half milk.

1) With a foul stomach, purgative and acid drinks are highly recommended. For example, lemon water, and barley water with honey. Hot compresses of hayseed decoction should be placed on the abdomen for half an hour, two or three times throughout the day, alternating with a whole wash, knee watering and a half-bath.

2) Every morning and evening, take 3 tablespoons tea made from sage, mint, common wormwood and angelica.

3) Let ½ cup (15 grams) common chamomile and 1 tablespoon (7 grams) rhubarb powder steep for several days in a bottle of Rhine wine and drink a wineglass every morning and evening.

Stomach Pain (Gastralgia)

Stomach pain can be caused by heavy food which is too sour or too fatty, by immoderate eating and drinking, especially beer, by too many purgatives, etc. If the pain occurs after eating very fatty food, it is good to eat a dry rusk immediately after the meal. One should, moreover, refrain for some time from eating food which experience has shown to disagree with one's stomach. Washes, half-baths, vinegar and water compresses, or clay compresses, are recommended for alternate use. For stomach pain caused by a flood of gall, drink speedwell. If the stomach pain is accompanied by wind, see also Flatulence.

Stomach (Ulcerated)

Ulceration of the stomach occurs not infrequently in women. Anaemic, scrofulous people and consumptives are the first to be affected by this. The principal symptoms of stomach ulcers are: pain in the stomach region, not exclusively related to food which has been consumed; sometimes the pain decreases after food has been eaten; with stomach ulcers, pain is also commonly felt in the back. During the illness, the pain sometimes disappears completely so that the patient believes himself to be cured, while at the same time all other symptoms disappear, too. Very frequently, however, this apparent cure does not last long and the patient seems even worse; much of the blame for this must fall on a bad diet. Food is vomited and, in chronic cases, with blood, or only blood and sometimes in great quantities. Minor stomach bleeding can also be recognized by black stools, mixed with blood. Severe bleeding of the stomach can be very dangerous and can even be the cause of instant death. Apart from pain and vomiting, there are no specific symptoms to be observed with stomach ulcers. Some sufferers complain of swelling in the stomach region and repeated heartburn; they have no appetite; others, on the contrary, feel reasonably well, if they have no pain, and their appetite is quite good.

Should the ulcer perforate the abdominal cavity, peritonitis can immediately occur, followed by death: the air and contents of the stomach penetrate the abdominal cavity with acute pain; there are palpitations and the patient's strength at once begins to ebb.

Most stomach ulcers last for years although some sufferers experience a complete recovery. It may be taken as a favorable sign if, in the case of incessant pain, the food eaten by the patient does not increase the pain, or only a little, or does not cause discomfort. If the pain can no longer be felt, it may be seen as a favorable sign. Food which is taken should be light; milk is especially good and should be taken with a spoon (for example, 1 tablespoon every fifteen to twenty minutes). Do not drink too much milk at one time. Buttermilk is also highly recommended. Milk boiled with honey is invigorating and wholesome. If one begins to dislike milk, soft boiled eggs, thin tonic soup, or light beef tea may be taken.

1) An excellent remedy, especially at the onset of the illness is to take 1 tablespoon sanicle (*Sanicula europaea*) tea with honey every two hours; hot compresses of hayseed decoction or horsetail on the abdomen are highly recommended.

2) Mix 1 spoonful sauerkraut water with 8 spoonsful of cold water; take 1 tablespoon every hour; this is most efficacious. Soft cheese is also recommended.

3) If the stomach pain is caused by piles, drink hot chamomile tea and place hot compresses on the abdomen.

4) With stomach ulcers, as in obesity, it is advisable to drink a cup of hot water before every meal.

STROKE (APOPLEXIA)

The chief cause of a stroke is the bursting of veins, pouring out blood into the brain or between the cerebral membranes, causing sudden paralysis which can be followed by immediate death. If little blood penetrates the brain—which is frequently the case—death does not occur so quickly, but the patient becomes unconscious, while the pulse, heartbeat and breathing continues. In the case of less violent strokes, which do not cause loss of consciousness and only paralyze a few muscles, such as face, mouth and eye, there is generally only a loss of speech and memory and the patient can make a full recovery. The causes leading up to a stroke are varied; for example, a strong rush of blood to the head following a heavy meal, emotions, alcohol, etc.

1) If someone has had a stroke, he or she must be undressed immediately and put to bed; cold compresses should be constantly laid on the head—the colder the water, the better. The compresses must be renewed every five to ten minutes and the water changed at least every fifteen minutes. As soon as possible, the patient should be given a purgative or, still better, a purgative enema; for example, salt water, black soap, etc. Rub the spine and limbs well with spike oil. A doctor should be called as quickly as possible.

2) The paralyzed limbs should be wrapped in hot hay compresses twice a day and 1 cup rosemary or vervain tea should be given daily.

To avoid a stroke do the following. Three times a day take a sugarspoon of white, unbruised mustard seed in half a glass of water. Drink a glass of rosemary wine or 2 cups rosemary tea twice a day.

Should one feel a stroke approaching, immediately take 1 tablespoon salt in the mouth; this dissolves much mucous which must, of course, be expelled. I once had the opportunity of using this remedy on a lady of noble birth from Persia during my stay in Wörishofen, Bavaria. I saw from her singular features that an attack was approaching; she was no longer capable of either word or sign. I forced her mouth open and gave her a spoonful of salt; before ten minutes had elapsed, she had recovered. A year later she died from a stroke.

STUTTERING (BREAK THE HABIT)

1) Use mild water applications as for nerve-sufferers.

2) When speaking and reading, the child must say the sound "oo" before every word: for example, oo-you, oo-will, oo-not, oo-stutter, etc.

SUNSTROKE (HELIOSIS)

It is commonly known that sunstroke can cause death. A highly recommended treatment for sunstroke is to apply scrapings of raw potatoes as a plaster and to renew it frequently. Compresses of cold water and vinegar are also advised.

SWEAT (MALODOROUS)

Take salt baths or baths from aromatic herbs such as thyme, mint, common wormwood, chamomile flowers, etc. Instead of baths, one can also put on a shirt soaked in salt water and well wrung out; but one should also be well-wrapped in a dry sheet and a woolen blanket and stay in bed for 1½ hours. The shirt can also be soaked in an infusion of one of the aromatic herbs mentioned above. In addition, take 1 tablespoon charcoal powder in two doses in milk daily. When taking baths or wet shirts, four to six whole washes are also recommended each week. For sweaty feet, hands or armpits, use one of the following remedies:

1) Every two days place a hot compress of hayseed decoction around the feet for twenty minutes; then wash them with cold water.

2) First dry the feet thoroughly and paint them every morning and evening with French brandy.

3) If the sweating of the feet has been driven away or suppressed, and one wishes it to return, place the feet every evening in a bag filled with hot bran. This will make the feet sweat again.

4) Let 1 tablespoon thyme steep for twenty minutes in 2 cups (½ liter) boiling water; add ½ sugarspoon alum; let steep for a further twelve hours and strain through a cloth. Wash with this

remedy until the sweating stops. A second remedy to bring back sweating, if it is deemed necessary, is to take a hot footbath with 2 handsful wood-ash and 1 handful salt for twelve minutes. Afterward, the feet should be rinsed in cold water.

SWELLINGS ON ARMS OR LEGS

1) For watery swellings on arms or legs, boil potatoes without salt, mash them well, mix with unboiled buttermilk to a paste. Place this paste (without smearing on a cloth) very thickly on the affected areas. If there is any burning, the poultice will draw it out and the swelling will then soon subside.

2) Soft cheese has almost the same beneficial effect on watery swellings. It should also be placed (without smearing on a cloth) very thickly on the affected areas. One can also apply compresses of whey in which elder flowers have been boiled.

SWOLLEN JOINTS

1) Boil together equal quantities of lard and black soap, apply fairly thickly on the swollen joints.

2) Mix 2 teaspoons (5 grams) ox-gall with 3 tablespoons (25 grams) French brandy and smear this on the affected part three times a day.

3) Place scrapings of bryony root on the swollen area.

4) Apply a mustard plaster on the affected place.

TAPEWORMS

Special symptoms are: pallor, blue rims to the eyes, dull eyes, the tongue is always coated, indigestion, loss of weight, the appetite varies—there is sometimes hunger and sometimes no appetite at all, sometimes fainting in the mornings, also occasionally after eating—heartburn, attacks of dizziness, irregular bowel movements, frequent headaches, abdominal pain, palpitations, etc.

1) Take ½ cup (40 grams) peeled grapefruit seeds, pound them to a paste, mix with 3 tablespoons (30 grams) castor oil and 2

tablespoons (30 grams) honey. This should be taken in a glass of milk in one dose. Two hours later, the following mixture should be taken:

  3 tablespoons (30 grams) castor oil
  2 tablespoons (30 grams) honey
  1 tablespoon (10 grams) lemon juice

The patient should not leave the room until the tapeworm has appeared; this takes place after a thorough purging, accompanied by severe colic.

2) Take 4 tablespoons (32 grams) bark of finely pounded pomegranate roots. Leave this to steep for twenty-four hours in ½ bottle of white wine. Pour off the wine without straining it. The patient must drink this in three doses within 1½ hours. One hour after taking it, the patient must take 3 tablespoons (30 grams) castor oil, with the addition of a little lemon juice to flavor it.

3) Take 3 teaspoons (10 grams) freshly prepared fern root extract and 3 tablespoons (40 grams) ordinary sugar syrup. Mix these ingredients carefully and take it in the morning on an empty stomach, followed one hour later by 3 tablespoons (30 grams) castor oil. It is advisable to eat a herring the evening before. This is an efficacious remedy for tapeworms.

4) Every twenty minutes, take 2 spoons olive oil, this will expel the tapeworm.

5) Drink lemon balm tea, mixed with honey—start in the morning on an empty stomach with 1 tablespoonful of the mixture. Repeat the dose every half an hour.

TEETH AND GUM PROBLEMS
1) When the teeth are on edge, rub them with powdered chalk or magnesia.

2) To keep teeth healthy, boil 1 tablespoon rue with 2 tablespoons sage in 2 cups (½ liter) water. Use this to clean the teeth and rinse the mouth.

3) Loose teeth are helped if one boils 1 tablespoon dried, finely chopped bramble leaves (blackberry leaves) in 1 cup (¼ liter) water; strain and add a piece of alum the size of a pea. Rinse the mouth with this every day.

4) Chew a piece of calamus root continually throughout the day when teeth are loose.

5) Rinse the mouth four to six times per day with tea made from sage, goldenrod, or oak decoction to aid loose teeth.

6) Mix 1 sugarspoon of tincture of myrrh in a glass of cold water and rinse the mouth with this several times a day when teeth are loose. This is also an excellent remedy for a coated or dry tongue and swollen gums.

7) To remove tartar from teeth, clean them with heavily salted water or finely ground salt and a toothbrush.

8) Place a bag of hot salt on the cheek for toothaches.

9) Take a little powdered chalk, sprinkle with rum and immediately sniff into the nose. Keep the nose closed for approximately one or two minutes; the toothache then generally subsides.

10) A missionary from China gave me the following remedy for toothache and decayed teeth. Pound a handful of henbane seed to a powder; mix with a little water to a paste; heat a stone in the fire; place this on an iron plate (or even better in an iron pot) and place the paste on top of it. Now make a paper funnel to conduct the vapor to the ear. Do this twice until the ears begin to ring, then stop immediately. This remedy should cure toothache and decayed teeth for good.

11) For ulcerated gums, rinse the mouth several times a day with the following infusion. Boil 1 tablespoon sage in ¾ cup (150 grams) wine, or rinse with goldenrod tea; this is excellent.

12) Fry barberry bark in oil; smear the gums with this two to four times a day. Also drink 2 cups of tea made from sanicle with honey, or cinquefoil without honey to alleviate ulcerated gums.

13) Throughout the day chew calamus root and swallow the sap to cure ulcerated gums.

14) For foul, rotten teeth in the mouth, drink a large quantity of cold water with a little tartar.

THROAT INFECTIONS/SORE THROAT (LARYNGITIS, PHARYNGITIS)

1) Mix freshly pounded rue with a couple of egg yolks and place this around the throat. This is an excellent remedy for a severe throat infection.

2) An efficacious remedy for inflammation of the throat is as follows: carefully mix together 2 parts slaked lime and 1 part lard. Smear this fairly thickly on linen cloth and place it around the neck. As soon as it begins to dry, it must be renewed.

3) Place cold compresses around the neck and renew them as soon as they begin to get warm. This kind of compress should never be left on for longer than twenty to thirty minutes.

4) Gargle four times a day with the following mixture: ½ cup (124 grams) water, 3 teaspoons (7 grams) unburnt alum. This remedy should be used at the onset of a throat infection.

5) Take 1 quart (1 liter) decoction of carrots, 2 spoons honey, 1 spoon vinegar, ⅛ ounce (4 grams) sal ammoniac (ammonium chloride). This should be used as a gargle three or four times a day but should always be used hot.

6) Gargle several times a day with tea made from bramble leaves (blackberries), or agrimony, or medlar leaves.

7) For ulceration of the throat: drink tea made from sanicle with honey and also use it as a gargle. This tea is highly recommended.

8) Pellitory (*Parietaria officinalis*) with an equal quantity of cultivated wild strawberry leaves, taken as tea, is an excellent gargle for an inflamed throat.

9) A sugarspoon kitchen salt dissolved in 1 cup (¼ liter) water is a very good gargle for throat infections and hoarseness.

10) Put 3 teaspoons (5 grams) alum in 2 cups (½ liter) sage tea and gargle with this throughout the day.

11) Boil 1 tablespoon honey in 2 cups (½ liter) water; add 1½ teaspoons vinegar. Gargle with this several times a day.

12) Boil 1 tablespoon linseed in 2 cups (½ liter) water and take 1 tablespoon every hour.

Thrush (Aphtha)

1) Rinse the mouth with hot tea made from plantain leaves or watercress.

2) Mix an egg yolk with 1 tablespoon sugar and 1 tablespoon rapeseed oil; smear the mouth with this several times a day.

3) Every morning and evening drink 1 cup of sanicle tea with honey.

4) Rinse the mouth several times a day with goldenrod tea and also drink 1 cup goldenrod tea daily.

Tongue (Paralysis, Stiffness, Dry or Split)

1) Gargle with a strong infusion of sage, valerian, thyme, or with the following tincture: 1 tablespoon mustard seed steeped in 1 cup (¼ liter) French brandy for twenty-four hours.

2) Put 5 or 6 drops lavender spirits on sugar in the mouth, allow it to dissolve slowly and swallow.

3) Smear the tongue with houseleek sap or chew calamus root.

4) For inflammation of the tongue, take 10 drops valerian tincture in 2 teaspoons water four times per day.

Tonsils (Swollen)

Add a pinch of alum to a cup of sage tea and gargle with this six to eight times a day.

Tubercular Abscesses or Swellings

Take a hot bath of chemically pure soda water for twenty minutes, four times per day. If the patient's body cannot be bathed, apply a hot soda compress for about half an hour six times a day. If the swellings are severe, a poultice made from potatoes and buttermilk should be applied. See also Bones and Sores.

TUBERCULOSIS

The signs of the onset of tuberculosis are as follows: a dry cough in the morning and evening especially, loss of weight, pallor, sweating in the mornings, diarrhea, blood-flecked sputum. Although the face is pale, the cheeks are a beautiful red; there is also a light fever. The best remedies for tuberculosis are hardening the body through cold water and walking in the fresh air. No consumptive will recover unless he hardens himself, stays in the fresh air and takes exercise. We shall mention here a few good home remedies which have been highly recommended for tuberculosis; but one should not forget the essential points mentioned above.

1) Rub the chest morning and evening for five to ten minutes with bacon rind on which there is still a little fat.

2) Every day drink 2 cups of tea made from equal quantities of white horehound, coltsfoot and ground ivy.

3) Boil a pot of turnips with the skin on; squeeze them out well in the water in which they were cooked; add 1 cup (160 grams) sugar to every 2 cups (½ liter) decoction; bring to the boil again briefly and take 1 tablespoon every hour. If no turnips are available, carrots may also be used.

4) Drink 2 cups knotgrass tea daily.

5) If there is thick, purulent phlegm, drink tea made from buckbean, sloe blossom or oak bark.

6) Mix 80 drops Peruvian balsam with 13 ounces (360 grams) treacle[30] and take 1 tablespoon three times a day. This remedy, like the previous one, is recommended for third degree tuberculosis. In America they drink tea from Aaron's rod.

---

[30] Treacle was a medicinal compound used in the 1800's, a kind of salve used against malignant diseases. It is no longer used.

7) Mix to a paste: 2 tablespoons rye flour, 1 tablespoon oil (rapeseed or olive oil), 1 tablespoon powdered vervain, and the whites of 4 eggs. Smear this paste on a linen cloth and apply on the bare chest; firmly bind with a bandage and renew the poultice after five days. This causes a rash on the chest; this is a very good sign. The cough will soon disappear if it is merely the beginning of tuberculosis. In addition, drink tea made from hyssop with honey, or knotgrass tea as mentioned above.

8) The lemon remedy was given to me by a lady who recovered from consumption after taking numerous medicines without the slightest success. I gave it to a consumptive whom I personally considered a hopeless case, in view of the fact that the phlegm was thick, the appetite nil and there was regular night-sweating. Put 10 lemons in cold water, boil until they are not too soft, then immediately squeeze them; add sugar to taste to the juice and take this quantity every day. In the case I treated, the patient was feeling better after a few days. The appetite had picked up, prospects looked more cheerful and healthier. After ten days the quantity of lemons was reduced by taking one less each day, until there were three, with which she continued until fully recovered. If this remedy causes diarrhea, one should take only 5 lemons until the full quantity can be managed.

9) A very good remedy for consumptives is as follows: take betony (flowers and leaves), common St. Johnswort, flowers of Aaron's rod and speedwell, a ½ tablespoon of each plant. Let all ingredients steep for half an hour in 4 cups (1 liter) boiling water in a well-closed pot. Strain through a cloth, boil a little longer with 4 tablespoons honey and meanwhile remove the scum. Take 1 tablespoon every hour or two.

10) A very good remedy for sweating in consumptives is 1 cup milk boiled with 1 sugarspoon sage. Rubbing the chest and back thoroughly with lard, morning and evening, cannot be praised highly enough. This not only stops the sweating but also strengthens the patient to an amazing degree. I experienced this both personally and in many others. The sage milk can be alternated each week with 1 cup chamomile tea with sugar.

11) The final remedy for lung diseases is the following: a mixture of herbs which truly deserves the honorary title of "Lung herbs." Take ⅓ cup (10 grams) sage, 4 tablespoons (10 grams) hyssop; boil in 1 quart (liter) water until reduced by half, squeeze well out, then add ⅓ cup (100 grams) honey; allow it to boil a few more minutes, skim and remove from the fire. Take 1 tablespoon every morning at seven o'clock, in the afternoon at three o'clock and in the evening at six o'clock.

12) The best remedy for fever in consumptives is to apply hot compresses of hayseed decoction on the abdomen.

TYPHOID

This dangerous disease may be caused by chills, particularly by living in damp, unhealthy houses or marshy regions, or by bad drinking water. Characteristic symptoms are general tiredness, restless sleep, nosebleeds, lack of appetite, attacks of dizziness and fever, diarrhea, pain on the lower right side of the abdomen, etc. One sign that always appears at the onset of the illness is an extraordinary change of complexion and swelling on the lower right-hand side of the abdomen. As soon as typhoid breaks out, the patient complains of severe headache, especially in the mornings; the hands and feet are usually cold, and there is a total lack of sleep. This dangerous disease must be treated by a doctor.

The principal aim in this illness is to combat the fever. This can best be done by cold whole washes; these must be repeated every time the fever rises. At the beginning, they should be given every hour; later on, four whole washes per day are sufficient. The patient should never be dried after the wash. He should be given tea made from fenugreek, or sage and common wormwood, and every morning and evening 1 tablespoon olive oil.

At the onset of this illness, cold half-baths are even more effective than whole washes; the patient can be given a half-bath for three to four seconds every two hours; in addition, upper body washes. These half-baths can best be given if there is very high fever or anxiety. After the bath, the patient should immediately return to bed where he should be well covered over, although not too heavily. The feet should be especially well covered; if they are cold, hot vinegar and water compresses should be aplied for half an hour and repeated until the feet get warm.

Fresh air should be provided by leaving a window slightly ajar. The patient should eat little. The best food is tonic soup, or gruel and milk given with a spoon—for example, 1 tablespoon every hour. Cold water is the best for the thirst, 1 tablespoon every hour or half hour. The patient should never drink too much at once.

URINATION PROBLEMS

1) Every hour take 1 tablespoon of tea made from stinging nettle. Boil 2½ cups (50 grams) stinging nettles in 2 cups (½ liter) water for half an hour for difficult urination.

2) Drink tea made from horsetail, oatstraw, rosehips or knotgrass. In addition, apply hot compresses of horsetail or oatstraw for difficult urination.

3) Every day drink 1 to 2 cups of tea made from goldenrod, meadowsweet, club moss, or one of the following: salad burnet, glabrous rupturewort, lady's bedstraw, parsley, linseed, cattail, skullcap, asparagus, currant, or ground ivy, for difficult urination.

4) Difficult or impossible urination: drink 2 cups stinging nettle tea daily.

5) For urinary incontinence: before retiring take 1 sugarspoon powdered agrimony in a glass of Bordeaux wine.

URINE (TO REMOVE THE SMELL)

Place a small bag of charcoal under the mattress.

VARICOSE VEINS

Obstruction of the blood circulation causes the veins to dilate; twisted bag-shaped distension occurs, sometimes the size of an egg. These are called varicose veins. It mostly occurs in the legs and feet through standing for long periods; also in pregnancy, with stubborn constipation, and from wearing elastic stocking garters, etc. Piles are also caused by distended veins at the end of the rectum. The bloodstream is obstructed by the pinched knots of blood and causes a rash of ulcers to develop on the legs. Sometimes a vein bursts and this is particularly exhausting for the patient. To effect a cure, the causes must first be removed; for example, by treating the constipation, leaving off garters and putting the legs up. The blood circulation can be improved by treating the whole body.

Varicose vein sores are cured by boiling a handful of wheat bran with a pinch of chamomile flowers for ten minutes and constantly applying in the form of compresses. If there is severe itching, smear with lily oil; the leg should be well bandaged. With varicose veins, only a little meat should be eaten. Eat plenty of vegetables, barley, oats, rice dishes, fruit, milk and farinacous foods. Coffee, tea and spirits are forbidden.

One usually begins with four weekly whole washes, three hot short compresses of hayseed decoction, and a clay, water and vinegar poultice for one hour twice a day around the legs or varicose veins. Every day one should drink a cup of tea made from yarrow, horsetail and meadowsweet.

VOMITING (VOMITUS)

1) If the vomiting occurs after eating, it may generally be assumed that hardening, ulceration or degeneration is present in the stomach, particularly if food is also vomited. In this case, hot hayseed compresses on the abdomen are highly effective. Take 1 tablespoon sanicle tea with honey every two hours. Alternate whole washes and upper body washes. You can also take 1 tablespoon milk every hour in the mornings.

2) If there is vomiting with severe pain and cramps in the stomach region and abdomen, and if the patient subsequently turns a yellow color, gallstones could be the cause; if the pain is more in the back, kidney stones could be causing it. The

person should drink a large amount of lemon water. Three times a day take 1 tablespoon of the following wine: let 1⅓ cups (20 grams) of greater celandine (*Chelidonium majus*) leaves and stems steep for twenty-four hours in a bottle of white wine. Put a hot hayseed compress on the abdomen every day; each week take four whole washes and two or three half-baths. If the vomiting is a consequence of kidney stones, drink 2 cups knotgrass tea; then take a sugarspoon of the following mixture twice a day:

> ½ cup (100 grams) old walnut oil
> ½ cup (100 grams) sweet almond oil

Mix these ingredients thoroughly. When using this remedy, it is also advisable to drink 2 cups of tea made from boiled oats and licorice every day. In addition, use a hot compress of hayseed decoction around the loins and abdomen, and every two days take a whole wash.

3) Vomiting with constipation demands a careful abdominal examination; there could be a rupture, so a doctor should be consulted.

4) Vomiting in children, before eating or drinking in the morning, is a sign of worms.

5) In the case of women there can be other causes of vomiting—pregnancy for example. When a pregnant woman vomits, try the following: a piece of preserved quince is an excellent remedy against this. Tea from common centaury is also most efficacioous. If neither of the above remedies is effective, take 2 spoons gin mixed with 3 spoons seltzer water before eating at midday and again before the evening meal (Dr. Crasson).

6) Vomiting in hysterical people may be recognized by the accompanying nervous irritability and tension; this vomiting generally follows emotion, or occurs in the morning on an empty stomach, or is accompanied by a severe headache. A good remedy is tea made from mint and lemon balm. In addition, every two days put a hot hayseed compress on the abdomen for half an hour; each week take four whole washes; every day take an upper body wash.

Vomiting Blood

1) Drink 1 cup of yarrow tea daily with a spoon.

2) Taking 15 to 20 drops of spirit of turpentine in a glass of cold water swiftly stops the vomiting of blood. This remedy is also recommended for spitting blood (Dr. Baille).

3) The application of ice and consumption of small pieces of ice is always beneficial in cases of blood-spitting. See also Spitting Blood.

Warts (Verruca)

Rub the warts four to six times a day with one of the following remedies:

1) Fresh greater celandine sap.

2) The fresh sap from haricot bean leaves.

3) Houseleek sap.

4) Marigold sap.

5) Petty spurge (*Euphorbia peplius*) is a most efficacious remedy for warts.

6) Rub the warts with a piece of chalk for a few days before sleeping; they will disappear.

7) If there are very many warts, a sugarspoon of magnesia should be taken three times a day over a period of two or three months.

8) Rub a piece of flannel with black soap and place on the warts.

9) Apply well-bruised leek leaves at night.

10) Smear four times a day with olive oil in which salt has been dissolved or mixed.

11) Apply vinegar compresses.

12) Make a strong solution of chemically pure soda water and moisten the warts with it several times a day, or apply as compresses.

13) Rub a piece of flannel with green soap and apply twice a day.

WASP OR BEE STINGS

1) Brush the place with the sap of a plant with a very strong fragrance such as thyme, sage, mint, lemon balm, rosemary, or parsley.

2) A drop of spirits of ammonia, or compresses of salt water or lemon juice give swift relief. These remedies should be applied as quickly as possible.

WHITLOW (INFLAMMATION AROUND THE FINGERNAIL)

Take 1 cup (50 grams) of potash and dissolve it in 3 cups (¾ liter) boiling water; take ⅓ part of this solution and add to it ⅔ part hot water. Dip the finger into this four to six times a day, each time as long as the pus continues to run out. Bathing in this solution should be continued and alternated with the application of fenugreek poultices.

If the finger has not yet opened, this process can be speeded up: take a raw egg yolk, mix it with a sugarspoon of salt and apply this to the finger for one day; it will then be open.

Usually, indeed nearly always in the case of a whitlow, fleshy excrescences appear, impeding the healing process. Sprinkle these with finely ground alum powder or powdered walnut septa; this will remove the fleshy excrescences. At night a poultice of fenugreek should be applied to the festered finger. In this way the whitlow will be cured in eight to ten days, but the finger must not be cut; if it is cut open, it will be three to six weeks before it heals.

A whitlow may be recognized by a hard leathery patch or point, and by the acute pain, especially if the hand is held downwards. The pain is so severe that the sufferer cannot sleep and walks around as though crazed.

Instead of the fenugreek poultice, a plaster of the following excellent ointment can be applied twice a day. Melt 60 grams yellow wax and ⅓ cup (60 grams) olive oil in a double-boiler; stir until the wax has thoroughly melted; remove from the fire, leave to cool and then add 7 tablespoons (80 grams) of Peruvian balsam.

Instead of potash, the finger can also be bathed six times a day in hot, chemically pure soda water; use two handfuls of soda per quart (liter) of water. After bathing, a plaster of the above mentioned ointment or a fenugreek poultice should immediately be applied.

WHOOPING COUGH

1) Monseigneur Kneipp prescribed a daily hay-shirt for one and a half hours and 6 to 8 drops fennel oil in syrup or on sugar *internally* twice a day.

2) Take mistletoe tea three times a day ⅛ to ¼ cup (30 to 50 grams).

3) Tea made from thyme taken thoughout the day is very effective. Hot beer with elder syrup is also.

4) Take an eggshell, remove the skin from the inside, grind it to a very fine powder; beat an egg yolk with 1 tablespoon sugar, add the juice of a lemon and the powdered eggshell. Take 1 tablespoon of this mixture every hour.

5) Take 2 tablespoons coarsely broken sugar, add 2 sugarspoons of good wine vinegar and give a sugarspoon of this mixture every two hours.

6) Drink tea made from equal quantities of sage and mint.

7) Many a child has been cured by the following prescription: every day a hot hay-shirt for 1½ hours; three times a day take 5 drops fennel oil with honey or sugar and water, and every two hours drink 1 tablespoon thyme tea with honey. For 1 cup of tea, use 2 sugarspoons thyme and 1 tablespoon honey.

WRITER'S CRAMP (MOGIGRAPHIA)

With writer's cramp, one should refrain from writing for some time, but if this is not possible, one should use a thick penholder and a soft nib. Good remedies are:

1) Take arm-baths of hot sage decoction followed by a cold arm-bath.

2) Every day bathe the hand two or three times in hot soda water and take an arm watering every day.

LIST OF REMEDIES

Abscesses: Fenugreek, Pimpernel, Comfrey.

Abdomen (hard, swollen): Goldenrod, Motherwort, Myrrh, Rhubarb.

Abdominal Complaints: Greater Celandine.

Abdominal Incisions: Aniseed.

Abdominal Infection: Sweet Clover, Hop, Coriander.

Acne: Heartsease.

Anasarca: Broom, Meadowsweet.

Anemia: Common Centaury, White Horehound, Thyme.

Anti-Decay: Charcoal.

Antispasmodic: Yarrow, Cinquefoil, Common Chamomile, Chestnut Tree, Cabbage, Linseed, Mint, Olive Oil, Orange Rind, Peppermint.

Appetite Stimulant: Elecampane, Wild Strawberry, Common Wormwood, Winter Cress, Betony, Broom, Dog's Mercury, Buckbean, Carline Thistle, Polypody Root, Narrow-leaved Water Parsnip, Corn Marigold, Gentian, Hyssop, Caraway, Cornflower, Lavender, Linseed, White Horehound, Mustard, Wood Avens, Leek, Rosemary, Watercress, Grapevine, Sorrel.

Ascites: False Hellebore, Broom, Pellitory, Juniper, Meadowsweet, Olive Oil, Rosemary, Haricot Beans.

Asthma: Elecampane, Aniseed Oil, Spignel, Nightshade, Purple Dead-nettle, Speedwell, Oak, Polypody Root, Celery, Germander-speedwell, Goldenrod, Common St. Johnswort,

Motherwort, Coltsfoot, Ground Ivy, Hyssop, Catmint, Chervil, Scurvy Grass, Garlic Mustard, White Horehound, Lovage, Sow Thistle, White Mustard, Olive Oil, Parsley, Pimpernel, Rosemary, Sage, Great Burnet, Valerian, Fennel, Bindweed, Bugle.

Bad Breath: Charcoal, Caraway.

Backache: Goldenrod.

Bedsores: Sage.

Bed-wetting: Agrimony, Oak, Houseleek.

Bilious Fever: Wood Sorrel, Carrot.

Bladder (inflammation): Asparagus, Stinging Nettles, Goldenrod, Horsetail.

Bladder Catarrh: Bearberry, Goldenrod, Common St. Johnswort, Heather, Juniper Berries.

Bladder Stones: Asparagus, Stinging Nettles, Goldenrod, Common Chamomile, Toadflax, Lovage, Parsley.

Bleeding: Bistort, Agrimony, Aloe, Common Wormwood, Alum, Blackberry, Stinging Nettles, Sanicle, Selfheal, Ploughman's Spikenard, Spotted Dead-nettle, Yarrow, Oak, Cinquefoil, Mouse-ear Hawkweed, Marshmallow, Orpine, Cinnamon, Chamomile flowers, Common Lousewort, Horsetail, Meadowsweet, Toadflax, Mistletoe, Wood Avens, Walnut, Long-stalked Cranesbill, Parnassus Grass, Sandalwood, Sage, Comfrey, Tormentil, Knotgrass, Lady's Mantle, Plantain, Willow, Bindweed, Ground Pine.

Bleeding (painful): Lady's Mantle.

Bleeding (to staunch): Alum, Shepherd's Purse.

Blood (loss of): Long-stalked Cranesbill, Knotgrass.

Blood (sharpness in the): Bugloss, Common Alkanet.

Blood (vomiting): Alum, Stinging Nettles, Sanicle.

Blood Poisoning: Hayseed.

Blood-Spitting: Agrimony, Thrift, Southernwood, Betony, Shepherd's Purse, Blackberry, Selfheal, Stinging Nettles, Rupture

Wort, Yarrow, Speedwell, Oak, Cinquefoil, Germander-speedwell, Goldenrod, Heath Spotted Orchis, Common St. Johnswort, Hart's Tongue Fern, Ground Ivy, Orpine, Teasel, Horsetail, Common Poppy, Meadowsweet, Aaron's Rod, Common Milkwort, Lungwort, Linseed, Periwinkle, White Horehound, Chickweed, Wood Avens, Olive Oil, Parnassus Grass, Moneywort, Purslane, Comfrey, Flixweed, Tormentil, Knotgrass, Plantain, Willow, Grapevine, Ground Pine, Bugle.

Bowel Movement (difficult): Barberry, Hayseed (Greek), Castor Oil.

Bowel Movement (very bad smell): Rhubarb.

Breasts (swollen): Chestnut Tree, Chickweed, Herb Robert, Nipplewort.

Broken Bones: Yarrow.

Bronchitis (infection of the windpipe): Angelica, Hop, Catmint, Aaron's Rod, Knotgrass, Onion.

Burns: Hedge Woundwort, Dead-nettle, Orpine, Common Chamomile, Ivy, Cabbage, Carrot, Comfrey.

Cancer: Common Figwort, Betony, Stinging Nettles, Blessed Thistle, Speedwell, Horsetail, Clay, Biting Stonecrop, Myrrh, Long-stalked Cranesbill, Carrot, Rhubarb, Sarsaparilla, Lady's Bedstraw.

Caries: Yarrow.

Catarrh: Chamomile Flowers.

Catarrh (chronic): Hemp-agrimony, Speedwell, Germander-speedwell, Goldenrod, Common St. Johnswort, Ground Ivy, Hyssop, Scurvy Grass, Garlic Mustard, Watercress, Bindweed.

Catarrh (mucus): Common Marjoram, Lemon Balm, Carline Thistle, Aaron's Rod, Mint, Peppermint, Sage, Sassafras, Knotgrass.

Cerebral Disorders: Hyssop, Sage, Ground Pine.

Chapped Hands and Feet: Camphor, Turnip.

Chest Catarrh: Elecampane, Speedwell, Chicory.

Chest Complaints: Polypody Root, Germander-speedwell, Heath Spotted Orichis, Oats, Marshmallow, Downy Hemp Nettle, Coltsfoot, Ground Ivy, Lungwort, Linseed, Mustard, Myrrh, Hedge Mustard, Vervain.

Chest (mucus): Speedwell, Germander-speedwell.

Chest (to cleanse): Motherwort, Knotgrass.

Chest Infection: Sow Thistle.

Chest Pain: Parsley, Lady's Bedstraw.

Chest Strengthening: Incense.

Colds: Nightshade, Yarrow, Common St. Johnswort, Coltsfoot, Lime Tree, Moneywort, Sunflower.

Colic: Hedge Woundwort, Asparagus, Blessed Thistle, Yarrow, Wild Angelica, Sweet Clover, Holly, Chamomile Flowers, Chestnut Tree, Cloves, Aaron's Rod, Lime Tree, Long-stalked Cranesbill, Tansy, Fennel, Vervain.

Colic (in children): Aniseed, Lemon Balm.

Colic (miserere): Linseed.

Colic (nervous colic): Common Wormwood, Ragged Robin.

Congestion of Blood in the Head: Aloe, Ash, Speedwell, Lavender, White Mustard, Valerian, Rue, Quassia.

Congestion of Blood in the Lungs: False Hellebore.

Constipation: Greater Celandine, Linseed, Magnesia, White Mustard, Olive Oil, Peach Tree, Chicory.

Constriction of the Chest: White Mustard Seed, Knotgrass.

Consumption: Wild Strawberry, Agrimony, Lemon Tree, Speedwell, Polypody Root, Germander-speedwell, Greater Celandine, Heath Spotted Orchis, Downy Hemp Nettle, Common Mallow, Chervil, Turnip, Aaron's Rod, Lady's Mantle, Lungwort, Garlic Mustard, White Horehound, Chickweed, Carrot, Parsnip, Fine-leaved Dropwort, Knotgrass.

Contusions: Common St. Johnswort, Clay, Common Daisy, Wallflower, Solomon's Seal, Arnica.

Convalescents: Common Centaury, Angelica, Heath Spotted Orchis, Chickweed, Quassia, Grapevine, Bran.

Convulsions: Lemon Balm, Motherwort, Lime Tree, Mistletoe, Grapevine.

Corns: Orpine, Ivy.

Cough: Almonds, Hemp-agrimony, Speedwell, Polypody Root, Germander-speedwell, Goldenrod, Heath Spotted Orchis, Oats, Marshmallow, Ground Ivy, Hyssop, Common Poppy, Lime Tree, Linseed, White Horehound, Mustard, Parsnip, Carrot, Burnet Saxifrage, Sage, Comfrey, Hedge Mustard, Thyme, Knotgrass, Plantain, Vervain, Licorice.

Cramp Colic: Linseed, Castor Oil.

Cramp Spasms: Lemon Balm.

Cramps (stomach or intestinal): Common Marjoram, Cinquefoil, Motherwort, Hayseed, Common Chamomile, Mint, Peppermint, Tansy, Fennel, Vervain.

Croup: Common Figwort, Goldenrod, Fenugreek, Honey.

Crusta Lactea (in children): Fumitory, Heartsease.

Cysts: Ground Ivy.

Dandruff: Mustard, Elder.

Deafness: Houseleek.

Depuratives: Fumitory, Wild Strawberry, Winter Cress, Stinging Nettles, Speedwell, Corn Marigold, Honey, Juniper Berries, Burdock, Meadowsweet, Bugloss, Groundsel, Periwinkle, Common Daisy, Sow Thistle, White Mustard, Common Alkanet, Dandelion, Dock, Carrot, Purslane, Sarsaparilla, Spruce, Thyme, Heartsease, Elder, Bugle.

Diabetes: Bilberry, Selfheal, Goldenrod, Sow Thistle, Tormentil, Knotgrass.

Diaphoretic: Currant, Alder Tree, Marigold, Juniper, Burdock, Rosemary, Heartsease, Elder.

Diarrhea: Bistort, Mugwort, Bilberry, Blackberry, Sanicle,

Blessed Thistle, Dead-nettle, Reed Mace (cattail), Oak, Raspberry, Canadian Fleabane, Cinquefoil, Goldenrod, Heath Spotted Orchis, Mouse-ear Hawkweed, Common St. Johnswort, Hare's Foot Clover, Marshmallow, Hart's Tongue Fern, Juniper, Aaron's Rod, Coriander, Purple Loosestrife, Parnassus Grass, Moneywort, Quassia, Rosemary, Sage, Comfrey, Meadowsweet, Knotgrass, Lady's Bedstraw, Plantain, Willow, Bindweed, Club Moss.

Digestive Organs (weak): Agrimony.

Diuretic: Currant, Winter Cress, Spignel, Broom, Common Honeysuckle, Goldenrod, Hemp, Motherwort, Ground Ivy, Hyssop, Juniper, Bladder Cherry, Burdock, Milk Thistle, Long-stalked Cranesbill, Common Alkanet, Leek, Haricot Beans, Lady's Mantle, Heartsease, Pepper Saxifrage, Sorrel, Speedwell, Bugloss, Garlic Mustard.

Dizziness: Aniseed, Betony, Speedwell, Germander-speedwell, Coriander, Caraway, Lavender, Mustard, Tansy, Rosemary, Sage, Thyme, Valerian, Grapevine, Ground Pine.

Drink (invigorating): Bran.

Dropsy: Currant, Agrimony, Asparagus, Elecampane, Common Wormwood, Barberry, Hemp, Agrimony, Stinging Nettles, Blessed Thistle, Common Centaury, Pea, Canadian Fleabane, Marigold, Hop, Juniper, Bladder Cherry, Meadowsweet, Common Milkwort, Sea Holly, Toadflax, Scurvy Grass, Woodruff, Daisy, Milk Thistle, Horseradish, Mustard, Long-stalked Cranesbill, Parsley, Tansy, Rosemary, Sassafras, Haricot Beans, Elder Flowers, Dwarf Elder Flowers, Lady's Bedstraw, Club Moss.

Dysentery: Bistort, Agrimony, Thrift, Shepherd's Purse, Bilberry, Blackberry, Mugwort, Ploughman's Spikenard, Oak, Raspberry, Goldenrod, Heath Spotted Orchis, Common St. Johnswort, Common Chamomile, Meadowsweet, Cornelian Cherry, Lady's Mantle, Periwinkle, White Horehound, Wallflower, Wood Avens, Long-stalked Cranesbill, Purple Loosestrife, Moneywort, Burnet Saxifrage, Comfrey, Knotgrass, Plantain, Club Moss, Grapevine, Bugle.

Earache: Greater Celandine, Cabbage.

Ears (running): Ivy.

Ears (swelling): Almond Oil.

Eczema: Fumitory, Elecampane, Nightshade, Blackberry, Buckbean, Hemp, Coltsfoot, Hayseed, Charcoal, Ivy, Burdock, Garlic, Aaron's Rod, Toadflax, Garlic Mustard, Mustard, Dock Carrot, Tansy, Spruce, Heartsease, Buckthorn, Watercress, Lady's Bedstraw, Soapwort, Bran.

Ejaculation (involuntary): Mouse-Ear Hawkweed, Hop, Toadflax, Wallflower, Quassia, Plantain.

Emetic: Sweet Violet, Buckthorn.

Enteritis: Linseed, Castor Oil.

Erysipelas: Chervil, Meadowsweet.

Epilepsy (falling sickness): Cow Parsley, Mugwort, Blessed Thistle, Alder Tree, Wild Angelica, Goat's Rue, Woodruff, Chervil, Ragged Robin, Groundsel, Lime Tree, Mistletoe, Mustard, Chickweed, Biting Stonecrop, Sage, Viper's Bugloss, Meadowsweet, Valerian, Knotgrass, Lady's Bedstraw, Hedge Bedstraw, Grapevine, Ground Pine.

Eye Complaints: Galangal, Chestnut Tree, Mustard, Eyebright, Grapevine.

Eye Inflammation: Ash, Sweet Clover, Clover, Plantain, Grapevine.

Eye Tonic: White Horehound, Fennel.

Eyes (burning): Galangal, Elder.

Eyes (painful): Elder.

Eyes (red, running, suppurating): Aloe.

Eyes (weakened, in old people): Valerian.

Facial Neuralgia: White Mustard.

Fainting: Rosemary.

Fatty Degeneration of the Heart: False Hellebore, Hyssop.

Febrifugal Remedies: Bistort, Common Wormwood, Almonds,

Spignel, Betony, Stinging Nettles, Blessed Thistle, Buckbean, Common Centaury, Alder Tree, Angelica, Raspberry, Gamander, Gentian, Hedge Hyssop, Marigold, Common St. Johnswort, Holly, Hyssop, Meadowsweet, Coriander, Linseed, White Horehound, Biting Stonecrop, Myrrh, Wood Avens, Long-stalked Cranesbill, Orange Rind, Quassia, Rosemary, Valerian, Knotgrass, Corn Salad, Willow, Vervain.

Fistula: Sanicle, Yarrow, Goldenrod, Long-stalked Cranesbill.

Fleshy Excrescences: Walnut.

Fluids (thickened): Motherwort.

Food (poisonous): Angelica, Charcoal Powder.

Frostbite: Sage.

Gall: Glabrous Rupture Wort, Quassia, Chicory, Thyme.

Gallstone: Common Centaury, Greater Celandine, Common St. Johnswort, Olive Oil.

Gangrene: Dead-nettle, Carline Thistle, Walnut.

Genital Organs (diseases): Goldenrod.

Goiter: Lady's Bedstraw.

Gout: Wild Strawberry, False Hellebore, Asparagus, Betony, Nightshade, Stinging Nettles, Buckbean, Common Centaury, Duckweed, Angelica, Ash, Good King Henry, Hedge Hyssop, Greater Celandine, White Bryony, Motherwort, Ground Elder, Honey, Hayseed, Birthwort, Hop, Juniper, Cowslips, Burdock, Cod Liver Oil, Common Daisy, Mustard, Olive Oil, Sage, Sarsaparilla, Sassafras, Noli Me Tangere, Corn Salad, Dwarf Elder, Licorice.

Gravel: Wild Strawberry, Almonds, Stinging Nettles, Glabrous Rupture Wort, Speedwell, Mouse-ear Hawkweed, Cinquefoil, Pellitory, Hart's Tongue Fern, Couchgrass, Dog Rose, Juniper, Bladder Cherry, Horsetail, Sea Holly, Woodruff, Linseed, Magnesia, Horseradish, Mustard, Wallflower, Long-stalked Cranesbill, Parsley, Sage, Meadowsweet, Meadow Saxifrage, Knotgrass, Lady's Bedstraw, Grapevine, Licorice.

Green Sickness: Elecampane, Common Centaury, Angelica, Marigold, Common St. Johnswort, Motherwort, Hyssop, White Horehound, Lovage.

Guinea Worm: Coltsfoot, Cornflower, Heartsease, Watercress.

Gums (ulcerated, loose): Bistort, Blackberry, Sanicle, Selfheal, Goldenrod, Charcoal, Wood Sorrel, Privet, Garlic Mustard, Biting Stonecrop, Myrrh, Galangal, Cinquefoil.

Hair (falling out): Bilberry, Stinging Nettles, Burdock, Walnut.

Hands (chapped): Yarrow, Tansy.

Hands (sweating): Sage, Thyme.

Head (congestion): Galangal, Mustard.

Headache: Aniseed, Ash, Lemon Balm, Duckweed, Galangal, Chestnut Tree, Cabbage, Lavender, Clay, Mayflower, Mustard, Wallflower, Vervain.

Headlice: Ivy, Red Rattle.

Heart (dilation of): False Hellebore.

Heartburn: Elecampane, Blessed Thistle, Common Centaury, Cinnamon, Linseed, Purslane.

Heart Complaints: False Hellebore, Motherwort, Rosemary.

Heart Strengthening: Common Marjoram, Bugloss, Hyssop, Woodruff, Lime Tree, Mint, Wallflower, Wood Avens, Common Alkanet, Peppermint.

Hematuria: Bearberry, Shepherd's Purse, Sanicle, Selfheal, Speedwell, Ground Ivy, Cinnamon, Horsetail, Meadowsweet, Parsley, Ground Pine.

Hemorrhoids (Piles): Figwort, Aloe, Asparagus, Stinging Nettles, Enchanter's Nightshade, Yarrow, Greater Celandine, Horsetail, Common St. Johnswort, Aaron's Rod, Toadflax, Linseed, White Horehound, White Mustard, Myrrh, Flixweed, Plantain.

Housemaid's Knee: Southernwood.

Humors (bad): Chervil, White Horehound.

Hydrothorax: Carrot, Rosemary.

Hypochondria: Fumitory, Black Horehound, Blessed Thistle, Hedge Hyssop, Calamus, Common Chamomile, Lavender, Lime Tree, White Horehound, Mustard, Biting Stonecrop, Lettuce, Valerian.

Hysteria: Common Wormwood, Black Horehound, Spignel, Mugwort, Pyrethrum, Hemp-Agrimony, Lemon Balm, Carline Thistle, Wild Angelica, Marigold, Common St. Johnswort, Calamus, Chamomile, Catmint, Ragged Robin, Woodruff, Lime Tree, White Horehound, Mistletoe, Tansy, Lettuce, Valerian, Lady's Bedstraw, Hedge Bedstraw, Grapevine.

Indigestion: Currant, Elecampane, Common Wormwood, Aniseed, Lemon Balm, Yarrow, Common Centaury, Devil's-Bit Scabious, Speedwell, Wild Angelica, Gentian, Hayseed, Hop, Charcoal, Juniper, Common Chamomile Flowers, Wild Chamomile Flowers, Garlic, Coriander, Cloves, Lime Tree, Lovage, Mustard, Mint, Myrrh, Wood Avens, Peppermint, Leek, Rosemary, Sage, Great Burnet, Chicory, Onion, Fennel, Grapevine.

Infection Complaints: Good King Henry, Gum, Ground Ivy, Chamomile Flowers, Linseed, Myrrh, Parsley, Purslane, Solomon's Seal, White Stonecrop.

Inflammation of Limbs: Nipplewort.

Influenza: Hazel Catkins, Fennel.

Injuries: Comfrey.

Insomnia: Common Wormwood, Yarrow, Goldenrod, Lime Tree, Linseed, Mustard.

Intermittent Fever: Hedge Hyssop, Skullcap, Greater Celandine, Juniper, Calamus, Coriander, Linseed, Wood Avens, Quassia.

Intestinal Bleeding: Sanicle.

Intestinal Blockage: Fumitory, Agrimony, Hop, White Horehound.

Intestinal Mucous: Sanicle, Blessed Thistle, Cabbage, Myrrh, Great Burnet.

Intestines (diseases of): Sanicle, Carline Thistle, Yarrow, Gum, Common St. Johnswort, Oats, Marshmallow, Honey, Calamus, Caraway, Coriander, Myrrh, Olive Oil, Quassia, Rhubarb, Castor Oil.

Intestines (weakness of): Agrimony, Yarrow, Quassia, Rhubarb, Great Burnet.

Itching: Speedwell, Goldenrod, Yellow Iris, Sage.

Jaundice: Fumitory, Southernwood, Barberry, Betony, Blessed Thistle, Buckbean, Common Centaury, Duckweed, Pea, Hedge Hyssop, Marigold, Greater Celandine, Common St. Johnswort, Hemp, Honey, Bladder Cherry, Catmint, Chervil, Wood Sorrel, Cornflower, Groundsel, Toadflax, Woodruff, White Horehound, Lovage, Milk Thistle, Walnut, Long-stalked Cranesbill, Dandelion, Carrot, Parsley, Quassia, Tansy, Rhubarb, Lady's Bedstraw, Vervain, Ground Pine, Bugle.

Joint Pain: Coriander.

Kidney (ulceration): Ground Ivy.

Kidney (bleeding): Sanicle.

Kidney Complaints: Common Wormwood, Asparagus, Southernwood, Bearberry, Broom, Carline Thistle, Common Centaury, Speedwell, Pellitory, Goldenrod, Oats, Motherwort, Dog Rose, Hayseed, Horsetail, Sea Holly, Long-stalked Cranesbill, Burnet Saxifrage, Purslane, Rosemary, Sage, Haricot Beans, Knotgrass, Fennel, Water Lily, Pepper Saxifrage, Vervain.

Kidney Stones: Common Wormwood, Asparagus, Stinging Nettles, Glabrous Rupture Wort, Heath, Magnesia, Gromwell, Knotgrass, Meadow Saxifrage, Club Moss, Grapevine.

Laxative: Annual Mercury, Elder, Castor Oil.

Legs (swollen): Leek.

Leucorrhea: Bistort, Agrimony, Elecampane, Common Wormwood, Blackberry, Dead-nettle, Reed Mace, Yarrow, Oak, Milk Thistle, Myrrh, Wood Avens, Walnut, Parnassus Grass, Moneywort, Rosemary, Lady's Mantle, Plantain, Willow, Bugle.

Limping: Goldenrod.

Liver Complaints: Wild Strawberry, Fumitory, Agrimony, Common Wormwood, Barberry, Hemp-Agrimony, Common Centaury, Polypody Root, Ash, Hedge Hyssop, Greater Celandine, Hemp, Hayseed, Charcoal, Bladder Cherry, Juniper, Chamomile Flowers, Sea Holly, Woodruff, White Horehound, Lovage, Mistletoe, Mustard, Myrrh, Parsley, Burnet Saxifrage, Rosemary, Lettuce, Chicory, Knotgrass, Fennel, Willow, Vervain.

Liver (atrophy and hardening): Mustard Seed, Chickweed.

Liver (blockage): Groundsel, White Horehound, Carrot.

Liver (hardening): Bugle.

Liver (inflammation): Chervil, Toadflax, Sow Thistle.

Loins (pain): Sanicle, Goldenrod.

Loss of Voice: Valerian.

Lung Complaints: Elecampane, Nightshade, Sanicle, Selfheal, Yarrow, Speedwell, Greater Celandine, Common St. Johnswort, Ground Ivy, Charcoal, Catmint, Chervil, Common Poppy, Lungwort, White Horehound, Mistletoe, Myrrh, Burnet Saxifrage, Comfrey, Thyme, Knotgrass, Sweet Violet, Lady's Mantle, Licorice.

Lung Catarrh: Common Calamint, Polypody Root, Celery, Common Honeysuckle, Sage, Hedge Mustard, Fine-leaved Water Dropwort, Knotgrass, White Water Lily.

Lungs (inflammation): Hazel Catkins, Common St. Johnswort, Marshmallow, Common Milkwort, Periwinkle, White Horehound, Milk Thistle, Olive Oil, Carrot, Viper's Bugloss, Chicory.

Lungs (phlegm): Blessed Thistle, Angelica, Coltsfoot, Spruce, Licorice.

Lungs (ulcerated): Germander-speedwell, Ground Ivy, Toadflax, Periwinkle, Moneywort, Bugle.

Lupus: Oak, Clay, Chickweed, Walnut, Lady's Bedstraw.

Lymphatic Disorders: Common Calamint, Lady's Bedstraw.

Maggots (threadworms): Garlic.

Mania: Common St. Johnswort.

Marsh Fever: Heath Spotted Orchis.

Measles: Bistort, Borage, Stinging Nettles, Raspberry, Hayseed, Viper's Bugloss, Sweet Violet, Licorice.

Melancholy: Fumitory, Common Centaury.

Menopause: Shepherd's Purse, Buckbean.

Menstruation Disorders: Elecampane, Aloe, Common Wormwood, Hedge Woundwort, Thrift, Pyrethrum, Shepherd's Purse, Sanicle, Lemon Balm, Dill, Blessed Thistle, Yarrow, Oak, Angelica, Raspberry, Marigold, Greater Celandine, Common St. Johnswort, Motherwort, Common Chamomile Flowers, Cinnamon, Catmint, Coriander, Sea Holly, Lavender, White Horehound, Lovage, Myrrh, Wood Avens, Tansy, Great Burnet, Marsh Cudweed, Lady's Mantle, Grapevine.

Mentagra (beard eczema): Haricot Bean.

Mental Faculties (disturbance of): Sage.

Migraine (nervous headache): Currant, Common Marjoram, Betony, Lemon Balm, Blessed Thistle, Speedwell, Angelica, Germander-speedwell, Ground Ivy, Juniper, Lime Tree, Mint, Wood Avens, Peppermint, Thyme, Valerian, Grapevine, Vervain.

Mother's Milk (to dry it up): Parsley, Chervil.

Mother's Milk (to improve): Aniseed, Dill, Periwinkle, Sow Thistle, Mint, Peppermint.

Mouth Disorders: Bistort, Agrimony, Thrift, Selfheal, Gum, Cinnamon, Wood Sorrel, Goldenrod, Privet, Myrrh.

Mouth (burnt): Olive Oil.

Mucous Membrane: Yarrow, Sandalwood.

Mucus: Quassia.

Mucus Dissolvent: Common Marjoram, Lemon Balm, Carline Thistle, Polypody Root, Pea, Germander-speedwell, Juniper,

Catmint, Garlic Mustard, White Horehound, Lovage, Rhubarb, Rosemary, Plantain.

Mucus forming: Mint, Peppermint.

Muscle (to Strengthen): Common Centaury.

Nasal Catarrh: Galangal.

Nausea: Common Centaury, Angelica, Gentian, Cinnamon.

Nephritis: Cinquefoil, Gum.

Nerve pains (neuralgia): Mugwort, Clay, Wallflower, Dwarf Elder, Lady's Bedstraw.

Nerve Tonic: Gentian, Juniper, Mustard, Wallflower, Rosemary, Sage, Ground Pine.

Nervous Colic: Common Wormwood, Ragged Robin.

Nervous Complaints: Balsam, Common Marjoram, Lemon Balm, Yarrow, Wild Angelica, Angelica, Marigold, Chamomile Flowers, Woodruff, Lime Tree, White Horehound, Magnesia, Lovage, Mint, Wallflower, Peppermint, Rosemary, Valerian, Willow.

Nervous Cramp: Common St. Johnswort.

Nervous Vomiting: Common Marjoram, Mugwort, Mint.

Nipples: Nipplewort, Houseleek, Comfrey.

Nose Bleeding: Shepherd's Purse, Sanicle, Horsetail, Mayflower, Knotgrass.

Nose Complaints: Galangal.

Obesity: False Hellebore, Hawthorn.

Palpitations: False Hellebore, Common Marjoram, Lemon Balm, Motherwort, Cabbage, Mayflower, Mint, Wood Avens, Peppermint, Valerian, Grapevine.

Paralysis: Betony, Mustard, Rosemary, Sage, Dwarf Elder.

Phlegm Discharge: Charcoal, Aaron's Rod.

Phlegm Tuberculosis: Nightshade, Downy Hemp Nettle.

Pituitous Fever: Angelica, White Horehound.

Pituitous Stroke: Valerian.

Podagra (foot gout): Common Wormwood, White Bryony, Ground Elder, Garlic, Noli Me Tangere, Sweet Violet, Elder, Dwarf Elder, Bugle.

Poisoning: Charcoal.

Polyps: Polypody Root, Ivy.

Poultices: Greek Hayseed, Common Mallow, Linseed Meal.

Psoriasis: Lady's Bedstraw.

Pulmonary Consumption: Common Milkwort, Periwinkle, Common Daisy, Carrot, Licorice.

Purgatives: Aloe, Betony, Broom, Box, Buckbean, Polypody Root, Flowering Ash, Hedge Hyssop, Charcoal, Holly, Nasturtium, Ivy, Peach Tree, Plum Tree, Senna Leaves, Rhubarb, Heartsease, Dwarf Elder, Buckthorn.

Purpura: Goldenrod, Horsetail.

Rectum: Lady's Mantle.

Renal Colic: Agrimony, Wild Angelica.

Respiratory Organs: Honey, White Mustard, Fine-leaved Water Dropwort, Licorice.

Rheumatism: Currant, Wild Strawberry, Agrimony, Borage, Nightshade, Stinging Nettles, Common Centaury, Yarrow, Alder Tree, Flowering Ash, Hedge Hyssop, Common St. Johnswort, Oats, Heath, Hemp, Ground Elder, Birthwort, Hop, Juniper, Chestnut Tree, Cowslip, Burdock, Common Milkwort, Lily, Linseed, Mustard, Wallflower, Leek, Tansy, Rosemary, Sage, Sassafras, Sarsaparilla, Bistort, Great Burnet, Corn Salad, Dwarf Elder, Licorice.

Rickets, Rachitis: Motherwort, Hayseed, Hop, Cod Liver Oil, Rhubarb.

Ringing in the Ears: Almond Oil, Greater Celandine.

Ruptures: Sanicle, Glabrous Rupture Wort, Hare's Foot Clover, Comfrey, Knotgrass, Lady's Mantle, Castor Oil.

St. Vitus' Dance: Mugwort, Sanicle, Ragged Robin, Mistletoe, Valerian.

Scabies: Elecampane, Garlic, Cornflower, Clay, Solomon's Seal, Lady's Bedstraw.

Scarlet Fever: Fumitory, Raspberry, Hayseed, Mustard, Sweet Violet.

Scars: Aloe, Solomon's Seal.

Sciatica: False Hellebore, Common St. Johnswort, Ground Elder, Poplar, Dwarf Elder, Ground Pine.

Scrofula: Common Figwort, Fumitory, Hedge Woundwort, Nightshade, Blessed Thistle, Oak, Polypody Root, Coltsfoot, Hop, Meadowsweet, White Horehound, Mustard, Walnut, Butterbur, Parsley, Sassafras, Heartsease, Dwarf Elder, Angelica, Hedge Hyssop, Goldenrod, Scurvy Grass, Cod Liver Oil, Common Daisy, Lady's Bedstraw.

Scrofulous Tumors: Common Figwort, Hare's Ear, Dead-nettle, Greater Celandine, Chervil, Butterbur, Parsley, Meadowsweet, Heartsease.

Scrofulous Ulcers: Tormentil.

Scurf in Children: Juniper, Ivy, Garlic, Cornflower, Clay, Meadowsweet, Walnut Tree, Tansy, Heartsease.

Scurvy: Fumitory, Bistort, Common Wormwood, Winter Cress, Barberry, Shepherd's Purse, Sanicle, Lemon Tree, Yarrow, Common Centaury, Angelica, Celery, Hart's Tongue Fern, Lime, Nasturtium, Calamus, Groundsel, Wood Sorrel, Ragged Robin, Scurvy Grass, Privet, Garlic Mustard, White Horehound, Mustard, Biting Stonecrop, Moneywort, Purslane, Sage, Sassafras, Corn Salad, Elder, Sorrel.

Self-Abuse: Yarrow.

Seminal Discharge at Night: Bearberry.

Shaking (trembling): Common Marjoram, Betony, Mint, Common St. Johnswort.

Shivering: Lime Tree.

Side (pain in the): Goldenrod, Heath, Lady's Bedstraw.

Skin Complaints: Fumitory, Nightshade, Stinging Nettles, Speedwell, Germander-speedwell, Good King Henry, Common Honeysuckle, Hedge Hyssop, Hayseed, Lime, Ivy, Burdock, Chervil, Garlic, Meadowsweet, Toadflax, White Horehound, Dock, Rosemary, Solomon's Seal, Sarsaparilla, Lady's Bedstraw, Soapwort.

Small Pox: Fumitory, Bistort.

Snuff: Chestnut Tree.

Sore Throat: Blackberry, Stinging Nettles, Selfheal, Pellitory, Hare's Foot Clover, Marshmallow, Turnip, Plantain.

Sores (internal): Bistort, Glabrous Rupture Wort, Goldenrod, White Horehound, Mistletoe, Wintergreen.

Sores (old): Aloe, Nipplewort, Blackberry, Blessed Thistle, Hare's Ear, Glabrous Rupture Wort, Dead-nettle, Corn Marigold, Common Honeysuckle, Greater Celandine, Goldenrod, Horsetail, Turnip, Common Lousewort, Cabbage, Clay, Lady's Mantle, Biting Stonecrop, Myrrh, Carrot, Sage, Flixweed, Heartsease, Bindweed, Bugle.

Spleen Complaints: Fumitory, Agrimony, Asparagus, Thrift, Selfheal, Barberry, Polypody Root, Ash, Greater Celandine, Sea Holly, White Horehound, Lovage, Carrot, Parsley, Chicory, Watercress, Willow, Vervain.

Spleen (blocked): Hemp-Agrimony, White Horehound.

Sprains, Dislocations: Agrimony, Betony, Mugwort, Tansy.

Stomach (acid): Common Wormwood, Juniper, Cinnamon, Linseed, Mistletoe, Quassia.

Stomach (cramps): Aniseed, Yarrow, Speedwell, Cinquefoil, Hyssop, Chamomile Flowers, Cloves, Mustard, Olive Oil, Valerian, Willow.

Stomach (foul): Ground Ivy.

Stomach (inflammation): Marshmallow, Sow Thistle, Olive Oil.

Stomach (mucus): Sanicle, Blessed Thistle, Yarrow, Glabrous

Rupture Wort, Fenugreek, Coriander, Myrrh, Parsley, Rosemary, Great Burnet, Chicory, Willow.

Stomach (oppression): Quassia.

Stomach (weakness): Aloe, Common Wormwood, Asparagus, Lemon Balm, Blessed Thistle, Buckbean, Juniper, Calamus, Cinnamon, Myrrh, Dandelion, Burnet Saxifrage, Quassia, Rhubarb, Rosemary, Sage.

Stomach Complaints: Blessed Thistle, Common Centaury, Angelica, Greater Celandine, Oats, Ground Ivy, Hayseed, Caraway, Lovage, Mustard, Carrot, Parsley, Burnet Saxifrage, Rosemary, Sandalwood, Knotgrass, Sorrel.

Stomach Ulcers: Sanicle, Yarrow, Honey, Hayseed (Greek), Moneywort, Knotgrass.

Stomachache: Lemon Balm, Yarrow, Speedwell, Cinquefoil, Gum, Lovage, Valerian, Lady's Bedstraw, Hedge Bedstraw, Cow Parsley, Raspberry, Heather, Hyssop, Caraway.

Stomachic: Southernwood, Spignel, Common Marjoram, Carline Thistle, Blessed Thistle, Devil's Bit Scabious, Speedwell, Gentian, Hyssop, Caraway, Catmint, Coriander, Horseradish, Mint, Wood Avens, Walnut, Eyebright, Orange Rind, Peppermint, Quassia, Fennel.

Stones: Wild Strawberry, False Hellebore, Goldenrod, Oats, Dog Rose, Juniper, Horsetail, Linseed, Mustard, Wallflowers, Knotgrass, Lady's Bedstraw, Licorice.

Strangulated Hernia: Castor Oil.

Stroke: Coriander, White Mustard, Wallflower, Rosemary, Sage, Ground Pine.

Swelling of the Limbs: Chervil, Orpine, Mustard.

Teeth (caries): Mustard Garlic.

Teeth (loose): Goldenrod, Garlic Mustard.

Tendons (strengthen): Common St. Johnswort.

Thighs (pain, paralysis): Goldenrod.

Throat Complaints: Selfheal, Pellitory, Oats, Mouse-ear Hawk-weed, Honey, Hayseed (Greek), Houseleek, Periwinkle, Long-stalked Cranesbill, Sage, Hedge Mustard, Carrot.

Throat Infections: Currant, Common Figwort, Agrimony, Black-berry, Sanicle, Alder Tree, Pellitory, Skullcap, Gum, Golden-rod, Houseleek, Wood Sorrel, Rampion Bellflower, Turnip, Periwinkle, Sweet Violet.

Thrush: Bistort, Gum.

Thrush in Children: Bistort, Blackberry, Gum, Houseleek, Sage, Watercress, Plantain Leaves.

Tongue (paralysis or stiffness): Pyrethrum, Valerian.

Tonic: Plantain.

Tonsillitis: Selfheal, Common Honeysuckle, Mouse-ear Hawk-weed, Field Scabious.

Toothache: Bistort, Ash, Galangal, Cinquefoil.

Trembling, Shaking: Common Marjoram, Betony, Common St. Johnswort, Mint.

Tubercles: Coltsfoot.

Tubercular Throat: Sanicle, Turnip, Carrot.

Ulceration: Blessed Thistle, Dead-nettle, Yarrow, Alder Tree, Greek Hayseed, Hayseed, Charcoal, Lime, Horsetail, Aaron's Rod, Field Scabious, Nightshade, Sarsaparilla, Sassafras, Bur-Marigold, Lady's Mantle.

Ulceration (internal): Field Scabious.

Ulceration (internal and external): Blackberry, Carline Thistle, Yarrow, Good King Henry, Mouse-Ear Hawkweed, Hart's Tongue Fern, Honey, Hayseed, Horsetail, Garlic Mustard, Comfrey, Flixweed, Marsh Cudweed, Lady's Bedstraw.

Ulceration of the Intestines: Lime, Knotgrass.

Ulcers (in the bladder): Agrimony.

Unhealthy Matter in Stomach and Intestines: Angelica.

Urinary Incontinence: Bistort, Agrimony, Bearberry, Oak.

Urination (difficult): Currant, Asparagus, Cow Parsley, Glabrous Rupture Wort, Celery, Skullcap, Gum, Greater Celandine, Goldenrod, Marshmallow, Heath, Ground Ivy, Horsetail, Meadowsweet, Cornflower, Sea Holly, Sow Thistle, Linseed, Olive Oil, Parsley, Burnet Saxifrage, Poplar, Carrot, Lady's Mantle, Noli Me Tangere, Lady's Bedstraw, Bugle, Licorice.

Urine (cold): Burnet Saxifrage, Noli Me Tangere.

Urine (stoppage): Broom, Bladder Cherry.

Venereal Disease: Nightshade, Sarsaparilla, Lady's Bedstraw.

Vomiting: Asparagus, Lemon Balm, Common Centaury, Wild Angelica, Angelica, Linseed, Mint, Peppermint, Quassia, Fennel, Grapevine.

Vomiting in Hysterical Patients: Mugwort, Cinnamon, Mint, Peppermint, Valerian.

Vomiting in Pregnant Women: Common Centuary, Cinnamon.

Warts: Greater Celandine, Euphorbia, Rampion Bellflower.

Wasp or Bee Stings: Lily, Leek.

Water Vessels (blockage): Soapwort.

Watery Gall: Mistletoe.

Weak Limbs: Chicory.

Weakness (general): Wild Angelica, Angelica, Pea, White Horehound, Quassia, Marigold, Cinnamon, Grapevine.

Whooping Cough: Greater Celandine, Common Poppy, Mistletoe, Thyme, Fennel.

Wind: Agrimony, Elecampane, Lemon Balm, Blessed Thistle, Angelica, Honey, Sweet Clover, Juniper, Calamus, Chamomile Flowers, Coriander, Lavender, Lily, Lovage, Mustard, Mint, Myrrh, Peppermint, Rhubarb, Rosemary, Sage, Great Burnet, Fennel, Grapevine.

Wind-Colic: Aniseed.

Worms: Clay, Walnut, Heartsease, Lady's Bedstraw, Common Wormwood, Common Marjoram, Betony, Blessed Thistle, Pea, Goat's Rue, Hedge Hyssop, Common St. Johnswort, Motherwort, Honey, Ground Ivy, Hop, Cowslip, Garlic, Groundsel, Mustard, Mint, Peppermint, Quassia, Tansy, Sage, Thyme, Valerian.

Wounds (fresh): Sanicle, Yarrow, Common St. Johnswort, Orpine, Ivy, Ivy-leaved Toadflax, Daisy, Solomon's Seal, Comfrey, Arnica, Lady's Bedstraw.

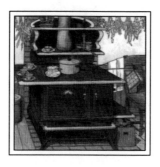

Part II

Medicinal Plants
& Healing Agents

(Includes Herbal Recipes, Prescriptions, and Draughts)

MEDICINAL PLANTS AND HEALING AGENTS

AARON'S ROD

Verbascum thapsus   Fam. Scrophulariaceae
Mullein

Aaron's rod is a biennial, herbaceous plant with a thick, ascendant stem which grows to a height of at least 3 feet (meters). Aaron's rod is found on wasteland, alongside railways, on the verges of woodlands and sometimes on old walls. The leaves which grow from the rootstock form a large rosette; these leaves are very large, larger than those on the stem, oblong, terminally acute, wooly on both sides, rather thick and grayish in color. The yellow flowers are rather large and form a spike on the stem terminal. The flowering period begins in July and lasts the whole summer. These flowers are used medicinally; they are collected throughout the summer. The infusion of the flowers consists of 1¼ to 1¾ cups (10 to 15 grams) per 2 cups (½ liter) boiling water. The leaves contain palliative properties and are used externally for ulcers, piles and eczema. Boil 5 cups (60 grams) of leaves in 1 quart (liter) milk and apply in the form of a poultice; this is most efficacious—both pain and inflammation rapidly subside.

The flowers discharge phlegm and are recommended for bronchitis and catarrh. In North America they are used for consumption; they are also useful for blood-spitting, painful diarrhea, colic, internal piles, and bladder complaints. A good remedy for blood-spitting, chest complaints, coughs, abdominal incisions, dysentry, consumption, bleeding and painful piles is made by boiling 1 to 1½ cups (10 to 15 grams) of leaf and flower

mixture in 2 cups (½ liter) water for twenty minutes and taking
1 cup twice a day. It can also be used internally for jaundice,
difficult urination and to stimulate the appetite. Boil 1½ cups
(15 grams) in 2 cups (½ liter) water; 1 to 2 cups to be taken
daily.

ACONITE (POISON)

Aconitum napellus   Fam. Ranunculaciae
Monks Hood, Blue Rocket

This poisonous, perennial plant has a long, ascendant, hairy
stem with palmate, divided, glossy leaves. The blue flowers are
hood or helmet-shaped. The oblong, fleshy roots are black on
the outside, white inside; it has little smell, bitter sap and blooms
from August to September. It does not grow here in the wild.
The whole plant is poisonous but the root, in particular, is
extremely poisonous. It is used medicinally for various complaints but only according to a physician's prescription. Careless
use can easily cause death.

AGRIMONY

Agrimonia eupatoria   Fam. Rosaceae
Church Steeples, Sticklewort

Agrimony is a perennial, herbaceous plant which may be found
on the edges of woodland and sunken roads. It grows to the
height of at least three feet (one meter). The stem is thin, pliant
and very hairy. The leaves resemble those of the bramble (blackberry); the upper side is light green and the underneath white
and silky, and they have a salty taste. The yellow flowers grow
around the stem and form a spike. The root is reddish-brown
and rather thick, fibrous and decumbent. The plant itself has
a sweet, spicy smell when it is in bloom. The sap is bitter and
astringent. Agrimony flowers from June to the end of July and
must then be gathered for winter storage.

The infusion of the plant contains ⅓ to ½ cup (15 to 20
grams) per 2 cups (½ liter) water. This tea has a pleasant taste
and is used with success for disorders of the liver and spleen,
abdominal blockage, pharyngitis, mild ulceration of the mouth

and throat, swollen tonsils, and is recommended as a tea and a gargle for all throat complaints. If a little honey is added, the efficacy is increased. It is also highly recommended in cases of chronic rheumatism, heavy bleeding, weakness of the digestive organs and blood-spitting. Mix 2 to 4 tablespoons (2 to 4 grams) of the powdered plant in wine and take in the evening to cure bed-wetting, also urinary incontinence in women, cold urine, blockage and weakness of the liver. The infusion is also recommended for consumption, skin complaints, rheumatism, gravel, intestinal weakness, dropsy, renal colic caused by gravel, dysentry, hematuria, prolonged fever, flatulence, leukorrhea, and ulcers in the bladder. Take 2 to 3 cups of tea from the infusion daily. If this herb is boiled with honey and wine and applied as a poultice, it is an excellent remedy for sprains and dislocations; the poultice should be renewed as soon as it becomes dry.

ALDER TREE (COMMON)

Alnus glutinosa   Fam. Betulaceae
English or Common Alder, Owler

This tree is commonly found in moist, marshy places, along river banks and, in general, wherever there is water. There is a saying that alder never grows on good ground. Although the alder prefers to grow in moist places, it also flourishes on dry ground. The wood is a reddish color, the bark dark gray, the branches are round and brittle, the leaves nearly round, serrated, dark green, with a strong resemblance to those of the hazel tree. The flowers are a greenish color and appear before the leaves in February-March. The male catkins are round, long, drooping; the female short, straight and reddish. Alder bark is very rich in tannin, which makes it very astringent and febrifugal.

The dose is ¼ cup (25 grams) powder in a glass of white wine, taken in the mornings on an empty stomach while the patient is in bed, as this remedy causes excessive sweating. Decoction of alder is an excellent remedy for inflammation of the throat and tonsils. One should gargle four to six times a day.

The fruit (alder buds) should be picked in October and bottled in gin; 1 tablespoon taken twice a day is a recommended remedy for epilepsy (falling sickness). The bluish colored buds, picked in the spring, dried and taken in the form of tea, are highly recommended for rheumatism. The fresh leaves, pounded and applied to ulcers, take away the burning and cause them to suppurate and heal.

ALMOND (SWEET)

Amygdalus dulcis   Fam. Rosaceae

These are the fruit of an almond tree widely cultivated in France. The fruit contains oil and mucilage. Its medicinal use especially lies in the preparation of almond milk. For this purpose take ⅓ cup (30 grams) peeled almonds which are pure white, 1½ tablespoons (15 grams) white sugar, ¾ cup (180 grams) hot water. These ingredients should all be pounded in a stone mortar and squeezed through a linen cloth. Almond milk is particularly used for intestinal inflammation, bladder complaints, gravel, dry cough, hoarseness and fever.

Almond oil is obtained by extracting it from sweet almonds. This oil is slightly rancid and must therefore be used as fresh as possible. It has the same properties as olive oil. Take 1 to 4 sugarspoons daily for *internal* use. The oil dissolves hardened earwax as well. Take 5 drops, one at a time, in the ears for ringing and swelling.

ALOES

Aloe vera   Fam. Liliaceae

Aloes, which is used as a purgative in medicine, is a gluey liquid extracted from the leaves of the aloe plant and is used as a tonic, a stomach strengthening purgative. As a tonic and stomach strengthening remedy, only ⅛ to ¼ of a teaspoon (10 to 15 centigrams) should be taken just before meals. As a purgative, the dose varies from ½ teaspoon (40 centigrams) to 1 teaspoon (1 gram). The same dose is also given to bring on late menstruation. Aloe is also most highly recommended for congestion of blood in the head, to make the head a little lighter.

A knife-point of aloe, 2 sugarspoons fenugreek, a sugarspoon of fennel powder in 2 cups of elder tea is a good purgative (Kneipp). Drink one cup daily. For red, running, purulent eyes, take ½ sugarspoon of aloe dissolved in ⅓ cup (100 grams) water and wash the eyes with this four times a day. Old, purulent sores, rotting flesh, or deep scars that exude pus, are cleansed and healed by aloe water. It should be applied in the form of compresses. Fresh wounds can also be successfully treated with this.

If aloe is misused, if too high a dose is taken internally, too much blood is driven to the large intestine, causing piles or bleeding. Those who suffer from bladder complaints, piles or complaints of the womb, should not take aloe.

ALUM

Alumen

Alum, a salt with a very astringent taste, is a well-known styptic and is therefore highly recommended for bleeding, particularly in the womb. Burnt alum should be used in this instance. Ordinary alum is only used *externally* as a gargle, for a mucous throat infection, for rotting ulcers, dirty purulent sores, festered ingrowing nails, fleshy excrescences, etc. In these instances, finely ground alum powder should be sprinkled directly on the sores. In such cases it can also be dissolved in water and the solution used to wash the sores or applied as compresses. Once the sores are clean, the alum swiftly heals them. Alum water is also an excellent remedy for swollen, bleeding gums. It is sufficiently well-known as a gargle or mouth rinse.

Internally alum is for bleeding. Let ⅛ cup (30 grams) burnt alum steep for twenty-four hours in a bottle of Bordeaux wine. With severe bleeding, the patient should take a sugarspoonful of this every ten minutes; after two or three hours, the heavy bleeding decreases and the patient should then take a sugarspoonful every fifteen minutes. The bleeding is generally followed by leukorrhea so the dose should be continued until the third or fourth day and the patient should remain in bed. During this period, the sufferer should only take lukewarm drinks, no hot food, no coffee, beer, or other strong drinks; a little wine is permitted. If the bleeding is very severe, cold compresses should also be placed on the abdomen and renewed every ten minutes.

ANGELICA

Angelica archangelica   Fam. Umbelliferae
European or Garden Angelica

Angelica is a perennial, herbaceous, large, strong, beautiful plant that is cultivated in gardens for its medicinal properties. The stems are gathered in June, the root in September. The stem is thick, herbaceous, round, hollow, reddish-green, white inside; the leaves are large, green on top, whitish beneath. The white umbels are very numerous. They appear from July to August. Angelica has a thick, fleshy root, green on the outside, white on the inside, with many numerous root fibers. This root cannot be recommended highly enough on account of its beneficial properties. If, for example, you have eaten poisonous food, or there is unhealthy matter in the stomach or intestines, and you are plagued by wind, take refuge in this root as it is most efficacious. All you poor people who suffer from nerves, try angelica—you will not regret it. The root can be mixed with the seed.

The remedy is also recommended for all chronic illnesses, intermittent fever, green sickness, absence of menstruation through illness, general weakness, cramplike vomiting, colic, nervous headaches, nervous complaints with lack of strength, chronic inflammation of the wind-pipe, gout, scurvy, lungs and chest affected by phlegm. Kneipp quite rightly called angelica an excellent home remedy which cannot be recommended highly enough. The decoction of the roots, or roots mixed with seed, or stems alone, consists of 2 to 3 tablespoons (10 to 15 grams) per 2 cups (½ liter) water.

A powder can also be prepared from the roots, leaves and stems: 1 sugarspoon of this can be taken three times a day instead of tea. Angelica wine can also be prepared; this has an even stronger effect than tea and powders. Take ½ to ¾ cup (50 to 70 grams) of stems or roots and let them steep in 4 cups (1 liter) of wine for several days. Take 2 wineglasses daily; it is best to take this in small quantities; for example, 1 tablespoon every hour. Kneipp usually gave 1 tablespoon every two hours. Take 1½ to 3 teaspoons (4 to 6 grams) of the powder described above daily, in some kind of liquid (honey or syrup). This is very effective for convalescents, and for a coated tongue, stomach complaints, scrofula, and pituitous fever.

ANGELICA (WILD)

Angelica sylvestris   Fam. Umbelliferae
Jack-jump-about

This is a strong biennial plant with a thick, hollow, grooved stem, covered with large leaves from top to bottom. It has a thick, swollen sheath. The lower leaves are very large and triangular; the upper leaves double pinnate. The white or reddish umbels are a blaze of glory from July to September. The fleshy root is gray on the outside, white on the inside, and has a strong, aromatic smell and taste. The plant grows in swampy places on the verges of water and woodland. The root is medicinally used for falling sickness, hysteria, nervous complaints, especially chronic nervous conditions, general weakness, vomiting, colic, etc. It is used in the same instances as angelica (*Angelica archangelica*) but must be made stronger. The root decoction contains 3½ to 4 tablespoons (20 to 25 grams) per 2 cups (½ liter) water. The seed, steeped in gin, is a recommended remedy for renal colic and indigestion.

ANISE

Pimpinella anisum   Fam. Umbelliferae
Aniseed

This annual herbaceous plant is indigenous to Africa, but also grows in France. It has an ascendant, round, branched, ribbed stem, and grows 18 inches high. The flowers are white, small (double umbels) with ten to twelve radiating flowers. The fruit is oval and hard. It blooms in June and July. The seed, which must be fully ripe, is gathered in August. It is tied in bundles, threshed like rye or wheat, cleaned and stored in a dry place.

Aniseed can be successfully used for indigestion, cramplike wind colic, colic in children, headaches caused by indigestion and dizziness from the same cause. It is recommended for nursing mothers as it improves and increases the milk. If an infant is suffering from colic, the nursing mother should simply take some aniseed and the child will recover. Children who are bottle-fed can be given aniseed syrup, or aniseed can be boiled in the milk or some other drink; this prevents abdominal gripe and facilitates bowel movements. Half an ounce of aniseed is sufficient to purge a newborn infant.

Aniseed is used in many preparations and medicines, sometimes to take away the bad taste, other times to prevent the colic caused by some purgatives. Aniseed infusion contains 2½ to 3½ teaspoons (4 to 7 grams) per 2 cups (½ liter) boiling water. If you use the powder use 1 teaspoon to 1 tablespoon (1 to 7 grams) mixed with sugar, water, wine, or milk. For aniseed syrup use 1½ to 3 tablespoons (30 to 60 grams). To use aniseed oil put 2 to 6 drops on sugar or in mixtures. Or put 6 to 8 drops of aniseed oil on sugar (or even better in old wine or liqueur) and take in the mornings on an empty stomach. It is very invigorating and a phlegm dissolvent for asthmatics; also recommended for dysentery.

ARNICA (POISON)

Arnica montana   Fam. Compositae

Arnica is an herbaceous, perennial plant; it can be found on fenlike heath and in wet meadows. It has a short, horizontal rootstock, a root rosette of oval, oblong or lanceolate leaves; these are very similar to the Plantago lanceolata. The flower stem shoots up from the center of the root rosette, bears two opposite leaves and ends in a flowerhead; the flowers are orange-yellow. Arnica is covered with soft hairs and has a pleasant, aromatic smell; the sap is bitter. The medicinal strength lies in the flowers; there is little in the leaves and roots. Arnica herb is little used nowadays; the tincture, on the contrary, which is very well known, cannot be recommended highly enough for fresh wounds. Tincture of arnica can be obtained from any dispensary; it can also be prepared at home by letting one part arnica flowers steep in 5 parts of 75% alcohol. Arnica tincture is used externally, diluted by half with water and applied on fresh wounds in the form of compresses. These compresses are also highly recommended for injuries, bruises caused by a knock or fall, blood-blisters, etc.

ASARABACCA (POISON)

Asarum Europaeum   Fam. Aristolochiaceae

Asarabacca is an herbaceous, perennial plant with a creeping rootstock, short, decumbent stem, which has two long-petiolate, kidney-shaped, smooth-edged, evergreen leaves, between which a single, short-petiolate dark red flower can be found. It has a strong, penetrating, aromatic smell; the sap is nauseating and bitter. Take 2 to 3 teaspoons (3 to 4 grams) of the root to cause vomiting and purging. On account of its poisonous properties, I find it advisable not to mention the beneficial properties of the plant.

ASH (FROM WOOD)

Cinis

The remains of burned plants, principally wood, are called ash. It purifies and dessicates. Ash from oak is an excellent styptic; when mixed with vinegar it is even more efficacious. Footbaths of wood ash and salt are highly recommended if the sweating of the feet has been suppressed or expelled; in addition footbaths can be used for congestion of blood in the head and to draw the blood away from the chest. Ash is also recommended for inflammation of the eyes, headache and toothache. Put 2 handsful wood ash and 1 handful salt in a bucket of warm water and keep the feet in it for ten to twelve minutes. Note: Footbaths should never be taken hot; lukewarm is the best and the best time is before retiring.

ASH TREE

Fraxinus excelsior   Fam. Oleaceae

This beautiful tree, with its grayish colored bark and long, pliant branches, is very well known and found everywhere in woodland and along roadside verges. The flowers appear before the leaves on the branch terminals in clustered red bundles. The leaves are opposite and decussate, developing from black buds. The fruit consists of flat nuts, winged at the top. Ash leaves are used medicinally. The infusion consists of 1½ to 2½ cups (15 to 25 grams) per 2 cups (½ liter) boiling water. Take 2 cups daily for gout and rheumatism. It also acts as a purgative. The decoction of the bark and the young wood, 2 to 3 tablespoons (10 to 15 grams) per 2 cups (½ liter) wine, is beneficial for blockage of the liver and spleen.

ASPARAGUS

Asparagus officinalis   Fam. Liliaceae

This is a well-known perennial which is cultivated in gardens. It has a decumbent rootstock from which grow a number of many-branched stems that are round and a fine shade of green. The numerous leaves are thread-like; the flowers are small, greenish, clustered in pairs. The fruits are round berries which are first green and later red. The roots are long and composed of many small ones, while the young shoots are a highly sought after food. This plant is recommended for dropsy, poor urination, bladder and kidney stones, gout and piles, gravel, jaundice, stones, liver and lung complaints. Podagrists (those who suffer from foot gout) are not advised to take it as its use could cause a fresh attack.

A knife-point of the dried, powdered herb taken with a little sugar three or four times a day is very good for vomiting, colic, stomach weakness, hardening of the kidneys, spleen and liver diseases. A tincture can be prepared from freshly grown asparagus by pressing it and adding an equal quantity of alcohol to the sap. This should be left to steep for two weeks; the clear liquid should then be poured off and kept for use. Take 2 drops twice a day. For dropsy, bruise and squeeze fresh asparagus, add a little sugar and take 1 tablespoon three times a day.

Autumn Crocus (poison)

Colchicum autumnale   Fam. Liliaceae
Meadow Saffron

In early autumn, these flowers can be found in abundance in moist meadowland. The short, petiolate, bell-shaped flower is a beautiful pink, with a rather violet tinge. The leaves are broad, oblong, lanceolate, acute and stiff. It only flowers for a few days. The green, smooth, glossy leaves appear in the spring; the seed is enclosed in a small, oblong-round fruit full of grains. These are all gathered at the end of June or beginning of July when the fruit splits open. Autumn crocus is used medicinally in the form of wine for gout and rheumatism. Due to its poisonous nature, it should only be used on a physician's prescription.

Baneberry (poison)

Actaea spicata   Fam. Ranunculacae
Herb Christopher

Baneberry is a perennial, poisonous plant with an ascendant stem, little branched, which reaches a height of two to three feet (6 to 9 decimeters). The three-lobed leaves are smooth, long-petiolate, ovate or obovate, regularly serrated and terminally acute. The small, white flowers are clustered in more or less hanging racemes, giving way to shiny black berries. The fleshy, fibrous root is black on the outside and yellow on the inside. It has a disgusting smell and bitter-sour sap. The berries are extremely poisonous. The flowering period is from May to June. The root was once used as a purgative and for asthma, but the plant is no longer used medicinally on account of its poisonous properties.

BATS-IN-THE-BELFRY

Campanula trachelium   Fam. Campanulaceae
Nettle-leaved Bellflower, Throatwort

Bats-in-the-Belfry is a perennial plant. The stems are erect, hairy, single or lightly branched; the leaves are coarse, hairy, irregularly dentate; the central leaves, with a heart-shaped base, are oblong and petiolate; the upper leaves are oval, pointed, lanceolate and short-petiolate or sessile. The blue flowers, growing singly or in pairs, have a rough calyx which is always erect. The flowering period is June. The thick roots are woody and without shoots. The plant grows in woodland and grassy places. The roots are used in the form of decoction as a gargle for external use for inflammation of the throat.

BEARBERRY

Arctostaphylos uva ursi   Fam. Ericaceae
Mountain Box

Bearberry is a shrub commonly found in Northern Europe on high, sandy soil and in woodlands. The leaves are thick, leathery, smooth, oblong-acute, lightly dentate, glossy green and have much in common with those of the bilberry. They have a smell similar to licorice, but this is mostly lost in drying. Bearberry has a bitter, astringent taste. The pink flowers grow in racemes on the stem terminals. The berries are red, sour and astringent; they are apparently much sought after by the bear, hence the name. The leaves are highly recommended for failure of the urinary organs caused by weakness, stones, ulceration, etc. They do not, however, have stone-breaking properties, but they are tonic and astringent. They are used for kidney complaints, hematuria, night-time pollution, urinary incontinence and bladder catarrh. The decoction contains 3 to 6 tablespoons (8 to 15 grams) per 2 cups (½ liter) water. Take 1 cup daily.

BETONY (WOOD)

Betonica officinalis   Fam. Labiatae

This plant is widely spread; it is found in shady woodlands and thickets, on dry and infertile ground. It is shrub-like, perennial and attains a height of a foot and a half (30 to 40 centimeters). The stem is erect, quadrangular, hairy, has no side-branches, bears a strong resemblance to the large nettle. The leaves are long, narrow, hairy and serrated; the flowers are red, small and form a spike on the stem terminals. The flowering period is July and August. It has a strong smell and its sap is sour and bitter. The dried, powdered leaves are an excellent snuff. A tea can be prepared from the leaves for epilepsy and acidity. This tea, mixed with honey and wine, is highly recommended for chest complaints accompanied by blood spitting.

Boiled leaves or, still better, boiling water poured on the leaves and left to steep a while, applied to sprained limbs serve a useful purpose. Betony roots are emetic and purgative. The whole plant can be used medicinally. The infusion of leaves and flowers is also recommended for worms, poor appetite and fever. The infusion of leaves and flowers consists of ¼ cup (10 grams) per 2 cups (½ liter) boiling water.

Betony is recommended for fits of dizziness, brain disorders, blockage of the liver and spleen, trembling, paralysis, gout, severe headaches, jaundice, gravel. The fresh leaves pounded with a little salt are good for cancerous sores. The freshly crushed plant is very good for sores on the head. Sugar should always be added to the decoction for internal use; 1 tablespoon should be taken every two hours.

BILBERRY

Vaccinium myrtillus   Fam. Vacciniaceae
Whortleberry, Huckleberry, Blueberry

This small shrub grows in abundance on dry, sandy soil. Some-times whole woods are covered with it. There is hardly a child who does not know the bilberry. It has quadrangular, pale green stems, is very branched and reaches a height of 2½ feet (60 to 70 centimeters). The oval-round, finely serrated leaves are very numerous and a beautiful color of green. The April flowers are pink, single and drooping, and greatly resemble the blackcur-rant. The fruit is a small berry, first green, then red, and when ripe, blue. Fruit and leaves are used medicinally; a tincture is prepared from the fruit by leaving a ⅓ part dried fruit to steep for some time in ⅔ part good gin. The leaves, which are picked in May and June and dried, are highly recommended for di-abetes. (Note: European bilberry not American blueberry.)

The infusion of the leaves should contain 1 cup (15 grams) per 2 cups (½ liter) boiling water. Bilberry tincture is an ex-cellent remedy for dysentry and diarrhea. Use 1 cup of leaf decoction daily. The dose of the tincture is, according to cir-cumstances, 2 or 3 sugarspoons per day in hot water or Bor-deaux wine. Children should be given 10 to 12 drops in hot water, hot wine, or on sugar. The fruit decoction is very good for hair which is falling out; the scalp should be rubbed with it every evening.

BINDWEED

Convolvulus arvensis   Fam. Convolvulaciae
Field Bindweed

Bindweed[1] is an herbaceous, perennial plant. It is a weed that causes much damage. It has a twining stem, with many side branches, and creeps along the ground and twines itself around

---

[1] We were unable to locate this herb in our source material, but it does grow locally in Maine and probably in many other places! It's a backyard weed.

surrounding plants. It is commonly found on sandy soil but also in the grass on clay soil. The leaves are sagittate. The flowers, which grow in the leaf axils, are much smaller than the white convolvulus which has larger, white flowers. Those of lesser bindweed are pale pink, occasionally white, and have five purple stripes on the outside. They bloom throughout the summer. The long, thin, creeping root has a pleasant, aromatic smell like bitter almonds. The leaves of the lesser bindweed should be gathered in August for use in the treatment of asthma and indigestion. The infusion contains 1 to 2 teaspoons (2 to 4 grams) per 2 cups (½ liter) boiling water; the dose should not be increased. Instead of this infusion, 2 teaspoons (3 grams) powder from the dried leaves can also be taken. Only ½ teaspoon (1 gram) of the powdered root should be taken. All parts of the lesser bindweed are laxative.

BIRTHWORT (POISON)

Aristolochia longa   Fam. Aristolochiaceae
Long Aristolochy

This plant, with its thin, long, brittle, hairless, curved twigs, attains a height of 3 feet (80 centimeters). The heart-shaped leaves are long-petiolate and grow alternately along the stems. The light-green flowers grow in the axils of the upper leaves in cymes of two to three each. The flowering period is May to June. The plant is perennial and grows on wasteland, under hedges and on stony ground. On account of its poisonous properties, it is inadvisable to use this herb except with the greatest of care, so definitely never more than the stated dose. The root, which is coarse on the outside and yellowish in the inside, 10 inches (25 centimeters) long and a finger thick, is used medicinally for gout and rheumatism. The decoction of the dried roots consists of 2 tablespoons (8 grams) per 2 cups (½ liter) water. Take 6 tablespoons every morning and evening. Never more than this quantity.

BISTORT

Polygonum bistorta   Fam. Polygonaceae
Snakeroot, Snakeweed.

This plant is called the snakeroot because the root is twice twisted, more or less resembling a snake. It is found in damp places, meadows and fields. It is perennial, herbaceous, and attains a height of 2 feet (70 centimeters). The radical leaves are rather large, oblong-ovate. The pink flowers grow in a dense spike on the stem terminals. The root is gathered in the autumn. The root is used medicinally: 2 to 4 tablespoons (10 to 20 grams) per 2 cups (½ liter) boiling water.

Internally: the root decoction can be successfully used for dysentry, bleeding, and internal sores.

Externally: To staunch bleeding boil ¼ to ⅓ cup (20 to 30 grams) in beer. This is one of the best astringent remedies for diarrhea, excessive mucus, leukorrhea, urinary incontinence, and intermittent fever. The powder can be used for smallpox, measles and fever: 1½ to 2 teaspoon (3 to 4 grams) per day. The root decoction, 3 to 4 tablespoons (15 to 20 grams) in wine, can be used as a gargle for throat infections, thrush, ulcerated gums, toothaches and all kinds of mouth ulcers. In addition, 2 tablespoons of the decoction should be taken three times a day.

BITING STONECROP

Sedum acre   Fam. Crassulaceae

Biting stonecrop, or common stonecrop, is found on grassy, sandy soil, old walls and roofs; it is a perennial, herbaceous, beautiful plant, with yellow flowers, almost sessile, which bloom in June and July; it attains a height of 4 to 5 inches (12 to 13 centimeters). This plant is only used externally and fresh for medicinal purposes. For example, for old sores or cancerous sores it is especially successful. The plant should be finely powdered for use and applied directly on the sores. For scurvy, boil ¼ to ⅓ cup (10 to 12 grams) of the fresh plant in 2 cups (½ liter) beer: take 1 spoonful every two hours. The decoction of biting stonecrop is also very good as a gargle for scurvy and rotting gums. Take ½ to 1 teaspoon (20 to 30 centigrams) daily for epilepsy.

BLACK NIGHTSHADE (POISON)

Solanum nigrum   Fam. Solanaceae

Black nightshade is an annual, poisonous plant which grows about a foot high. It is much branched; the leaves are ovate, long-petiolate, hairless and have an unpleasant, intoxicating smell. The flowers form short-petiolate cymes and give way to round, green berries which turn completely black when ripe. It can be found in uncultivated fields, rubbish tips and in gardens. For medicinal purposes it is only used externally on painful ulcers. Freshly pounded leaves should be applied.

BLACKBERRY

Rubus fructucosus   Fam. Rosaceae
Brambleberry

This shrub is commonly found almost everywhere in old hedges and on the edges of woodland. It has long, pliant stems which are densely covered in curved thorns. The leaves are ovate round, finely dentate and dark green in color; the flowers are pink or white, giving way to berries which are black throughout when fully ripe. Preserves are made from these berries.

The leaves have a very astringent effect. They should be picked before the shrub blooms. The infusion contains ½ cup (15 grams) per 2 cups (½ liter) boiling water. Take 1 cup per day. The infusion of the leaves and young stems is very good for diarrhea, dysentry, leukorrhea, sore throat, swollen gums, inflammation of the tonsils, and thrush. For external use as a mouth wash and gargle: use ¾ cup (25 grams) per 2 cups (½ liter) boiling water. Fresh, bruised leaves are very beneficial on old sores and eczema; the bruised herb should be placed on the affected area.

BLACK CURRANT

Ribes nigrum   Fam. Saxifragaceae

The black currant is frequently grown in gardens. It can be recognized by the leaves and the hanging bunches of black currants. The former have numerous small glands on the underside which, when touched, exude an aromatic perfume. Both leaves and fruit are used medicinally. The infusion of the former consists of 4 teaspoons (15 grams) to 2 cups (½ liter) boiling water; the fruit should be bottled in gin. Both remedies are diuretic and recommended for painful urination. Take 1 to 2 tablespoons of the fruit tincture daily. Black currant remedies are a stomachic, diaphoretic, and good for throat infections, migraine, indigestion, dropsy and rheumatism.

BLADDER CHERRY

Physalis alkekengi   Fam. Solonaceae
Red Winter Cherry, Morelberry

This herbaceous, perennial plant is found in the south of France on dry, sandy, stony ground. The stem is erect, single, soft-haired; the green stem later turns red. The leaves are heart-shaped and dull. The flowers grow singly, are white or pale-yellow, and grow along the stem. The berries are round, red, and the size of an ordinary cherry; they also strongly resemble cherries; they have a sweet-sour taste. All parts of the plant are used medicinally. The entire plant is gathered in September when the cherries have ripened. The infusion of the leaves and stems contains ½ to 1 cup (15 to 30 grams) per 2 cups (½ liter) boiling water. The decoction of the cherries also contains ½ to 1 cup (15 to 30 grams) per 2 cups (½ liter) water. One can also eat 2 to 4 teaspoons (10 to 20 grams) of fresh cherries. Bladder cherry is a good diuretic, and can be usefully taken for gravel, dropsy, jaundice, liver complaints and stoppage of the urine.

BLESSED THISTLE

Cnicus benedictus   Fam. Compositae
Holy Thistle

This is an annual plant from southern Europe, grown in many gardens, and attains a height of 1½ to 2 feet (30 to 60 centimeters) and has branched stems with deeply grooved leaves. The herb must be gathered before it blooms in the month of June. The scent is pleasant but the taste bitter. The decoction of the herb contains 5 tablespoons (10 grams) per 2 cups (½ liter) water and is recommended for intermittent fever, stomach complaints caused by weakness and accompanied by formation of wind, etc. In addition, it can be used for dropsy, jaundice, hypochondria and irregular menstruation.

In years gone by, so many important properties were attributed to this herb that it was given the honorable name of blessed thistle. Mathiolus writes that there is probably no remedy more efficacious than this splendid plant. The sores should be washed four times a day with an infusion of the plant and after each wash the sore should be sprinkled with powder from the dried leaves. This can also be used for old, deep-rooted sores.

The infusion of the plant in wine—5 tablespoons (10 grams) per 2 cups (½ liter) wine—is beneficial for lymphatic persons, for scrofula, scrofulous tumors and ulceration. 1 wine glass should be taken in the mornings on an empty stomach. For phlegm in the chest, 2½ teaspoons (3 grams) powder should be taken in wine every day.

When mixed with an equal quantity of common centaury, the infusion is even stronger and is recommended for epilepsy, intermittent fever, stomach complaints, abdominal cramp, migraine, cancer, etc. Drink 1 cup of tea daily. No sugar should be added to this tea.

Blessed thistle is a stomachic, particularly excellent for weak stomachs, mucous stomachs, intestines, and lung and liver complaints. Its tea cures diarrhea caused by weakness, also chronic diarrhea. Worms are killed by it for good and prevented from multiplying as it stops the formation of mucus in the intestines.

The following tincture can also be used for the complaints mentioned above: 1 part blessed thistle steeped for several days in 4 parts good gin; 8 drops to be taken two or three times daily in water or on sugar. It is best to keep to the infusion for the treatment of worms.

BORAGE

Borago officinalis   Fam. Borraginaceae
Burrage

Borage is an annual plant with an herbaceous stem and grows a foot and a half high (30 to 40 centimeters). It has a round, pale green, branched and hairy stem. The leaves are also hairy, thick and oblong, the lower ones are largest. The flowers are heavenly blue, very numerous and strongly resemble those of the potato, although they are rather larger and hang in racemes on the stem terminals. The root grows straight down into the ground, is rather thick and whitish in color. Both leaves and flowers are used medicinally. The flowers are picked as soon as they open, every day throughout the summer. The flowering period is May to October. The leaves are gathered from mid-July to August. The tea or infusion of the flowers is very refreshing and palliative. Use 3 to 4 tablespoons (5 to 8 grams) flowers per 2 cups (½ liter) boiling water. Use ½ to ⅔ cup (20 to 25 grams) of the leaves per 2 cups (½ liter) boiling water. It is most efficacious for painful rheumatism and measles. Take 1 cup daily.

BOX TREE

Buxus sempervirens   Fam. Buxaceae

Box is frequently used for edging flowerbeds. This is an evergreen shrub, blessed on Palm Sunday and placed in houses, stalls and on farmland with the aim of warding off illness, etc. The leaves of the plant are used medicinally as a purgative. The decoction contains ⅛ to ¼ cup (8 to 12 grams) per 2 cups

(½ liter) boiling water. Or, steep 3 parts box leaves for several days in 12 parts gin for a very good remedy for pneumonia; 1 tablespoon should be given two or three times a day with a little water.

For chronic rheumatism, boil ½ cup (10 grams) of wood or root for fifteen minutes in 2 cups (½ liter) water and take 1 tablespoon three to five times a day. A larger dose makes a good purgative. In addition, the powdered leaves, 1 to 2 tablespoons (3 to 4 grams) per day taken in some kind of fluid, are recommended for chronic rheumatism. For epilepsy and toothache, 10 or 12 drops of box oil should be taken with sugar; this oil is extracted from the wood. When mixed with melted butter, the oil can be used as a rub for rheumatism, scabies, acne, eczema, psoriasis, mealy eczema, and gout, with good results.

BRAN

Furfur

Bran is the husk of grain. Wheat bran, boiled in water and used in the form of compresses, is excellent for the treatment of hardening, eczema and old sores. Internally, the decoction of wheat bran, with the addition of a little honey, is a pleasant tonic drink for children and convalescents. Hot bran bags have been of good service many a time for cramps, colic, etc.

BROWN-RAYED KNAPWEED

Centaurea jacea   Fam. Compositae
Meadow Knapweed

The brown-rayed knapweed should not be confused with the *Centaurea nigra*, commonly found on roads and dykes and rugged places. The brown-rayed knapweed grows in the same places but is not so abundant. It is a perennial plant with purple flowers; the marginal florets are larger than the inner ones and the fruits have no whorl of rays on the outer florets; it has ascendant, grooved, branch-like, hairy stems. The lower leaves are undivided, sinuous, oblong; the upper leaves are oblong-round and the flowering period is July to September. This plant has astringent properties; the flowers are used medicinally for pneumonia.

Bryony (white, poison)

Byronia dioica   Fam. Cucurbitaceae
English Mandrake

A long, thick root, white in color, can be found under old hedges and bushes on rich soil. From this root sprouts an angular, branched stem, with palmate, five-lobed leaves, which are very hairy, as is the whole plant. Thread-like tendrils grow next to the leaves. This is bryony or English mandrake, an exceedingly poisonous plant. The flowers are greenish-white and produce red berries the size of a pea. This plant smells rather intoxicating and unpleasant. Although the root is used in the treatment of many illnesses, in the interests of safety I shall not give any instructions for internal use. The grated root applied externally in the form of a poultice relieves the most severe pain caused by gout (podagra) within a short time; if this treatment is continued for some time, the malady is cured forever.

Buckbean

Menyanthes trifoliata   Fam. Gentianaceae
Bog-bean, Marsh Trefoil

Buckbean is a perennial plant and grows on marshy ground, especially on peat-moors. It is usually very common. It has a creeping rootstock, three-lobed, obovate, smooth-edged leaves and pale pink flowers gathered in racemes which grow on thick stems. It is in bloom in May. The flowers are used medicinally. They are gathered in May and June.

The decoction contains ⅓ to ½ cup (10 to 15 grams) per 2 cups (½ liter) boiling water and can be successfully used for gout, eczema (but never if the eczema is inflamed), jaundice, weak stomach, poor appetite, and fever. If the dose is too high, it causes vomiting and acts as a purgative. A daily cup of buck-bean tea is certainly worthy of recommendation. It is also excellent during the menopause when a cup of tea should be taken every morning and evening. It causes the headaches to subside and after a few days the patient feels much better. The same tea is also recommended for chronic gastric complaints.

Boil a small handful in 1 cup (¼ liter) milk or wine until reduced to a third; this is an efficacious remedy for heavy bleeding and a dry cough. Take 2 to 3 tablespoons in the morning.

BUCKTHORN (ALDER)

Rhamnus frangula   Fam. Rhamnaceae

Buckthorn is a shrub that is found abundantly in woodlands. The wood is black, rather flecked and produces red berries which later turn black. The inner rind of the buckthorn is used medicinally. When fresh, it is a strong emetic and purgative and can be considered poisonous. When it is dry, there is nothing to fear as it loses much of its potency in the drying process. The infusion contains 2 to 3 tablespoons (10 to 15 grams) per 2 cups (½ liter) boiling water and is a good purgative. Take 3 to 3½ teaspoons (2 to 3 grams) of the powder in syrup or honey. When making a decoction, add 2 teaspoons of aniseed, but this should not be boiled with the decoction, merely steeped in it for twenty minutes. Instead of aniseed, 1 teaspoon common wormwood can be added. The rind, freshly crushed with vinegar, can be applied to eczema with good result, even if it is deep-rooted.

An excellent laxative, which is never injurious, can be made by drawing 2 teaspoons of dried rind for twenty minutes in boiling water with a sugarspoon of aniseed or common wormwood. It should be taken in the evenings. Another good laxative can be prepared by toasting 1 sugarspoon of dried, ripe fruit or berries, grinding them fine and letting them steep in 2 cups (½ liter) boiling water for twenty minutes. Take 1 tablespoon every two hours.

BUGLOSS (BORUGE)

Lycopsis arvensis   Fam. Boraginaceae
Small Bugloss

This annual, coarse-haired plant with either broad or narrow lanceolate leaves and pale blue flowers from June to September is found on sandy wastelands and on roadside verges. It has much in common with common alkanet; the difference between the two lies in the corolla which in bugloss is curved and in common alkanet is straight. A decoction of the leaves is a recommended remedy for sharpness in the blood; it strengthens the heart, is palliative and diuretic. Take 4 to 5 tablespoons (10 to 15 grams) per 2 cups (½ liter) water.

BURDOCK

Articum lappa   Fam. Compositae

Four varieties may be found growing wild: *A. Lappa Major* (greater burdock), *A. Lappa Minus* (lesser burdock), *A. Lappa Intermedia* (wood burdock or common burdock), and *A. Lappa Tomentosa* (wooly burdock). Burdock is commonly found as a weed along roadsides, uncultivated fields and meadows. It is a biennial plant with coarse, thick stems, quadrangular, red in color, very branched and three feet (one meter) or more high. The leaves grow very large, have a long tail, are dark green on top and white and knotty underneath. The rather dense flowers are a violet-red color and hook on to clothing. The root is thick and grows vertically down into the ground, is black on the outside and white inside. It has no smell, the sap is rather sweet, bitter and astringent. This root is used medicinally; it is gathered in October, but first year burdock should be gathered in the spring when the leaves are beginning to bud. Burdock root must be gathered fresh every year since it only retains its potency for one year.

For internal use, the decoction of the root contains 2 to 4 tablespoons (15 to 30 grams) per 2 cups (½ liter) water and is used as a diaphoretic, a depurative and a diuretic; in addition, for rheumatism and gout, skin complaints such as eczema, scrofulous complaints. Burdock leaf tea is an excellent remedy for gastric ulcers. The infusion is 1 to 3 tablespoons (10 to 20 grams) per 2 cups (½ liter) water; 2 cups should be taken daily. The decoction of the root with half water and half vinegar is an excellent hair tonic and is highly recommended to prevent hair from falling out. The scalp should be rubbed with it twice a day.

BUR-MARIGOLD

Bidens tripartita   Fam. Compositae

Bur-marigold (water agrimony) is an annual water plant with red, ascendant, hairy stems, usually with three- sometimes five-lobed, coarsely serrated leaves. The yellow flowerheads appear on the stem terminals with several sharp points, usually in the form of a trident. The root is fibrous. The flowering period is July to September. This plant may be found in wet, marshy places. The decoction of the plant is used externally in the form of compresses on foul, gangrenous ulcerations.

BURNET SAXIFRAGE

Pimpinella saxifraga   Fam. Umbelliferae

Burnet saxifrage is a perennial, herbaceous plant with a fleshy root; it is found abundantly along roadsides, on high-lying meadows and woodland. The stems are round, striped and usually bare at the top; the stem leaves are coarse and blunt, the leaves pinnate, oval-round and irregularly serrated; the flowers white. The flowering period is July through September, when the whole plant is gathered. The plant has an unpleasant smell, resembling that of a goat. It is gathered during the flowering period and used medicinally for kidney and lung complaints, difficult urination, cold urine, coughs, stomach disorders, asthma, liver disease, dysentery and pneumonia. The decoction is ¼ to ⅓ cup (10 to 12 grams) per 2 cups (½ liter) boiling water. The plant root, fried in butter, is a good remedy for ulcers.

BUTTERBUR

Petasites vulgaris   Fam. Compositae

This plant can be abundantly found in moist clay soil, alongside dykes, on farmland, etc. It has a knotty rootstock and a rosette of large heart-shaped leaves, gray-green underneath. The flower stem appears before the leaves in April; it has numerous dirty-red flowerheads that form a long, pyramid-shaped raceme. The fresh leaves applied to scrofulous tumors and sores are of great benefit; the sores are cleansed and the lumps subside. They are also recommended for colds on the chest; a fresh leaf should be placed on the bare chest.

CABBAGE

Brassica oleracea   Fam. Cruciferae

Cabbage is so well-known that it is unnecessary to describe it. Preserved cabbage is called sauerkraut. This is a very good food and also an efficacious medicine; it cleanses the stomach and intestines and increases the gastric juices. If sauerkraut is applied for a headache, the pain soon subsides; it is also recommended for burns, injuries and old sores. Compresses of sauerkraut water can also be used in the same cases. For internal burning, 2 tablespoons sauerkraut water should be taken every morning and evening. Fresh cabbage leaves, applied for the treatment of severe burning in the head, headaches, earaches, cramps and palpitations, are an excellent remedy.

CALAMINT (COMMON)

Calamintha officinalis   Fam. Labiatae

Calamint is an annual plant that almost entirely resembles thyme. It reaches a height of one and a half to two feet (4 to 6 decimeters), has relatively large leaves and a pleasant fragrance. The pink flowers grow in branched cymes in the leaf axils. The flowering period is June to September. The plant is used medicinally. Use 1⅔ cups (10 grams) per 2 cups (½ liter) boiling water for chronic lung catarrh and lymphatic complaints. It is also highly recommended for disorders of the womb, consumption, asthma and indigestion. It is also a diuretic, and for this purpose, 1 cup of tea should be taken daily.

CALAMUS

Acorus calamus   Fam. Araceae
Sweet Flag, Sedge

Calamus is an herbaceous, perennial plant, abundantly found in marshy areas, near ponds, etc. The creeping rootstock is the thickness of a thumb and more than 20 inches (½ meter) long. The leaves are grass-green, lanceolate and long. The flowers are dark yellow. They bloom in June and July. The root is used medicinally. It is jointed, dark brown, and covered with a large number of scars underneath. It has a pleasant, spicy smell, and a bitter, sharp taste. It is used for nervous and pituitous fevers, especially if accompanied by exhausting dysentry; for intermittent fever, weakness of the stomach and intestines, mucic acid, wind, hypochondriacal and hysterical complaints, phlegm in the chest, leukorrhea, scurvy; its use for the latter is highly recommended. In addition, for abdominal pain, mucous stomach, swollen spleen and to promote menstruation. It is used externally on old, soft ulcers. For internal use, take 4 teaspoons (6 grams) per 2 cups (½ liter) boiling water.

Tincture of calamus is prepared by dissolving 3 tablespoons (30 grams) calamus oil in 2 quarts (liters) alcohol. The dose is 10-20-30 drops. For internal use, 1 cup of tea should be taken daily, or 1 tablespoon calamus tincture, or 3 teaspoons (3 grams) calamus powder mixed with honey or some other kind of fluid. For ulceration of the breast, take a sugarspoon of calamus powder mixed with honey every day.

Canadian Fleabane

Erigeron canadense   Fam. Compositae

This annual plant is found on wasteland and rubbish tips. Its
stem is erect, the upper part branched, attaining a height from
one to three feet (4 to 10 decimeters). The narrow, lanceolate
leaves are coarse, with stiff bristles. The numerous small flower
heads are clustered in an elongated raceme and are a white,
yellowish color. The flowering period is July to October. The
scent is pleasant, the sap astringent and bitter. The infusion
consists of ½ to ⅔ cups (20 to 30 grams) per 2 cups (½ liter)
boiling water, and is used for diarrhea and dropsy. Drink 2
cups per day.

Caraway

Carum carvi   Fam. Umbelliferae

This is a biennial plant and is commonly found in fertile meadows. It has a striped, branched stem with double pinnate leaves.
The fruit is oblong. The aromatic taste of caraway seed is the
reason it is used in cakes in Germany and in cheese in Holland
(the well-known caraway cheese). The ethereal oil contained in
the seed has a beneficial effect on the digestive system and
expels wind. Caraway seed warms and strengthens a cold stomach and weak intestines, alleviates abdominal pain, takes away
dizziness, stimulates the appetite, purifies the breath and is very
good for stomach complaints. The decoction contains 2 tablespoons (10 grams) per 4 cups (1 liter) water. Take 1 teaspoon
(1 gram) of powder daily.

Carline Thistle

Carlina vulgaris   Fam. Compositae

The carline thistle is a biennial plant which is found on dry,
rocky wasteland. Large, long, broad, lanceolate, leathery,
deeply cut leaves, covered with strong prickles grow from the

root. The stem is only about a finger's length. The flowers are white or purplish, and form a kind of umbel. The root grows vertically into the ground, is sometimes two feet long, as thick as a thumb, dark on the outside and white on the inside. It has a strong, aromatic scent; it tastes rather pleasant and spicy.

This root is used medicinally as a stomachic; it also dissolves mucus, especially in cases of catarrh, pain in the side and nervous complaints, cleanses the intestines and kidneys, stimulates the appetite and is an efficacious remedy for hysteria, blockage of the liver and spleen, stones and above all promotes menstruation. The decoction is ⅓ to ⅔ cups (30 to 60 grams) per 2 cups (½ liter) water. A stronger decoction, for example 1⅛ cup (100 grams) per 2 cups (½ liter) water, is highly recommended for external use as compresses for sores, ulcers and gangrene. The sores should be washed with it three or four times daily, and compresses of the same decoction should also be applied throughout the day. For internal use for the complaints mentioned above, take 1 to 2 cups with a spoon, or 2½ teaspoons (3 grams) of the powdered root in wine or some other liquid.

CARROT

Daucus carota   Fam. Umbelliferae

This is one of the most well-known plants in the vegetable garden. The seed and roots are used medicinally. The roots are palliative and used for throat complaints, consumption, tubercular throats and old sores. The decoction should be used for tuberculosis of the lungs and throat. A dish of peeled carrots should be boiled in water until they are quite soft; they should then be thoroughly squeezed out in the water in which they were boiled. Add 1½ cups (300 grams) brown sugar-candy per 4 cups (1 liter) of liquid and give the patient 1 tablespoon every hour. For tuberculosis of the throat, it is also advisable to gargle with it several times a day.

Carrots cooked in milk are an excellent remedy for old sores; they should be applied very thickly and lukewarm in the form of a poultice three times a day. The decoction—with or without sugar—is also a good depurative and highly recommended for jaundice and bilious fever; it should be taken over a long period. For hydrothorax with swollen feet, 2 to 2½ teaspoons (4 to 5 grams) of carrot seed powder should be taken daily in wine; this powder is also highly recommended for stomach complaints, difficult urination, throat disorders, blockage of the liver and spleen, consumption, pneumonia and coughing. The dose should be ½ teaspoon (1 gram) powder with a little wine or honey four times a day. Scrapings of fresh carrot is a well-known remedy for burns or cancer sores; it is also good for eczema. For internal use, the powder can be taken in wine instead of dry; the seed can also be boiled in water. Boil 3 to 4 teaspoons (10 to 12 grams) in 2 cups (½ liter) water and take 2 cups of this tea daily.

CASTOR OIL

Ricinus communis   Fam. Euphorbiaceae
Palma Christi

This oil is extracted from the seeds of the castor oil plant or wonder tree which grows in India. It is cultivated in gardens as an ornamental plant. Castor oil (*Oleum ricini*) is used medicinally as a very mild, almost infallible, laxative. It is an excellent remedy for inflammation and cramp-like contractions of the intestines, if the stools are dry and hard. It is additionally highly recommended for cramp colic and strangulated hernias. Take 2 teaspoons to 2 tablespoons (4 to 20 grams) according to circumstances. It is best taken in milk.

CATMINT

Nepeta cataria   Fam. Labiatae
Catnip

This is the only variety found here in the wild and then only seldom; it is found on rubbish tips, old walls and rough places. It is a perennial, herbaceous plant with an ascendant, branched stem; the leaves are heart-shaped, the flowers form a spike on the stem terminals. They are purple or white. The flowering period is August and the herb should be gathered during this period. The sap is bitter and is used medicinally to strengthen the stomach and promote menstruation. It also renders a useful service for jaundice and hysteria. The infusion contains ⅓ to ½ cup (10 to 12 grams) per 2 cups (½ liter) boiling water. Take 1 cup daily. It is an especially good phlegm solvent in cases of bronchitis and asthma; it is a good remedy for scurf and spots around the genital organs: to be used in the form of compresses. The bruised herb poked into the nose helps nosebleeds. It can also be recommended for internal use for the treatment of piles, ulcerated kidneys, kidney diseases, bladder and intestinal complaints, hematuria and blood-spitting. Instead of the infusion, 2½ teaspoons (3 grams) of powder may be taken daily in wine or water.

CELERY (WILD)

Apium graveolens   Fam. Umbelliferae
Smallage

Celery is often grown in gardens, is a biennial plant, blooms from July to September and two varieties are cultivated: leaf and turnip-rooted celery. Celery, or wild celery, has a thin, woody root. The stems are straight, grooved, hollow, thick and woody. The leaves are rather large, glossy, deeply cut, the flowers are whitish-green, very numerous and grow in umbels on the stem terminals. The root is divided into a number of fibers, red on the outside and white on the inside. Wild celery has an aromatic, strong, rather pleasant smell; the sap is sour and bitter. The leaves are used medicinally for chronic lung catarrh and humid asthma. Use about ½ cup (10 to 12 grams) of fresh leaves per 2 cups (½ liter) of very fresh milk. This milk should be taken in the mornings on an empty stomach.

The freshly squeezed sap can also be used as a diuretic; take 3 to 4 tablespoons (20 to 30 grams) a day. You can also fry celery leaves in butter with an equal quantity of mint; then take powdered celery seed, sprinkle over the breasts and then apply a plaster of the ointment described above: this dries up the milk.

CHAMOMILE (COMMON)

Anthemis nobilis   Fam. Compositae
Roman Chamomile

Common chamomile originally came from the Orient and is now cultivated in our gardens; the flowers are used medicinally. They have a strong, spicy smell, a warm, very bitter taste and are used externally, like wild chamomile, in herb bags for intestinal cramps. Internally, they are used in powder form, from 3 teaspoons to 3 tablespoons (2 to 8 grams). The infusion for internal use contains 3 tablespoons to ¼ cup (8 to 12 grams) per 2 cups (½ liter) boiling water. It can be used with success in the treatment of intermittent fever and hypochondriacal or hysterical complaints; it is highly recommended for intestinal cramps caused by the accumulation of gas, for dysentery and diarrhea, for menstruation which is painful or has stopped, or for indigestion. Chamomile flowers must be picked as soon as they open in order to preserve their beneficial properties. They may be considered one of the best home remedies and no home should be without them.

CHAMOMILE (WILD)

Matricaria chamomilla   Fam. Compositae

The chamomile flower is an annual plant which is commonly found along roadsides, on rubbish tips and in cornfields. The leaves are small and narrow; the flowers white, yellow inside; the petals hang down and have a particularly strong smell and bitter taste. The decoction contains 2 to 3 tablespoons (5 to 7 grams) per 2 cups (½ liter) boiling water; it relieves cramps and is one of the best remedies for colic, stomach cramps and swelling from wind; it is also recommended for indigestion, heavy bleeding, liver complaints and nerves, for hysteria, kidney and bladder stones, and dropsy. When applied externally in the form of warm bags, chamomile relieves cramps, inflammation, etc. Burns should be constantly bathed with the decoction.

CHARCOAL

Carbo vegetabilis

Internal use of vegetable charcoal[2] is highly recommended as a purgative in the dose of 4 to 6 teaspoons (7 to 12 grams); in addition, for chronic lung disease, liver complaints, particularly in cases of excessive foul phlegm discharge, accompanied by consumptive fever. Externally, charcoal is an excellent remedy to draw severely suppurating, foul ulcers. It is also used as an antiseptic, and for wet eczema and ulcerated gums. Internally, it can best be taken with milk and sugar; this is also recommended for indigestion: 1½ teaspoons twice a day is sufficient. In cases of any kind of poisoning, 1 tablespoon of charcoal powder should be taken.

CHERVIL

Anthriscus cerefolium   Fam. Umbelliferae
Cow Parsley

This well-known plant can be found in every vegetable garden and is commonly used in the kitchen. It also grows wild alongside roads and on wasteland. Chervil also has a medicinal use for jaundice, swelling of the liver, and to dry up mother's milk; in addition, for erysipelas and swellings. For swellings and to dry up mother's milk, the bruised herbs should be applied externally. The juice extracted from the fresh plant can be used

---

[2] Carbo vegetabilis: is Carbon Vegetal Activado or activated charcoal which is the residue from the destructive distillation of various organic materials. It is used today as an adsorbent (not absorbent) for the purpose of flatulence. Also, useful as an emergency antidote for poisioning because of its adsorbent powers. But we think the author means carbo vegetablis, which is a common homeopathic remedy.

for pulmonary tuberculosis, the beginning of consumption, skin complaints, hardened glands and breathlessness, 2 to 3 cups (50 to 60 grams) daily. Dried, powdered chervil mixed with honey and applied as a plaster on cancer sores is highly recommended. Boiled chervil mixed with vinegar cures Guinea worm and rashes on the scalp. The infusion, which can be taken instead of the drops, contains ¾ to 1 cup (15 to 20 grams) per 2 cups (½ liter) boiling water.

CHICKWEED

Stellaria media   Fam. Caryophyllaceae

It grows in green clusters, which can be either dense or spread out, with decumbent and ascendant stems and small oval-round, acute leaves, growing opposite and decussate. Its flowers are white and grow on the stem terminals. This herb can be found everywhere in wasteland, rich fields and in gardens. When freshly crushed, the herb is very effective for lupus. Internally, it is highly praised as a diuretic. Dr. Kneipp used to give it to consumptives.

Chickweed, steeped in wine, is highly recommended for convalescents, exhausted by lengthy illness. For inflammation of the liver, apply the bruised herb or compresses of the decoction; likewise for piles and inflammation of the genital organs. In cases of consumption, pining away or emaciation, it is advisable to eat chickweed; likewise for epilepsy and blood-spitting. If the bruised herb is applied to the breasts, it makes them soft again. Take 3 tablespoons (30 grams) of the sap extract daily. The decoction is made from ½ cup (15 grams) per 2 cups (½ liter) water; 2 to 3 teaspoons (4 to 5 grams) of the powdered dried plant should be taken daily.

CHICORY (WILD)

Cichorium intybus   Fam. Compositae

Wild chicory grows abundantly on high ground, dykes and along roadside verges; it is an herbaceous, biennial plant, gray-green in color. The leaves are oblong, deeply cut, the radical leaves rather large. The pale blue flowers bear a great resemblance to the cornflower, but are larger. The long, yellowish root, like the leaves, contains bitter sap. Leaves and roots can be used medicinally; the former are gathered in June, the roots in September. The leaf infusion consists of ¼ to ½ cup (10 to 25 grams) per 2 cups (½ liter) boiling water; 2 cups should be taken daily. The root decoction contains ⅓ to ½ cup (15 to 25 grams) per 2 cups (½ liter) water; this should be reduced by half, and 1 tablespoon should be taken every two hours. The leaf infusion is recommended for constipation, mucous stomach and excessive gall; it cleanses the liver, spleen, kidneys, stomach and promotes digestion. A tincture of the root in 75% alcohol is used externally to rub weak limbs twice a day. Take 2 cups tea made from the leaf decoction as an excellent remedy for a mucous stomach, for it encourages digestion and puts the stomach in order again. The decoction of roots, leaves and stems is highly recommended for pneumonia and chest catarrh.

CINNAMON

Cinnamomum zeylanicum   Fam. Lauraceae

Cinnamon is the bark of the laurus cinnamomum, a tree that grows in Eastern countries. Cinnamon is available in the form of thin, rolled up pipes of a brittle substance, reddish in color, with a pleasant, spicy smell and a warm, sweetish, slightly astringent taste. Take 2 to 2½ teaspoons (3 to 4 grams) cinnamon powder, or a decoction of 2 tablespoons to 2 cups (15 to 300 grams) water, for diarrhea caused by intestinal weakness; in addition, for vomiting in pregnant and hysterical women, for chronic gastric weakness accompanied by wind, nausea and vomiting, heavy bleeding and hematuria. Cinnamon can also be used to improve the nauseating taste and harmful effects of certain medicines; for acidity, heartburn, gastric mucus, heavy menstruation, general weakness and loss of strength.

Cinquefoil

Potentilla reptans   Fam. Rosaceae
Five-Leaf Grass

Cinquefoil is a perennial, herbaceous plant with erect or ascendant, more or less silky, grayish stems, the tops of which bear golden-yellow flowers. The leaves are five-lobed, obovate, deeply serrated, green on top and silvery beneath. The root is black, long and fibrous; the sap astringent. It is found almost everywhere along roadsides and waterways. It blooms throughout the summer. The leaves and flowers can be gathered through the summer period.

The infusion of the leaves contains ¾ to 1 cup (10 to 15 grams) per 2 cups (½ liter) boiling water. It can be successfully used for diarrhea. The root is good for fixing loose teeth and avoiding toothaches; for this purpose, one should simply chew a root from time to time. The leaves are also highly recommended for blood-spitting and leukorrhea. This simple herb also cures cramps in the stomach or intestines quite easily. Boil 1 cup (15 grams) of dried leaves in 2 cups (½ liter) of milk and give to the patient to drink as hot as possible. This remedy seldom fails to give immediate relief. If the cramp is severe, or if it has not been fully effective, the same quantity may be safely taken three or four times a day. It is also used for bleeding, gravel, repressed menstruation, dysentery, jaundice, scurvy, dropsy, and alleviates infections of the kidneys, bladder, and bleeding gums.

The decoction of the leaves is an excellent eyewash for red, running eyes. It is also for ulcerated or suppurating sores, on which compresses of the infusion should be applied. In the case of fever, the fresh herb should be pounded with salt and vinegar and applied to the soles of the feet. When steeped in boiling milk and taken hot, cinquefoil is especially highly praised for cramps of the heart and chest.

CLAY

Clay is a yellow, greasy substance from the ground which can be found everywhere. Bricks are made from this substance, also earthenware. From a medical point of view, clay deserves great respect. After thorough cleaning, it is dried and finely ground, mixed with water and vinegar, sometimes also with herbs and arnica, and applied in the form of compresses for various complaints such as old sores, swellings, inflammation, cancer; it is especially efficacious for lupus; in addition for scurf, Guinea worm and eczema. It is also used for headaches, neuralgia, and bruising.

CLOVES

Eugenia caryophyllata   Fam. Myrtaceae

The use of cloves tends to be more culinary than medicinal. They contain an ethereal oil which is heavier than water. It can occasionally be used with success in cases of indigestion, stomach cramps and colic; about 2 to 4 drops of the oil should be given on sugar.

CLUB MOSS

Lycopodium clavatum   Fam. Lycopodiaceae

Club moss is a perennial, creeping plant, covered with side-branches from top to bottom; the whole plant is covered with long, mossy hair. It is found on moist heath. A rather long, thick spike grows on the stem; it is full of a yellow powder that can be applied to children's cut legs. The whole plant is used medicinally for dropsy. The infusion contains 4 to 8 teaspoons (7 to 15 grams) per 2 cups (½ liter) boiling water. Dosage: 1 cup daily. Some physicians also recommend this powder for dysentery and diarrhea. For this purpose, take 4 teaspoons (4 grams) club moss powder, ½ cup (125 grams) fennel water and 3 to 5 tablespoons of syrup. Club moss, boiled in wine, expels stones. All infestations in both people and animals can be cleared up by washing with club moss decoction. A quantity of club moss placed at the end of the bed draws cramps from the feet.

Cod-liver Oil

Cod-liver oil, extracted from the liver of the codfish, is a little rancid, has an unpleasant smell and a bitter taste. It is a remedy for complaints of a scrofulous nature, gout, and rickets. It can be used both internally and externally. Adults should take 2 to 3 tablespoons daily, children 1 to 2. It can be rubbed in externally twice a day. Since it has a harmful effect on the stomach, it is not recommended for internal use.

Coltsfoot

Tussilago Farfara   Fam. Compositae

Coltsfoot grows in abundance on moist clay soil. It is a perennial herbaceous plant with a creeping, branched rootstock and is difficult to eradicate in places where it has once taken root. The leaves are large, heart-shaped, dentate, glossy green on the upperside and covered with white felt beneath. The yellow flowers open before the flowers in April on a stem terminal covered with lanceolate scales. Each stem bears a single flower. From very early times, coltsfoot has been a well-known chest remedy, and is mainly used for chronic phlegm complaints of the lungs, chronic colds which very often degenerate into consumption, for tubercles of a scrofulous nature which sometimes start to suppurate, and after repeated suppuration develop into consumption. Coltsfoot can also be taken for scrofula, but it must be taken over a long period. Leaves and flowers are used medicinally. The leaves are gathered in May, the flowers in April. The infusion of the leaves and flowers consists of ⅓ to ½ cup (10 to 15 grams) per 2 cups (½ liter) boiling water. The sap extracted from the fresh plant deserves preference. The dose is 3 to 6 tablespoons (25 to 50 grams) per day and is used for eczema, Guinea worm and asthma. Take 1 cup daily.

COMFREY

Symphytum officinale   Fam. Boraginaceae

Comfrey grows abundantly in wet places, especially along the banks of the Meuse. It is a perennial, herbaceous plant, with a black, very slimy, thick root, white inside. The leaves are hairy, large, oblong and feel rough to the touch. The flowers hang in racemes on the stem terminals; they are purple, yellow or white in color. The root is used medicinally. It is gathered in the autumn, cut into slices and dried in the oven. It is highly recommended for blood-spitting, coughing, diarrhea and dysentery. The decoction contains ⅓ to ½ cup (15 to 20 grams) per 2 cups (½ liter) water. This root should be boiled in a glazed pot; an iron pot makes the decoction turn black. Fresh scrapings can be successfully used externally on ulcers; it soon brings them to a head and heals them; when comfrey is applied to burns, the pain immediately subsides. The finest results have been obtained by applying it on hernias. Split nipples (in women) are soon healed by the application of these scrapings.

COMMON ALKANET

Anchousa officinalis   Fam. Boraginaceae

This plant, with its branched, very hairy, prickly stem, grows along roadsides and on wastelands. Its leaves are lanceolate; the dark-blue or red flowers grow close to each other. The flowering period is May to September. An infusion of the leaves is recommended for melancholy, sharpness in the blood is sweetened by it; the remedy is also depurative, and strengthens the heart and is diuretic.

COMMON BROOM

Sarothamnus scoparius   Fam. Papilionaceae

This shrub is found on all wasteland; it sometimes adorns whole hills with its beautiful golden yellow flowers. These are fragrant, rather large and appear in the spring. The shrubs attain a height of 6 feet (2 meters) the leaves are oblong, narrow and the uppermost leaves are hairy. The seed is enclosed in small pods, resembling beans. These beans make very good chicken fodder.

Broom is used medicinally as a diuretic. The ash is especially useful for stoppage of the urine. Take a good handful of ash per quart (liter) of boiling water. This infusion is highly recommended for dropsy. The infusion of the tops and flowers, 3 to 4 tablespoons (15 to 20 grams) per 2 cups (½ liter) water, is beneficial for ascites, edema, and kidney complaints; it is a diuretic, a purgative, and stimulates the appetite. Take 1 cup daily.

Common Bugle

Ajuga reptans   Fam. Labiatae

This is a perennial plant with ascendant, quadrangular stems, with hairs on two sides and with long, creeping runners. The leaves are opposite, oblong-oval, hairy, lightly dentate and petiolate. The blue or red-colored flowers appear on the stem terminals; at first resembling whorls, later clustered in spikes. The numerous, white, fibrous roots have no smell; the sap is bitter and aromatic. It can be found in meadows and alongside ditches. The flowering period is May to June. A decoction of the leaves and flowers, containing 5 to 6 tablespoons (15 to 25 grams) per 2 cups (½ liter) boiling water, is a recommended remedy for jaundice, hardening of the liver, asthma, ulceration of the lungs, blockage of the urine, heavy bleeding, blood-spitting, leukorrhea and dysentery; it is also a depurative. The dosage is 1 to 2 cups of tea daily.

Common Centaury

Erythraea centaurium   Fam. Gentianaceae
Feverwort

This is an annual plant, growing in dry woodland, meadows, etc. The sap is very bitter and has hardly any smell. The flowers are a beautiful shade of pink and grow in racemes on the stem terminals. The stem is thin and quadrangular, the leaves are oblong, acute, narrow, light-green in color and generally have three main veins. The root is white, dry and very hard. The flowering period is July to August.

The flower heads are used medicinally. The infusion contains ⅛ to ¼ cup (5 to 10 grams) per 2 cups (½ liter) boiling water when used to strengthen the muscles. For high fever, ⅓ cup (15 grams) should be used per 2 cups (½ liter) water. A wine decoction can be made and this is even more powerful. Use ⅔ cup (30 grams) per 2 cups (½ liter) wine.

Common centaury is an excellent remedy and is used medicinally to restore the strength of weak convalescents. Anemic girls soon recover their color if they take the infusion for some time. Spring and autumn fever is also swiftly cured by means of this herb. It is additionally highly recommended for heartburn, gastric complaints, nausea, indigestion, liver complaints, melancholy, kidney disorders and even gallstones. It is also one of the best remedies for jaundice, rheumatism, gout, scurvy and dropsy. Take 1 cup of tea with a spoon every day. Instead of the infusion, powder from the dried plant can also be taken. It should be mixed with aniseed powder and 2 grams taken daily.

Common Figwort

Scrophularia nodosa   Fam. Scrophulariaceae
Knotted Figwort

Common figwort is a perennial, herbaceous plant. It grows fairly commonly in shady, damp places. The stem attains a height of about 3 feet (1 meter), is branched, quadrangular, and brown in color. The leaves are opposite and decussate, heart-shaped and have a serrated edge; the flowers are red-brown, grow on the stem terminals, and resemble a helmet or snail shell. The plant has an unpleasant smell, almost the same as the dwarf elder. The root consists of numerous knobbles. The flowering period is July to September. During this time, the plant is gathered, dried and stored for use. The root is gathered in the autumn. The whole plant and root is used medicinally. The sap is bitter and can be used in glandular disorders, scrofulous tumors, cancer and piles. The decoction of the plant consists of ⅓ cup (15 grams) per 2 cups (½ liter) water and is recommended for glandular complaints and croup, and as a gargle for throat infections.

For external use, the root is ground to a powder, fried in fresh butter and placed on the swollen glands. The same ointment may be used for piles, and 1 cup of tea from this plant should also be taken daily.

For swollen glands and croup, compresses of the plant decoction can also be successfully used, but the quantity should then be doubled to ⅔ cup (30 grams) per 2 cups (½ liter) water. A tincture can also be prepared from the roots, leaves and stems; this has a much more powerful effect when taken internally. Take an equal quantity of roots, leaves and stems, fill a quarter part of a wine bottle with them and then fill to the brim with good quality gin. Take 1 tablespoon daily. Instead of gin, the same quantity of wine can be used; 1 wineglass should be taken twice a day.

COMMON ST. JOHNSWORT

Hypericum perforatum   Fam. Hypericaceae

Common St. Johnswort is a perennial herbaceous plant, the stems are straight, elegant, branched, round, pliant and hard. The leaves are undivided, oblong, lanceolate, narrow and marked with small, translucent spots. These spots are an ethereal oil in which the true potency lies. The flowers are a beautiful golden yellow. If the fresh flowers are rubbed between the fingers, a blood-red fluid is produced, a sign of the true St.

Johnswort. They grow in racemes on the stem terminals. The flower heads are used medicinally. It is gathered in June and September. St. Johnswort is found in woodland and along roadside verges. The sap is bitter, salty and resinous. The infusion contains 3 to 4 tablespoons (10 to 15 grams) per 2 cups (½ liter) boiling water. It is used for lung complaints, chronic catarrh, asthma, chills, bladder catarrh, and if the urine is thick. It is also used for hysteria, jaundice, absence of menstruation due to illness, green sickness, blood-spitting, leukorrhea, pneumonia, rheumatism, fever, intestinal blockage, dysentery, nervous cramps, and uterine cramps.

For gall complaints, take 2 tablespoons (6 grams) powdered seed with honey water; this is also good for sciatica. Drink 1 to 2 cups of tea daily. Leaves and flowers boiled in olive oil are a good remedy for sores and contusions. For shivering and shaking in those who suffer from nerves, this oil should be rubbed in twice a day. For bruises, a cloth dipped in this oil should be placed on the affected area. To strengthen the tendons, rub them twice a day with this oil.

CORIANDER

Coriandrum sativum   Fam. Umbelliferae

Coriander is an annual plant with white or pink flowers and has single, pinnate leaves on the lower part of the stem, double pinnate higher up; the former are divided into broad leaflets and the latter into narrow leaflets. While unripe, the fruit, leaves, and stems exude an unpleasant smell. The fruit is totally round and yellow; the plant attains a height of 20 inches (½ meter) and has a very thin, curved root. If the seed is taken in the mornings on an empty stomach, the oil extracted from it expels wind and strengthens the stomach. The bruised herb can be used externally for inflammation, carbuncles, and ulceration. The seed steeped in sweet wine expels worms and promotes menstruation. Half a sugarspoon of coriander seed taken once a day after a meal is efficacious in the treatment of indigestion, mucous stomach, mucus in the intestines, wind,

nausea, diarrhea, dizziness, arthralgia, suppressed menstruation, intermittent fever and also as a preventative measure for
strokes.

Corn Marigold

Chrysantemum segetum   Fam. Compositae
Field or Wild Marigold

This is very commonly found on sandy, cultivated ground,
sometimes just as if it had been sown there. It is an annual
plant, with a hairless, branches stem, oblong, coarsely-serrated
leaves and round flowers; both the radial and disk florets are
golden yellow. The smell is not unpleasant. This plant is a very
good remedy for sores, and is used externally on sores in the
form of compresses; the infusion for this purpose should contain 1 cup (30 grams) per 2 cups (½ liter) boiling water. To use
internally: take 1 cup of tea daily made from ½ cup (15 grams)
per 2 cups (½ liter) boiling water, as it is a depurative and
stimulates the appetite.

Cornelian Cherry

Cornus mas   Fam. Cornaceae

The cornelian cherry is a shrub with grayish colored branches;
the leaves are oblong-oval; the yellow blossoms appear very
early in March (before the leaves) and grow in racemes; the
edible fruit is red and ovate. This shrub was formerly cultivated
more extensively in parks and gardens than it is today; in south
Limburg hedges and bowers of cornelian cherry are often encountered. The pliable wood can be trained in all shapes and
directions. The bark and fruit are used medicinally. The bark
is astringent and febrifugal; the fruit is astringent and dessicant.
Application of fresh, bruised leaves staunches bleeding. The
fruit decoction is used for feverish burning and dysentery; it
also stimulates the appetite. Take 2 to 4 teaspoons (10 to 15
grams) per 2 cups (½ liter) boiling water.

CORNFLOWER

Centaurea cyanus   Fam. Compositae

This grows abundantly, as its name reveals, in corn, and is biennial, quite hairy, has a greasy stem with stiffly ascendant branches and narrow, obovate leaves. The ovate flower heads grow singly on the branch terminals, and have large, blue, funnel shaped radiating flowers and paler disc florets. The flowers are used medicinally. Give 4 teaspoons (4 grams) powder internally for jaundice, or for menstruation and heavy bleeding with cramps and difficult urination. The decoction, about 7 tablespoons (10 to 12 grams) per 2 cups (½ liter) water, is a highly recommended internal remedy for scurf and Guinea worm. It should be applied in the form of compresses.

COUCHGRASS

Agropyrum repens   Fam. Graminaceae
Dog Grass, Twitch Grass

Couchgrass is a kind of thin, nodular grass that attains a height of three feet (1 meter). The leaves are long, acute, and rough to the touch. The flowers form corn-like spikes. The roots are long, creeping, nodular, red-white and almost scentless. The sap is bitter. This plant is much sought after by dogs; hence the name dog grass. The roots are used medicinally; they are gathered in the autumn, thoroughly cleaned, well beaten to remove the outer rind and then hung in a dry place. The decoction of the roots consists of 2 to 4 tablespoons (6 to 12 grams) per 2 cups (½ liter) water and is highly recommended for all infections. It is a very good diuretic and is therefore recommended for gravel and poor urination. This tea is also most refreshing. Take 1 cup daily.

Cow Parsnip

Heracleum sphondylium   Fam. Umbelliferae
Hogweed

This herbaceous, perennial plant attains a height of 20-60 inches (1½ meters), grows abundantly on moist, shady ground, has a fleshy, aromatic root which, when cut, reveals an oily, brown fluid. The stem is thick, deeply grooved and ridged; the leaves are rather large, pale green, with a three-lobed terminal leaf. The pale pink flowers form an umbel on the stem terminal in July and August. The seed is broad and oval. This plant is readily eaten by animals. Internally, the root is used for epilepsy; 3 teaspoons (8 grams) of the powdered dried root should be taken daily. The seed is used for abdominal pain and worms.

Cowslip

Primula officinalis   Fam. Primulaceae
Oxlip

The cowslip which is used medicinally should not be confused with the ordinary cowslip which is commonly found in abundance in moist meadows, woods and pastures and which has little or no smell. Only the dark yellow, fragrant cowslips are used medicinally; their leaves and flowers are much finer than those of the ordinary cowslip. *Primula officinalis* is seldom found here. It grows in meadows and woodland wherever there is grass. It is a perennial, herbaceous plant, with beautiful, grayish-green leaves which sprout in the spring and form a rosette, from which grow one or more flower stems; a beautiful raceme of yellow flowers appears, all hanging to one side. The flowering period is April to May. These flowers are highly recommended for rheumatism, especially articular rheumatism and gout. The decoction contains 1 to 2 tablespoons (6 to 7 grams) per 2 cups (½ liter) boiling water. The decoction of the roots, ⅓ cup (10 grams) per 2 cups (½ liter) water, is used for worms. The root is rather thick, and when fresh smells a little like aniseed.

CROSS-LEAVED HEATH

Erica tetralix   Fam. Ericaceae
Bell Heath, Common Heath

Cross-leaved heath is a low shrub that at first glance may be
confused with heather, but the difference is soon apparent,
especially during the flowering period. Cross-leaved heath is
found on lower lying, rather moist sandy ground; it has numerous, hairy, young branches that attain a height of two feet
(7 decimeters). Its leaves are narrow and oblong. The beautiful
purple flowers adorn the tips of the branches in racemes of six
to twelve wooly-haired stems. The calyx is bell-shaped, ovate
with four teeth, eight stamens and an ovary with four chambers.
Stems, leaves and flowers have medicinal properties; they are
gathered during the flowering period of August to September.
The decoction consists of ½ to ⅔ cups (15 to 20 grams) per 2
cups (½ liter) water, and is very efficacious for the treatment
of rheumatism, kidney stones, and promoting urination.

CUCKOO-PINT (POISON)

Arum maculatum   Fam. Araceae

Cockoo-pint is a perennial, poisonous plant, found in shady
places in woods and damp regions. It can be recognized by its
usually dark purple spotted leaves. The tuber is thick, round
and brown; the leaves are long-petiolate, saggitate, glossy green
and hairless on the upper side and pale underneath. The flower
stem grows about a foot high (2 to 3 decimeters), is a beautiful
shade of green and ends in a single flower in the form of a
white or pale green bugle. The flowering period is May. This
is followed by a spike of scarlet berries. The tuber, which is
used medicinally, is gathered in the autumn and dried; the
drying process removes much of the sharpness. When fresh, it
is extremely poisonous and when eaten causes a constricting
pain in the throat and stomach which may be followed by vomiting and death. For safety's sake, no directions for use are
included here.

Daisy

Bellis perennis   Fam. Compositae

The daisy is a perennial, herbaceous, attractive little plant which pushes up everywhere between blades of grass. The rather fleshy leaves have a medicinal use. They can be taken internally as a depurative remedy for consumption, scrofula, dropsy, gout, fevers, and intestinal burning. The infusion of the dried leaves should consist of ¼ to ½ cup (10 to 15 grams) per 2 cups (½ liter) water; sap extracted from the fresh leaves and flowers can also be used: ¼ to ⅓ cup (80 to 100 grams) daily. Take 1 to 2 cups of the infusion daily. A tincture can also be prepared from sap freshly extracted from the plant by mixing equal quantities of extracted sap and alcohol in the Spring. After two weeks, it is ready for use; 6 drops should be taken three times a day.

Dandelion

Taraxacum officinale   Fam. Compositae

The dandelion is a commonly known perennial plant; it is especially found in meadows in such abundance that during its flowering period almost nothing but yellow dandelions can be seen and the grass seems to be quite crowded out. The leaves are obovate and dentate; the hollow flower stems attain a height of 4 to 6 inches (12 to 15 centimeters). The flowering period is followed by a large quantity of seed in the form of a transparent ball of petiolate pappuses which blow away at the slightest breeze.

The leaves are much sought after in the spring as they provide a delicious salad that is both nourishing and depurative. The milky root is very bitter and is successfully used in the treatment of jaundice, bladder disorders, and a weak stomach. The root decoction contains 3 tablespoons (15 grams) per 2 cups (½ liter) water. The strongest action comes from freshly extracted sap, 2 to 4 tablespoons (20 to 40 grams) of which may be given daily. The roots boiled in milk are also very good for consumption, fevers, gravel, renal pain, scurvy, dropsy, glands, deep-rooted eczema, liver complaints, pneumonia, dysentery. The remedy is also diuretic. Take 1 cup daily with a spoon. A tincture can be prepared from the freshly extracted sap from dandelion roots; this is best done in August. Mix 2 tablespoons (18 grams) 90% alcohol, 2 teaspoons (15 grams) glycerine, 2 tablespoons (17 grams) water, and ⅓ cup (100 grams) sap. Let stand for a few days then filter and store for use in a well-corked bottle. Take 1 to 2 tablespoons daily.

Deadly Nightshade (poison)

Atropa belladonna   Fam. Solanaceae
Belladonna

Deadly nightshade is a very poisonous, perennial plant which is but seldom found here in wet woodland. It has thick, branched, round, hairy stems, and smooth-edged, dark-green, pointed oval, short-petiolate leaves. The red-brown flowers are long-petiolate and droop singly in the shape of quite large bells. The ripe berries bear a marked resemblance to black cherries; they are a glossy black color. The root is fleshy. The flowering period is June to July. Deadly nightshade is extensively used for medicinal purposes, but in spite of its beneficial properties, it is inadvisable to try even the smallest quantity without a doctor's prescription as it can have such very injurious consequences. I have described this and other dangerous plants in this work precisely so as to avoid their being confused with other plants.

Devil's-Bit Scabious

Scabiosa succisa   Fam. Compositae

Devil's-bit scabious[3] is a perennial, herbaceous plant with oblong, short-petiolate, hairy leaves. The flower heads are round and blue in color. The plant attains a height of 2½ feet (80 centimeters). It is found on hills, woods and fields. The

---

[3] We were unable to locate this herb.

rootstock is black and looks as though it has been bitten off. This root is used medicinally. A tincture is prepared from it by drawing a good handful of roots in 2 cups (½ liter) of gin. This tincture stimulates the appetite, aids digestion, strengthens the stomach and drives away pain from the womb.

The decoction of the plant, ¼ ounce (15 to 20 grams) per 2 cups (½ liter) water, is also recommended for the same complaints; in addition, for leukorrhea, ulceration of the liver, skin complaints, epilepsy, dropsy, coughs, asthma, pain in the side, blockage of the womb, eczema. It is also depurative. Externally, it can be used as a gargle for venereal ulceration of the throat and gums. Use ¼ ounce (25 grams) of the whole plant (leaves, stems and roots) per 2 cups (½ liter) water.

DILL

Anethum graveolus   Fam. Compositae
Dillweed, Dillseed

Dill, an annual plant, indigenous to southern Europe, has yellow flowers which appear in July. The leaves, like those of fennel, are divided into very fine, threadlike lobes. The strong scent of dill resembles that of fennel and aniseed. All parts of the plant are used medicinally in the same cases and the same dosage as fennel and aniseed. The seed combats the formation of wind, sluggish menstruation and increases mother's milk.

DOG ROSE

Rosa canina   Fam. Rosaceae

The dog rose is a shrub covered in prickles; it reaches a height of a good six to seven feet (two meters) and is found in the wild in woodlands and hedgerows. It is also cultivated in gardens to improve roses. The flowers (wild roses) are pale red with a pleasant fragrance and are followed by obovate, red fruits. These fruits, rosehips, are used medicinally. The greatest power lies in the pips or seeds of the rosehips. These fruits are most highly recommended for kidney complaints, gravel and stones, especially in elderly people. Boil 1⅓ to 2 cups (100 to 150 grams) in 4 cups (1 liter) of water for at least three-quarters of an hour; if milk and sugar are added, it is not only an excellent medicine, but a delicious, beneficial drink, too.

Dog's Mercury

Mercurialis perennis   Fam. Euphorbiaceae

This herbaceous plant is frequently seen on both farmland and wasteland, although mostly in gardens. It has an irregular stem with long-petiolate, ovate and blunt-serrated leaves. The male flowers appear in the leaf axils and protrude above the leaves; the female flowers, on the contrary, are short and have dry, shrunken cymes. The flowering period is June to August. This plant exudes an unpleasant, nauseating smell. Although its decoction may help in several illnesses, it is not, however, advisable to use it.

Duckweed

Lemna minor   Fam. Lemnaceae

This herbaceous, perennial plant floats on the water; it has two small, smooth-edged short-petiolate, obovate leaves. It grows amazingly fast in large quantities. The bruised fresh herb is used externally for gout and headaches caused by heat. The following tincture of the plant is used internally for jaundice. Take a good handful of the dried plant and let steep for 48 hours in a bottle of wine near the fire. Take 1 tablespoon every two hours.

Elder (common)

Sambucus nigra   Fam. Caprifoliaceae

This well-known shrub, which provides us with elder flowers, can be found here and there in old gardens and on the edge of woodlands; it is also cultivated in gardens for the pleasant smell of its flowers and the usefulness of the whole plant. Each leaf has five ovate, serrated leaflets. The flowers are very fragrant and adorn the branch terminals in racemes, followed in the autumn by black berries. Elder flowers are undoubtedly the most well known diaphoretic in use and can be successfully employed at the onset of all kinds of chills. The inner rind of one year old shoots, mixed with a half quantity of licorice, is an excellent remedy for dropsy. The leaves, drunk as tea, are a depurative. The infusion should contain ¼ to ⅓ cup (10 to 12 grams) per 2 cups (½ liter) boiling water.

The well-known elder syrup can be made from berries picked in the autumn. The infusion of elder flowers contains 4 to 5 tablespoons (8 to 10 grams) per 2 cups (½ liter) boiling water. Elder flowers boiled in milk with a slice of white bread soaked in it, applied between thin linen cloths on burning eyes, soon draws out all the burning; sore eyes are also soon healed by this remedy. A good laxative is 4 to 6 teaspoons (12 to 15 grams) of elder berries. Elder leaves, boiled in milk, are beneficial for scurf; they are depurative and laxative. The dosage is 1 to 2 cups daily.

ELDER (DWARF, POISON)

Sambucus Ebulus   Fam. Caprifoliaceae

Dwarf elder is a perennial, herbaceous plant that can be found in wet places on the edge of woodlands. Each leaf has five ovate, serrated leaflets. The flowers are white, appear in umbels on the stem terminals and are succeeded, like the common elder, by black berries. The long, white root grows very deep into the ground. This root is used medicinally and should be gathered in July. The decoction contains 1 to 2 tablespoons (10 to 15 grams) per 2 cups (½ liter) water and is very beneficial for the treatment of dropsy. A larger dose acts as a purgative. Gout and podagra are soon cured by the application of elder root, boiled for quite a long time in wine dregs. Flowers and leaves, boiled to a paste, are highly recommended for sciatica, rheumatism, and paralysis. This alone will cure these complaints. It can also be fruitfully used in the treatment of neuralgia.

ELDER (GROUND)

Aegopodium podagraria   Fam. Umbelliferae
Goutweed

This is a perennial herbaceous plant, a very troublesome weed, found in abundance under hedges, in shady places, roadsides, etc. The stem is erect, the upper part branched. The leaves are double-tri-partite. The flowers are white and form an umbel on the stem terminal. Ground elder has a horizontal, creeping rootstock from which the young plants grow. The flowering period is June to July.

For internal use, the infusion of the plant consists of ⅓ cup (15 grams) per 2 cups (½ liter) boiling water. Drink 1 cup daily. Externally, use 1¼ cups (50 grams) per 4 cups (1 liter) boiling water. It is used medicinally for gout, podagra, rheumatism, sciatica, and feeling of cold in the limbs. It is used externally in the form of compresses and hot baths made from the decoction of the plant.

ELECAMPANE

Inula helenium   Fam. Compositae
Scabwort

This is a perennial, herbaceous plant with a strong, erect stem which is lightly hairy and round, attaining a height of 4 to 5 feet (1½ meters). It is seldom found. It grows in rich, moist, shady soil, but is also cultivated in gardens. The leaves are rather large, irregularly dentate, woolly and have a long stem. The flowers are a beautiful yellow color, large, solitary, with much in common with the sunflower. The plant has a thick, long root, red on the outside and white on the inside. This root is used medicinally. It has a strong, aromatic, penetrating smell. Its sap is sour and bitter. The roots of two or three year old plants should be gathered in the autumn, finely chopped and dried in the oven.

The root decoction consists of 4 to 5 teaspoons (10 to 15 grams) per 2 cups (½ liter) water and may be fruitfully used for the treatment of leukorrhea and green sickness. Take 1 cup daily with a spoon. This decoction also stimulates the appetite and dissolves phlegm; it is recommended for asthma, lung complaints, flatulence, heartburn, catarrh, dropsy, indigestion and irregular menstruation in young girls. It can also be applied externally for itching eczema and scabies.

ENCHANTER'S NIGHTSHADE

Circaea lutetiana   Fam. Onagrariaceae

This is a perennial, herbaceous plant with a long, creeping root that is commonly found in moist woodlands and shady areas on the edge of woods. The erect stem has many branches near the top and reaches a height of 1½ feet. The long-petiolate leaves are acute-ovate, smooth, dentate and grow above each other. The flowers are white or pink, without bracts; they have two sepals and two petals, two stamens and two one-seeded compartments in the ovary. The flowering period is June through August. The decoction of this plant can be fruitfully used externally for piles. Steep 20 to 40 grams in 2 cups (½ liter) water. A cloth folded double twice should be dipped in it and applied several times a day.

EUPHORBIA

Euphorbia helioscopia   Fam. Euphorbiaceae
Sun or Wort Spurge

Euphorbia is an annual plant with an ascendant stem that grows abundantly in gardens and on farmland. The leaves are blue-green, hairless, smooth-edged, obovate. The main umbel has three rays with forked branches. When a leaf or stem is picked, it immediately exudes a white, milky sap. The sap can be used externally with good results for the treatment of warts. If they are moistened two or three times a day with the milk, they usually disappear within eight days.

EUROPEAN BARBERRY

Berberis vulgaris   Fam. Berberidaceae

This is a thorny shrub with woody, yellow roots, and erect yellow stems. The inner rind of the stems is golden yellow; the alternate, single leaves are hairless, ovate, acute-dentate, forming small rosettes with trifid spines. The flowers are yellow, hanging in racemes, later giving way to oblong, scarlet berries. The flowering period is June and July. Barberry is found in moist woodlands and in hedgerows; roots, leaves and berries are used medicinally. The root is very bitter and is used with the stem rind instead of rhubarb.

The inner rind of the stem and root is very good for liver and spleen diseases and dropsy. The decoction contains 2 tablespoons (4 grams) per 2 cups (½ liter) water; 1 cup should be taken daily with a spoon. The decoction of the leaves is 1 cup (10 to 15 grams) per 2 cups (½ liter) boiling water, and is a good laxative. The root is also used for jaundice. The leaves are recommended for scurvy and dropsy. The berries can be preserved. A refreshing drink which is very useful for fever can also be made from them. A decoction of the root is 3 tablespoons (8 grams) per 2 cups (½ liter) water and ensures good bowel movements.

EYEBRIGHT

Euphrasia officinalis   Fam. Scrophulariaceae

Eyebright is an annual plant, particularly found on sandy and chalky soil, sometimes in great abundance among the blades of grass. It has a slender, branched stem, sessile, ovate, serrated, opposite and decussate leaves, and sessile or short-petiolate flowers which only grow in the axils of the uppermost leaves. The corolla is white; there is a yellow fleck on the lower lip while the upper lip is finely crenulated. The flowering period is August and September. Eyebright should be gathered throughout the flowering period for medicinal use.

The infusion, ¼ to ⅓ cup (10 to 15 grams) per 2 cups (½ liter) boiling water, is used medicinally for weak, infected eyes; the eyes should be washed three times a day with this infusion. Taken internally, this remedy strengthens the stomach. To fortify the brain and the memory, a conserve can be made from the fresh herb and sugar. Take 1 eggspoonful every morning, or take a daily glass of wine in which the dried herb has been steeped. The decoction in water, filtered, is good for weak eyes. Take 1 cup of the infusion daily. The powder can also be boiled in wine for internal use. Use ⅓ cup (12 grams) to a bottle of wine.

False Hellebore (poison)

Adonis aestivalis   Fam. Ranunculaceae
Pheasant's Eye, Ox-eye

False hellebore is an annual plant, 1½ to 2 feet high (about 70 centimeters), which seldom grows here and in fact belongs to southern Europe where it grows abundantly in cornfields and cultivated calcareous and clay soil. It has fine-lobed, pinnate leaves, red or yellow flowers with five hairless sepals which are smaller than the petals. The ribbed pod fruits form a spike. The flowering period is from May to June.

A tincture can be prepared from the flowers; it is highly recommended for gout, sciatica, heart complaints, fatty degeneration of the heart, and stones. Take 5 to 6 drops three times a day in a spoon of water. It increases urination and gradually brings about recovery in cases of heart complaints and diseased cardiac valves. Ascites, caused by the heart complaint, likewise enlargement of the heart, can be cured by this remedy, while palpitations and fatty degeneration of the heart can be improved by this tincture, if not cured.

FENNEL

Foeniculum vulgare   Fam. Umbelliferae

The sweet, cultivated fennel is smaller than wild fennel, but the seed is larger, sweeter and more abundant; the taste and fragrance are also more pleasant. Fennel is an annual plant; the stem is thick, round and branched; the leaves are very divided. The small, yellow flowers form umbels on the stem terminals. Fennel seed is used medicinally. The decoction consists of 2 to 3 tablespoons (10 to 15 grams) per 2 cups (½ liter) water. It is highly recommended for gas, colic, cramps; it also strengthens the stomach and facilitates digestion. Fennel seed also has the beneficial property of increasing mother's milk; mothers who do not yet have sufficient milk should drink a daily cup of fennel seed tea and the lack of milk will soon cease. Fennel seed is also recommended for influenza; it warms and improves the stomach. For cramps, colic, etc, boil 1 sugarspoon fennel seed in 1 cup milk and drink while hot.

Fennel oil is given to children with whooping cough or who are vomiting: 5 to 6 drops on sugar or with honey twice a day. A knife-point of fennel powder, taken twice a day, expels gas, cleanses the kidneys and liver. Externally, fennel powder is recommended as an eye tonic; put a small sugarspoonful of fennel powder in an ordinary glass of water, briefly bring to the boil and you will have a good eyewater; the eyes should be washed with this two to three times a day. Fennel oil is also highly recommended for asthmatics; 12 to 15 drops should be taken with a glass of milk. Take 6 to 8 drops twice a day for wind colic.

FENUGREEK

Foenum-graecum   Fam. Leguminosae

It grows in the south of France and has a straight stem; the leaves are petiolate, oblong-ovate and serrated; the flowers are yellow and give way to long, narrow, curved pods containing yellow seeds with an unusual smell and a very bitter taste. Fenugreek blooms in July and August. A third of its weight consists of mucilage; 1 teaspoon (1 gram) of seed turns 2 tablespoons (16 grams) of water into slime when heated. A poultice can be prepared from the milled seed, which is an excellent remedy for swellings, callouses, ulcers, etc. There is no other remedy which has such a painless dissolvent effect as the poultice made from fenugreek. Taken internally, it is a mild laxative: use 1 sugarspoon of seed for 1 cup of tea; leave to boil for ten minutes. This decoction is also highly recommended for phlegm in the chest and as a gargle for throat infections; it is also a good gargle for croup. Take 1 tablespoon of the decoction every hour. In the case of stomach ulcers and mucous stomach, 1 tablespoon fenugreek tea should be taken every two hours.

FEVERFEW

Pyrethrum parthenium   Fam. Compositae
Common Pellitory

This perennial, herbaceous plant can be found on the edge of woodlands, on stony wastelands, on old walls and rubbish tips and grows about two feet in height. The lower part of the stem is bare, the upper part covered in soft hairs; the leaves are yellow-green and also hairy. The flowers, which are yellow inside, grow in racemes on the stem terminals. The flowering period is June to July. While in bloom, the plant exudes a strong, unpleasant chamomile-like smell. Since it has a bitter taste, it is not used very much any more. The root is used for hysterical complaints and menstrual disorders. For paralysis of the tongue, a piece of root should be chewed. The decoction contains 2½ to 4½ teaspoons (4 to 10 grams) per 2 cups (½ liter) boiling water.

FIELD SCABIOUS

Kanutia arvensis   Fam. Compositae

Field scabious is a perennial plant with a hollow, hairy stem. It has a short, apparently broken off root like that of devil's-bit scabious. The leaves, which are opposite and decussate and unserrated, have large terminal lobes and small side lobes. The whole plant is hairy; the pale blue flowers have long stems and grow singly. The flowering period is June to July. Field scabious is very commonly found along roadsides, in meadows and woodlands. It has no smell; its sap is a little bitter, astringent, stimulates the appetite and dissolves mucus. The whole plant is used medicinally. The decoction contains ¼ to ⅓ cup (10 to 15 grams) per 2 cups (½ liter) boiling water. Take 1 to 2 cups daily as necessary. It is a useful remedy for epilepsy, internal ulcers, tonsillitis and ulcers.

FINE-LEAVED WATER DROPWORT (POISON)

Oenanthe phellandrium   Fam. Umbelliferae

This perennial water plant has a tall, widely-branched, grooved, hollow stem with pinnate leaves with small, short lobes. The flowers bloom from July to September and are white, and form short-petiolate umbels. The fruits are black-red with an aromatic taste; the thick, white root has a sharp smell; the sap is bitter. The seed is used medicinally for consumption, chronic lung catarrh and disorders of the respiratory organs. Use ⅛ teaspoon (20 centigrams) of the powdered seed. The infusion contains ½ teaspoon (1 gram) per 2 cups (½ liter) boiling water. One should remember that the plant is poisonous and certainly never take more than the prescribed dose.

FLIXWEED

Sisymbrium sophia   Fam. Cruciferae

This is a biennial plant with ascendant, branched, hairy stems and finely divided, soft-haired leaves with pinnate leaflets. The small, yellow-green flowers appear from May to October. The petals do not grow above the calyx. The fruit racemes are long, growing on widely separated, flimsy stems with curved pods; the seeds are flat-oval and brown. Flixweed grows on sandy soil and wasteland; it has a bitter, astringent taste, similar to that of mustard. When placed on sores, the freshly crushed fruit heals them; even old, deep-rooted ulcers are cured. Internally, the decoction 4 to 8 teaspoons (5 to 10 grams) per 2 cups (½ liter) water is given for blood-spitting and severe bleeding from piles; while the powdered seed, 3 teaspoons (3 grams) daily taken in wine, is of benefit for diarrhea and dysentery.

FOXGLOVE (POISON)

Digitalis purpurea   Fam. Scrophulariaceae

This herbaceous, extremely poisonous, biennial plant can be found growing wild in woods and on mountainous, stony, ground. It has a gray-green stem and the purple-red flowers somewhat resemble a thimble and hang like bells on one side of the stem. The radical leaves are fairly large, oblong-ovate, crenate and long-petiolate; the stem leaves are narrower and shorter-petiolate. Although this plant contains a strong poison, it is still a potent medicine and widely used in the treatment of heart complaints and dropsy caused as a result of it. The leaves can be used for this purpose but beware of trying it. Only a physician can prescribe the treatment since too large a dose can cause paralysis of the heart.

FRANKINCENSE

Olibanum, Olibanum Gum   Fam. Burseraceae

Incense is the gum of the *Pinus sylvestris* (the fir tree). This gum strengthens the chest. Take 4 to 6 grains of incense daily.

FUMITORY

Fumaria officinalis   Fam. Fumariaceae

Fumitory is an annual, very wispy plant with quadrangular stems. It attains a height of about 20 inches (50 centimeters), grows in gardens, roadsides and on farmland, especially corn-fields. It flowers from May to October. The leaves are small, pinnate, and an ash-gray color. The small red flowers grow in racemes on the stem terminals. The plant is harvested during the flowering period. It is a depurative remedy and very effective in the treatment of eczema, crusta lactea in children, scrofulous complaints, swollen liver and jaundice. It is also recommended for hypochondria, melancholy, smallpox, scurvy, intestinal blockages, disorders of the spleen and to bring out scarlet fever quickly. Drink 1 to 2 cups of tea per day. The infusion consists of 4 to 5 tablespoons (15 to 25 grams) per 2 cups (½ liter) boiling water.

GALANGAL

Alpinia officinarum   Fam. Zingaberaceae/Scilaminae

Galangal is cultivated in the gardens of eastern India. There are two kinds commercially available—large and small. Only the latter is used medicinally. The root has the thickness of a small finger, is completely brown both inside and out and has a sharp, pleasant taste. Finely powdered galangal is taken as snuff for headaches caused by congestion of the head, for toothaches caused by watery swelling, also for catarrh of the head and nose. Galangal powder has an excellent dissolvent effect and is also recommended for ozena. Eye infections, particularly burning eyes, are sometimes cured by sniffing a little of this white powder twice a day. It is recommended for all eye complaints.

GARDEN BALSAM

Impatiens balsamina   Fam. Balsaminaceae

This plant comes from India and is frequently grown in gardens on account of its pleasant fragrance. It is a perennial, shrublike plant with erect stems to a height of 3 feet (1 meter) with many oblong, dentate, rather large, pale green leaves. The flowers are small and grow on the stem terminals. The flowering period is from June to September. The leaves are gathered before the flowering period. Balsam is recommended for hysteria and nervous complaints in general.

GARLIC

Allium sativum   Fam. Liliaceae

Garlic is a potent, stimulating stomachic; it facilitates the digestion of heavy, slimy food and disperses wind. A simple method of getting rid of the unpleasant smell it causes is to chew on some parsley or chervil. Three garlic onions boiled in 1 cup milk or sugar and water and then taken is an excellent vermifugal remedy, especially for maggots; 2½ teaspoons (20 grams) of garlic sap in 1 cup (200 grams) warm milk, taken in the morning on an empty stomach, expels the worms. A clove of garlic taken every morning cures gout. People with skin complaints, eczema, etc., should not take garlic; nursing mothers should likewise refrain from garlic. When used externally, garlic is an efficacious remedy for scurf. Garlic sap should be mixed with unsalted butter and honey and smeared on the affected areas twice a day. Garlic is highly recommended to those suffering from scrofula. When boiled in milk it expels kidney and bladder stones.

GARLIC MUSTARD

Alliaria officinalis   Fam. Cruciferae

Garlic mustard,[4] so called because the bruised leaves smell of garlic, is a biennial, herbaceous plant, abundantly found under old hedges, in woods, along roadsides and in shady places. It attains a height of 2½ to 3 feet (80 to 90 centimeters), generally has a round, branched, pale-green stem. The radical leaves are rather large, long-petiolate, irregularly dentate; the stem leaves are short-petiolate and heart-shaped. The white flowers grow in racemes on the stem terminals. The seeds are oblong, black and lengthways striped. Although the plant has an unpleasant

---

[4] We were unable to locate this herb.

smell, animals are fond of eating it. It flowers from April to June. This plant is used medicinally for scurvy; it strengthens the gums and tightens the teeth. In cases of the above mentioned complaints, the fresh herb can be chewed and then discarded; this should be done frequently if successful results are desired. The dried plant is also used as a diuretic in cases where it is necessary to increase the flow of urine. The infusion contains ¼ ounce (15 grams) per 2 cups (½ liter) boiling water; it is also a well known remedy for asthma as it is a particularly good phlegm dissolvent; in addition, for chronic catarrh, scurvy, and internal, cancer-like ulceration. Freshly bruised leaves can be applied on eczema.

GERMANDER-SPEEDWELL

Veronica chamaedrys   Fam. Scrophulariaceae

This is a perennial plant with a creeping rootstock, usually with an unbranched stem and ovate, hairy, coarsely crenulated leaves, lanceolate at the base. The blue flowers appear from April through June in relatively large racemes. This plant is found in woodland and hedgerows. The infusion contains ⅓ cup (15 grams) per 2 cups (½ liter) boiling water. Take 1 to 2 cups daily for asthma, chest complaints, chronic catarrh, especially for phlegm in the chest, spitting blood, dry coughs, migraine, dizziness, mucus, lung ulcers, consumption, skin complaints and eczema.

GERMANDER (WATER)

Teucrium scordium   Fam. Labiatae

This perennial plant, with creeping, fibrous roots and branch-like, quadrangular, hairy stems, has pale-green, ovate, coarsely serrated large, hairy, soft leaves. The small reddish flowers grow in a spike in the axils of the bracts. The smell resembles that of garlic, the sap is hot and bitter. The decoction, containing ½ to ¾ cup (15 to 20 grams) per 2 cups (½ liter) boiling water, is used for fevers, blockage of spleen and liver, and mucus in the lungs.

GLABROUS RUPTURE WORT

Herniaria glabra   Fam. Caryophyllaceae
Burstwort

Only two varieties of this plant grow in the wild. It is annual with decumbent stems which are very branched and which spread along the ground, one above the other. The yellow-green leaves are very small, strongly resemble those of thyme, and grow opposite at the base of the stems. There are numerous very small flowers growing along the whole stem; the sepals are green on the outside and yellow-green on the inside. The fruit contains only one glossy grain of seed. The glabrous rupture wort grows especially on dry sandy ground and heath and on wasteland, sometimes also along the verges of roads and water. It has a small root and bitter-sour, salty sap. It blooms from May to October.

This plant has very astringent properties and is highly recommended for kidney stones, gravel, hernias, bladder complaints, jaundice, and mucous stomach; it expels excessive gall, helps urination, cures internal and external sores and breaks up stones. The infusion consists of ⅓ to ⅔ cup (15 to 25 grams) per 2 cups (½ liter) boiling water. Take 1 to 2 cups daily, depending on the circumstances. The powdered plant is particularly used for kidney stones and gravel: 3 to 4 teaspoons (3 to 4 grams) should be steeped in white wine for several days and this quantity taken daily.

GOAT'S RUE

Galega officinalis   Fam. Leguminosae

Goat's rue is a perennial and indigenous to southern Europe, where it grows in damp, swampy areas. In our country, it is found in gardens. It attains a height of a good meter (3 feet), has many grooved, branched stems, long, lanceolate leaves bearing a soft thorn or prickle at the tip. The blue or lilac flowers stand above the stems in dense petiolate racemes. The seed is contained in narrow 2 inch (5 centimeter) long pods, the valves of which are striped in the most unusual way. The smooth, white roots are spread out. The flowering period is June to August. The sap which is extracted is highly recommended for falling sickness and worms; use 1 tablespoon per day.

The leaves should be gathered before the flowers open; 4 handsful of fresh leaves should be pounded in a china mortar and placed in a bottle of white wine (Mosel or Rhine). Let it steep for six days in a warm place, then filter and store for use in a well-corked bottle. A wineglass may be taken every morning for a year, with intervals of three months, for epilepsy.

GOLDENROD

Solidago virgaurea   Fam. Compositae

This is a perennial herbaceous plant that grows in woods and on mountains. Its stem is red, smooth, angular, more or less curved and attains a height of 3 feet (1 meter). The leaves are smooth, narrow, acute, pale-green, serrated and have an astringent, bitter taste. The upper part of the stem divides into branches on which grow yellow flowers, densely clustered, forming a long spike. The flowering period is August and September.

The infusion of this plant, ¼ to ⅓ cup (10 to 15 grams) per 2 cups (½ liter) boiling water is used externally as a gargle and is highly recommended for throat infections and ulceration of the throat. Immediate gargling with this remedy also cures an ulcerated mouth and tightens loose teeth. Take 2 to 3 cups of tea every day for fistulas, throat infections, neck complaints, croup, bladder and kidney complaints, blocked spleen, jaundice, dropsy, old sores, blood-spitting, diarrhea, rotting gums, dysentry, scrofula, asthma, swelling, insomnia, coughing, chronic catarrh with much expectoration, chronic pain in the side, back pain, diabetes, stones. For stones, three handfuls should be placed in a bottle of white wine and 2 wineglasses should be taken daily; this breaks up and expels the stones.

Sores can be healed by the application of freshly bruised leaves. Goldenrod cannot be recommended highly enough for kidney complaints; when there is no hope left, the infusion of this plant could still help. Women in confinement, who are unable to urinate properly following the birth, are greatly relieved by a few cups of this tea.

Good King Henry

Chenopodium Bonus Henricus   Fam. Chenopodiaceae
Goosefoot

Good King Henry is a perennial, herbaceous plant with an erect stem. Branches shoot from the axils of leaf rosettes. The leaves are triangular-lanceolate, with a smooth edge; the green flowers form a spike or raceme on the stem terminals. The plant is very widely spread on wasteland. The flowering period is May to August. The whole plant (especially the root which has the greatest potency) has a palliative, cleansing, solvent effect. The fresh, pounded herb is very useful for infections, sores, skin eruptions and ulcerations. The bruised herb relieves the pain of gout most wonderously; it should be boiled and applied as a poultice.

Gooseberry Bush

Ribes grossularia   Fam. Grossulariaceae

It can be recognized by its thorns and its white blossoms, clustered in twos or threes. The patch-like leaves are cut and serrated, the berries round or oval-round. They are red, yellow or white, hairy or hairless. It is found in almost every garden. The delicious fruit is very nourishing and excellent wine and vinegar can be prepared from it. People with acid stomachs should not eat gooseberries. It is highly recommended for those suffering from involuntary seminal discharge or leukorrhea; it also stimulates the appetite.

GOOSEGRASS

Galium aparine   Fam. Rubiaceae
Clivers

This annual herbaceous plant has long, quadrangular, creeping stems; the lanceolate leaves have prickles around the edge whereby they easily stick to clothing. The greenish-white flowers grow in three-forked inflorescences; the fruit is also covered in white prickles. The sap is sour-bitter and the plant is scentless. Stems and leaves are used medicinally and are highly recommended for lymphatic, scrofulous persons, for scurvy, kidney and bladder stones. The bruised plant can be applied with success for skin complaints, psoriasis, eczema, stubborn ulceration, scrofulous sores, even cancer sores and syphilis. The decoction of the dried plant is 1½ to 3 cups (20 to 40 grams) per 2 cups (½ liter) boiling water and, when applied in the form of a compress, has the same effect as the freshly bruised plant. In addition, take a daily cup of tea from the decoction of the dried plant, consisting of 1 to 1½ cups (15 to 20 grams) per 2 cups (½ liter) boiling water for all the illnesses mentioned above. The powdered, dried plant is also a very good remedy for sores and ulcerations. The sores should be sprinkled with it four to six times a day. Drinking 1 cup goosegrass tea daily is an excellent remedy for pain in the chest and side, and is also highly recommended for jaundice and dropsy.

GRAPEVINE

Vitis vinifera   Fam. Vitaceae

The grapevine belongs to the climbing plants; it comes from Asia and is now cultivated throughout almost the whole of Europe. It grows in the wild in the south of France, on the upper Rhine and along the Danube. Fruit, leaves, wood and sap are all used medicinally. The ripe, fresh fruit with its delicious juice is refreshing and nourishing, stimulates the appetite and is a mild purgative. Wine is prepared from it. White wine stimulates the appetite. It is frequently used in this book in decoctions with herbs (for kidney stones, gravel, etc.). Red wine causes less headache than white wine; when taken in moderation wine is generally invigorating, stimulating and good for the digestion. Immoderate use is very injurious and causes strokes, paralysis, gout, rheumatism and kidney disorders. Wine is recommended for illnesses caused by weakness, indigestion and for convalescents. Fresh vine leaves are very astringent and refreshing. The decoction is taken internally for dysentery, vomiting and blood-spitting. The sap from the wood stimulates the appetite and is beneficial in the treatment of gravel and kidney stones; it is also a tonic eyewash, especially for inflammation of the eyes.

GREAT BURNET

Sanguisorba officinalis   Fam. Rosaceae

Great burnet has a creeping root, an angular, grooved stem, divided, acute, dentate leaves and oblong-oval fruit. The flowers, which appear in June and July, are white or reddish. This perennial plant is scattered over hills and under hedges. Its root has an aromatic fragrance, it tastes sharp and hot. This root is used medicinally as a stimulant.

Salad burnet, *Poterium sanguisorba*, is an herbaceous, perennial plant. It is found all over Europe in wet meadows, along roadsides, etc. The leaves are both divided and ovate, short-toothed leaflets which are sometimes also double divided. The stem is round, the upper part leafless, or at least the leaves have not developed. The flowering period is June and July. The root is used medicinally; it is gathered in September. The decoction contains 4 teaspoons to 2 tablespoons (7 to 15 grams) per 2 cups (½ liter) water. The tincture is prepared by steeping 4 tablespoons (30 grams) coarsely crushed burnet root in 1 quart (liter) 75% alcohol for eight days. Take 20 to 60 drops daily for extremely weak intestines, indigestion with wind, mucous stomach and intestines, humid asthma, chronic rheumatism and weak menstruation. The herb of both burnets is highly recommended as a decoction, 3 to 4 tablespoons (20 to 30 grams) per 2 cups (½ liter) water, as one of the best remedies for heavy bleeding. In Spain it is eaten as a salad.

GREATER CELANDINE (POISON)

Chelidonium majus   Fam. Papaveraceae

The greater celandine is a well-known perennial herbaceous plant, which is commonly found in moist, shady places. It has several pale-green, round stems, very brittle and knotted, containing gold-colored sap with a very unpleasant smell. The yellow flowers grow on the stem terminals. It blooms through out almost the whole summer. The herb should be gathered in May; the root in April. The greater celandine is a poisonous plant.

Internally, an infusion of the fresh plant or the root is used: ⅓ cup (5 grams) per 2 cups (½ liter) boiling water. This quantity should be taken within twenty-four hours for liver and spleen complaints and especially for dropsy. The infusion with wine is more potent; ⅔ to 1⅓ cups (12 to 20 grams) of the fresh plant should be used per bottle of wine. Take 3 or 4 tablespoons daily for the complaints mentioned above, also for constipation and bladder complaints. Or, use 1 to 4 teaspoons (1 to 4 grams) of the sap mixed with honey or sugar for the same effect. It can be boiled with sugar and stored for winter use.

The sap or freshly pounded plant applied to scrofulous tumors makes them soon disappear. Eczema is sometimes cured by means of this when all other remedies fail. Greater celandine powder cures old sores and fistulas if it is sprinkled on them. For eye-spots and dark sight, ¼ cup (60 grams) greater celandine sap should be boiled for a few minutes with 2 teaspoons (15 grams) honey until it has been thoroughly skimmed; a little should be placed in the eyes twice a day.

The freshly bruised herb can be applied on piles. A tincture can be prepared from the freshly squeezed roots and herb by adding an equal quantity of alcohol to the sap; this should be stored in a well-corked bottle. Take 5 drops per day in a glass of water, or according to the circumstances, take 5 drops two or three times per day, but *never more*. This is a recommended remedy for suppressed menstruation, also consumption (even when in an advanced stage), chronic syphilis, intermittent fever, painful urination, burning in the bladder, constipation, earache, ringing in the ears, gallstones, complaints of the liver and stomach, gout, disorders of the spleen and piles. The fresh sap gets rid of warts.

GROMWELL

Lithospermum officinale   Fam. Boraginaceae

Gromwell is a perennial, herbaceous plant with a much branched, rough stem; the leaves are narrow, oblong, obovate; the small flowers are yellowish-white. The root is thick and fleshy, and it flowers from May to July. Gromwell grows on sandy farmland, on stony soil, in woodlands and along roadsides. The whole plant can be used for medicinal purposes. The decoction, ½ cup (15 grams) per 2 cups (½ liter) white wine, is highly praised for kidney stones. A wineglassful should be taken every morning on an empty stomach. One can also take 4 teaspoons (4 grams) powdered gromwell seed daily in white wine to break up the stone.

GROUND IVY

Glechoma hederacea   Fam. Labiatae

Ground ivy is a commonly known, perennial, herbaceous plant held in little esteem, but which has very valuable properties. It grows in shady places, in woodlands, under hedges and on rubbish tips. It has relatively long, creeping, quadrangular stems. The leaves are a beautiful color green, round and lightly dentate. The flowers are blue and grow in the leaf axils. One only needs to touch the plant for it to exude a rather pleasant, strong smell. The sap is bitter and sour. In April, ground ivy is in full bloom and is then gathered. The whole plant is used medicinally as a mucus dissolvent. It is particularly used for chronic catarrh and lung complaints. The infusion consists of ¼ to ⅓ cup (10 to 15 grams) per 2 cups (½ liter) boiling water and is recommended for consumption, blood-spitting, diarrhea and a bad stomach.

The fresh sap of the plant, 3 to 4 tablespoons (20 to 30 grams) daily is even more powerful. Ground ivy infusion is used *internally* for coughs, ulceration of the kidneys, cysts and scrofulous ulcers. It is used both *internally* and *externally* for worms, chest and lung ulceration, asthma and hematuria. Take 1 cup daily. The infusion sniffed or sprayed up the nose is very effective for migraines; the most severe headache is cured by this simple remedy.

GROUND PINE

Ajuga chamaepitys   Fam. Labiatae
Yellow Bugle

This hairy, gland-shaped, rather colorful, annual plant, with stems that spread from the rootstock all over the ground, has dentate, opposite leaves and yellow flowers, growing singly or in pairs in the axils of the leaves, which are much larger than the flowers. The flowering period is June to September. It is found on poor, sandy wasteland. The herb has a bitter taste and is used, above all, internally to prevent strokes, for the treatment of epilepsy, dizziness, brain disorders, blood-spitting and jaundice. Boil ½ to ⅔ cup (10 to 12 grams) in 2 cups (½ liter) white wine. The decoction in water is efficacious for the treatment of hematuria, weak nerves, podagra, dysentery, leukorrhea, difficult urination, asthma, lung ulcers, kidney complaints, sore throats. It is depurative. Good results can be obtained by the application of bruised leaves to sores. When boiled in apple vinegar, the herb can be used in the form of compresses for the treatment of sciatica.

GROUNDSEL

Senecio vulgaris   Fam. Compositae

An annual, herbaceous plant which grows in all vegetable gardens as a weed, it has oblong, pinnatified leaves, yellow-green, and very small florets on the stem terminals and branches. The decoction is used for epilepsy: take ¼ to ⅓ cup (10 to 15 grams) per 2 cups (½ liter) water. The sap extracted is beneficial in the treatment of worms, liver blockage, gravel, stones, suppressed menstruation, jaundice and scurvy; it is also a good depurative. When boiled, the flowers can be applied to the stomach region in cases of stomachache. One can take ⅛ to ¼ cup (40 to 60 grams) of the sap daily in spoonsful. If more of this sap is taken, it causes vomiting. If one takes ¼ cup (60 grams) of sap on an empty stomach, it is good for pain in the loins. Externally, the bruised herb mixed with incense and a little wine can be applied to burning swellings, the anus or genital organs. It can be applied on sores without the wine or mixed with lard.

Gum Arabic

Acacia senegal   Fam. Leguminosae

Gum arabic is the sap from various kinds of acacia trees, found in different parts of Arabia, Africa, etc. Gum arabic is used internally for spasmodic, painful complaints of the stomach and intestines, caused by sharp matter, acid, poison, or inflammation of the throat, thrush, ulcers in the mouth and split nipples. In cases of bleeding, the powder should be sprinkled on the wounds.

Hare's Ear

Bupleurum rotundifolium   Fam. Umbelliferae
Thoroughwax

This rather rare plant is an annual. It may be found in fields amidst the corn, on sandy ground and roadside verges. It has a branched stem; the small yellow flowers are clustered in racemes on the stem terminals and produce black, oblong grains of seed, grouped in pairs. The leaves are ovate or nearly round, smooth-edged, petiolate, as though the leaf stem had pierced the leaf. The plant was formerly used as an excellent remedy for sores and still deserves fame as such. It is also effective for scrofulous tumors; the fresh plant should be bruised and placed on the scrofulous tumor, which it will dissolve. In addition, hernias and protruding navels in children can be cured by means of this remedy; a little wine and flour should be added to it and applied as a poultice.

HARE'S FOOT CLOVER

Trifolium arvense　　　　　　　　　　　　Fam. Leguminosae
Hare's Foot Trefoil

This annual, herbaceous plant has a hairy, branched stem, 4 to 7 inches (1 to 2 decimeters) high, very narrow, lanceolate, hairy leaves and short-petiolate, pale pink flowers that resemble the feet of rabbits. The seed is small and round; the taproot woody, fibrous, twisted and white. The plant is found on grassy, sandy soil and cornfields. The flowering period is August to September. The leaves and stems are gathered during the flowering period. The infusion, ¾ to 1 cup (15 to 20 grams) per 2 cups (½ liter) boiling water, or, still better, wine, is useful for diarrhea, sore throats, hernia, dysentery and heavy menstruation. Take 1 glass of wine decoction or 1 cup tea daily in two doses.

HARICOT BEAN

Phaseolus vulgans　　　　　　　　　　　　Fam. Leguminosae

Haricot bean pods, like all varieties of beans, are an excellent diuretic. The decoction contains ⅛ cup (15 grams) per 2 cups (½ liter) water and is recommended for kidney complaints and dropsy. When the pods are thoroughly cooked, the decoction should be applied as hot as possible on ulcerated fingers, especially whitlow. Haircot beans ground to flour are excellent for eczema on the face; first smear the area well with lard and then sprinkle with bean powder. If this is done three times a day, the results will be amazing. Haricot beans boiled with milk are excellent when applied lukewarm to swollen breasts and glands (three times a day), especially if the glands are inflamed. In my opinion, the following remedy is the best for dropsy: boil haricot bean pods with an equal quantity of inner rind of elder, a handful in 1 quart (liter) water, until reduced by half; then add ½ sugarspoon of saltpeter and drink this throughout the day.

Hart's Tongue Fern

Scolopendrium vulgare   Fam. Filices

Hart's tongue grows in Italy, France, and Germany in shady, stony places, and is cultivated here and there in gardens. The beautiful, glossy green leaves grow from the rootstock on long, hairy stems; they are long, narrow and acute. The edges are smooth and heart or tongue-shaped; under the leaves, there are broad, brown lines, containing the plant seed. It has no smell, but an astringent taste, is perennial and has no stems. The decoction of the leaves, ¾ to 1 cup (15 to 20 grams) per 2 cups (½ liter) water, is a very pleasant drink and can be used with success for liver and spleen complaints, lung and bladder complaints, blood-spitting, dysentery, gravel and especially scurvy. Take 1 cup of tea daily. Compresses of the decoction can be applied externally to ulceration.

Hawthorn

Crataegus oxyacantha   Fam. Rosaceae

The hawthorn is a very common, shrub-like plant, which is often used in hedges. The leaves are smooth-edged, although sometimes also serrated or deeply lobed. The flowers are usually white, although there is one variety with pink flowers. They bloom in May and June. The flowers grow in the leaf-axils and have a very pleasant smell. Flowering is followed by the appearance of green fruit which, when fully ripe, are red throughout. This fruit is used medicinally for leukorrhea. Take 2 sugarspoons of fruit to make a cup of tea which can be taken daily for this complaint. The flowers are recommended for obesity. The infusion contains ½ to ¾ cup (8 to 10 grams) per 2 cups (½ liter) boiling water; 1 cup should be taken daily.

Hayseed (Hay Residue)

Semen herbae   Fam. Gramineae

Hayseed is taken here to signify the residue from hay: flowers, leaves, seed, stems, weeds—everything remaining after the hay has been removed. It is used externally for baths and compresses. The decoction consists of a good handful of hayseed per quart (liter) water. Hayseed compresses are recommended for skin rashes, eczema, scarlet fever, measles, chronic stomach complaints, ulcers, blood poisoning, liver complaints, indigestion, kidney complaints, etc. Hot baths of hayseed can also be taken: full baths, half-baths, footbaths, arm-baths, etc. In cases of blood poisoning or paralysis, where speed is essential, it is preferable to pour boiling water over a quantity of hayseed, let it steep for ten minutes, and bind the hayseed itself around the affected limbs; it should be applied fairly thickly and covered with linen and woolen cloths. The patient should retire to bed. The compress should be renewed after one to one and a half hours. Note: For a compress, take linen cloths folded double three or four times. After a hot bath, the patient should always take a cold wash. See water applications, in Part III.

Hazel Catkins

Flor. Corylus avellana   Fam. Betulaceae

These are the male flowers of the hazel tree. They are long, full, hanging catkins which grow in groups of three or more on young branches. They have a medicinal use. They are gathered in the flowering period, dried and stored in a dry place. The infusion contains ¼ to ⅓ cup (8 to 10 grams) per 2 cups (½ liter) boiling water. This is an excellent remedy for pneumonia; in particular, it causes sweating. It is also highly recommended for influenza. Taking 1 cup of this infusion is sometimes sufficient for thorough sweating. A Princess once wrote to me as follows, "My six children were cured from influenza in a few days by tea from hazel catkins. The sweat broke out after one cup. With gratitude, V.V."

HEARTSEASE

Viola tricolor   Fam. Violaceae
Wild Pansy

Heartsease is an annual plant and has much in common with the pansy that is grown in gardens, but its leaves, stems and flowers are smaller. It is commonly found in meadowland; it is in bloom almost the whole summer. The infusion consists of 1¼ to 2½ cups (20 to 40 grams) per 2 cups (½ liter) boiling water and is used for skin complaints. It is given to children for crusta lactea: 4 teaspoons to ½ cup (2 to 6 grams) per 2 cups (½ liter) milk. The crusts disappear after a few weeks. A little fennel powder should be added.

Too large a dose causes vomiting but can do no harm. It is particularly efficacious in the treatment of convulsions, glandular complaints, scrofula, crusta lactea, Guinea worm, scurf, eczema, asthma, fever, intestinal inflammation; it is also a diuretic, diaphoretic, purgative, and depurative. The decoction can be used externally with great success in the form of compresses on all skin complaints, especially crusta lactea in children. A handful should be used per 4 cups (1 liter) milk, without the addition of sugar or fennel powder. When used externally, 1 cup of tea made from the milk described above should be taken with fennel powder and sugar. Or take 3 to 4 teaspoons (3 to 4 grams) of the powder daily in honey.

HEATHER

Calluna vulgaris   Fam. Ericaceae
Ling

Heather is a well-known perennial evergreen shrub. Its twisted branches bear pale-green sessile leaves, growing opposite and decussate, close to the wood in four rows. The flowers are red-purple, sometimes white and nearly sessile; they produce large beans. The plant covers extensive areas, usually infertile sandy ground. The whole plant has astringent properties. The decoction is recommended as a wash for gout. The infusion of the flowers, ½ to ⅔ cup (15 to 20 grams) per 2 cups (½ liter) boiling water, is good for pain in the side, abdominal pain and bladder catarrh. Drink 1 cup of tea daily.

HEDGE BEDSTRAW

Galium molugo   Fam. Rubiaceae

Hedge bedstraw is a perennial plant with a quadrangular, pliant, much-branched stem. The flower stems are thicker than in other varieties of bedstraw and spread in all directions, supported by surrounding objects. The white flowers open wide. The plant can be found in the edge of woodland, in thickets, etc. The infusion, containing ⅓ to ½ cup (10 to 15 grams) per 2 cups (½ liter) boiling water, is used for stomachache, hysteria and epilepsy.

HEDGE HYSSOP (POISON)

Gratiola officinalis   Fam. Scrophulariaceae

This is a perennial herbaceous plant, found in moist places, meadows and heaths. It flowers from June to August. The flowers are yellow-red and grow in the leaf-axils. The lower part of the stem is round, the upper part quadrangular, unbranched and hollow. The leaves grow opposite and decussate, are sessile, lanceolate, serrated; the white root is decumbent. The plant flower heads are picked in June. The decoction containing no more then 5 to 7 teaspoons (3 to 4 grams) per 2 cups (½ liter) boiling water, must not be taken any stronger, as it would then be poisonous. It can be successfully used for dropsy, gout, intermittent fever, and worms.

For jaundice, take 2 teaspoons (1 gram) powdered leaves per day. It is also useful for chronic liver and spleen complaints, hypochrondia, scrofula, chronic rheumatism, skin complaints and syphilis. The decoction contains only 4 to 7 teaspooons (2 to 4 grams) per 2 cups (½ liter) boiling water; but a little sugar may always be added. Hedge hyssop is also a drastic purgative.

HEDGE MUSTARD

Sisybrium officinale   Fam. Cruciferae
English Watercress

Hedge mustard is an annual, herbaceous plant. Its ascendant
stem has wide-spread branches; the leaves are pinnate, rough,
with two or three pairs of irregularly dentate, oblong side-lobes
and a round, irregularly cut terminal lobe. The small, yellow
flowers bloom from May to October. It can be found in abundance along roadsides, in dry meadows and on wasteland. It
bears flat, brown, oval seeds. The whole plant is used medicinally for chest and throat complaints, lung catarrh, chronic
coughing, chronic hoarseness, asthma, phlegm in the chest,
jaundice. The decoction of the plant, which should be gathered
in June at the beginning of the flowering period, contains ½
cup (20 to 25 grams) per 2 cups (½ liter) water. Take 1 sugarspoonful powdered seed with honey three times a day.

HEDGE WOUNDWORT

Stachys sylvatica   Fam. Labiatae

A perennial, herbaceous plant with a very hairy, high stem and
long leaf-stems. Hedge woundwort[5] has coarse, hairy leaves that
are sometimes blunt and sometimes acute-serrated. The corolla
stands far above the calyx, and it usually bears six flowers,
without wool, reddish-purple in color, with whitish, wavy stripes
on the lower lip and a narrow tube, the same width throughout.
The smell is strong and unpleasant, the taste bitter. It is found
in woods and hedgerows. The flowering period is from July to
August. The flowers and leaves are gathered during this period.
The infusion for *external* use consists of ¼ to ⅓ ounce (15 to
30 grams) per quart (liter) of water and may be fruitfully applied in the form of compresses for burns. For *internal* use, the
infusion is ¼ ounce (12 grams) per quart (liter) water. It is used
for colic, scrofulous tumors, and to promote menstruation.

---

[5]We were unable to locate this herb.

HEMP AGRIMONY (POISON)

Eupatorium cannabinum   Fam. Compositae
Water Hemp

This perennial is easily recognized by its light red, small, cylindrical flower heads. The tall, branched stem, usually red, can be 3 feet high (1 meter). The leaves are opposite, usually 3 or 5-lobed palmate, with lanceolate, bordered lobes. The flowering period is June to September. Flowers and leaves are gathered during the flowering period, the roots in September. The plant is found along riverbanks and in moist places. The infusion of flowers and leaves, and the decoction of the roots, are both used medicinally. That of the flowers and leaves is ⅓ to ½ cup (15 to 25 grams) per 2 cups (½ liter) water; that of the roots is 2 to 4 tablespoons (15 to 30 grams) per 2 cups (½ liter) water. Take ⅓ cup (15 grams) per 2 cups (½ liter) water, reduce to one third, strain, add sugar and take 1 cup per day in two doses.

    The root decoction is a mild purgative, that of the flowers and leaves is a powerful remedy for hysteria, blockage of the liver, spleen and gall bladder, internal sores and injuries, cough, chronic catarrh, dropsy and worms. For worms take 2 to 2½ tablespoons (15 to 20 grams) sap with ¼ cup (60 grams) honeywater. For dropsy, compresses of the infusion should be placed on the swollen limbs; the same applies to liver and spleen complaints. Hemp agrimony boiled to a paste cures hydrocele and swollen testicles, if this poultice is applied three times a day.

HEMP, INDIAN (POISON)

Cannabis sativa   Fam. Urticaceae
Cannabis

Hemp is an annual plant cultivated here and there in our country. Its stem is coarse and pliant. The leaves have lanceolate, very serrated leaflets. There are two kinds of flowers. The male flowers form a small, branched raceme on the stem terminal; the female flowers, on the contrary, are clustered close together in a kind of spike which produces the so-called hemp seed. The flowering period is July and August. Hemp seed is used medicinally. The decoction consists of 3 to 4 tablespoons in 1 quart (1 liter) milk. This quantity should be drunk throughout the day to cure blockage of the liver and seminal discharge. Water is expelled by drinking 2 to 3 wineglasses per day of ¼ cup (25 grams) bruised hemp seed boiled in wine. The infusion of the leaves, ⅓ to ½ cup (15 to 20 grams) per 2 cups (½ liter) boiling water is a good remedy for chronic rheumatism and eczema.

HEMP NETTLE

Galeopsis tetrahit   Fam. Labiatae

Hemp nettle is an herbaceous, annual plant; its hairy stem has pale green, soft-haired, lanceolate or ovate, sharply serrated leaves and a pale yellow corolla. The flowering period is July to August. It is found in mountainous regions on sandy farmland in the Mosel and the Ardennes. It was formerly sold as best chest herbs, a remedy for chest complaints and consumption. It has a slimy, bitter taste and can be recommended for a cough with phlegm. The whole plant is gathered during the flowering period. The decoction consists of ¾ to 1 cup (20 to 30 grams) per 2 cups (½ liter) water, of which 2 cups should be taken daily. *Galeopsis ladanum*, hemp nettle with purple flowers, has the same action as the pale yellow hemp nettle.

HENBANE (POISON)

Hyoscyamus niger   Fam. Solanaceae

This is a poisonous, biennial plant with hairy, sticky leaves, undulating-dentate, half encompassing the stem; the dirty yellow flowers with purple veins grow on one side of the flower stem and have funnel-shaped corollas. The flowering period is June to September. The leaves are used medicinally as a narcotic. Henbane sometimes poisons animals that eat it and is therefore highly dangerous for the use of people. The plant exudes a nauseating, stupefying smell. For safety's sake, I shall not mention its good properties.

Herb Robert

Geranium Robertianum   Fam. Geraniaceae

Like all weeds, this plant grows in abundance; it is found under old hedges, on old walls and poor ground. It is an annual, red, hairy plant that attains a height of 12 to 16 inches (30 to 40 centimeters); the leaves are lightly hairy, divided and grow opposite in pairs. The flowers are a beautiful shade of pink, have five pistils and are succeeded by a hairy fruit which resembles a stork's bill. It is in bloom for a large part of the year and is gathered for medicinal use during the flowering period.

The infusion consists of ¾ to 1 cup (15 to 25 grams) per 2 cups (½ liter) boiling water and can be successfully used for jaundice and gravel; it cannot be recommended highly enough for gravel, above all. It is an efficacious remedy for dropsy and can be used with good results for dysentery, diarrhea, heavy bleeding, loss of blood, kidney disorders, colic, intermittent fever, and alleviates the pain of those suffering from cancer. Drink 1 to 2 cups daily. The boiled plant or the decoction can be applied to the bladder region in the form of compresses; it expels the water and alleviates the pain. It can be applied in the same way for fistulas, swollen breasts, glands and sore throat. The decoction can also be used as a gargle for a sore throat.

Hoary Plantain

Plantago media   Fam. Plantaginaceae

Hoary plantain has short-petiolate, elliptical, rather thick, soft-haired leaves. The flower stem is relatively long; the cylindrical spikes are not much shorter than those of the greater plantain; the white flowers have a very pleasant fragrance. The plant is usually found on sandy ground and meadowland, but it is rarer than the other varieties. It has the same properties as the other members of its family.

HOLLY

Ilex aquifolium   Fam. Aquifoliaceae

Who does not know holly with its prickly leaves which one can hardly touch without receiving scratches? It grows abundantly in woodland and hedges, and is also cultivated in gardens on account of the beauty of its evergreen leaves. As a shrub, it attains a scant height, about 3 to 6 feet (1 to 2 meters), but if it is grown as a tree, it can grow to a height of 42 to 45 feet (13 to 14 meters). The leaves, which are covered with sharp thorns on both sides, are oblong, pliant, leathery and glossy green. The white flowers grow in racemes along the stems; they are followed by red berries with a strongly purgative effect. The leaves are used medicinally. The decoction of holly, consisting of ⅓ to ½ cup (15 to 20 grams) per 2 cups (½ liter) water, is used for gout, colic and fever. Take 1 cup daily. The fruit also has a medicinal use: if 10 to 12 berries are taken, they will have a very purgative effect and are a very powerful remedy for colic. The leaves should be gathered at the beginning of the flowering period.

HONEY

Mel

Honey is produced by bees. The best is the white honey which drips of its own accord out of the honeycomb (called *schleuderhonig* in Germany). The yellow honey is obtained by squeezing the honeycombs. This has a browner color, not such a pleasant taste, is somewhat thicker than the white honey, but fully dissolves in water. It is used for intestinal blockage, jaundice, worms, etc. It is also used for respiratory complaints of an inflammatory nature, for wind, gastric ulcers, and green sickness. Honey is invigorating and depurative and gives a beautiful color. It is a recommended remedy for dangerous throat disorders; 1 sugarspoon of honey should be taken every ten minutes. If it begins to cause an aversion, it can be boiled in milk and given with a spoon.

Those who suffer from gout will do well to take 2 tablespoons honey daily. A tablespoon of honey boiled in 1 quart (1 liter) water is a good gargle for singers; it clears the voice. If some of it should be swallowed by mistake, it will do no harm. In cases of ulceration, take equal quantities of honey and pure flower, mix together well to obtain an excellent ointment. For inflammation of the respiratory organs, 3 parts honey should be briefly boiled with 1 part vinegar; the dose is 2 teaspoons to 1 tablespoon (15 to 30 grams). For mouth rinses and gargles: 2 teaspoons to 3 tablespoons (15 to 60 grams). The pain from gout is wondrously alleviated by the application of a honey plaster.

HONEYSUCKLE

Lonicera periclymenum　　　　　　　　　Fam. Caprifoliaceae
Woodbine

This shrub, which entwines itself around other objects and grows in the wild, is found in hedges, woodland and thickets. The weak stems bear opposite and decussate, ovate, short-petiolate leaves; the flowers grow abundantly in racemes on the stem terminals. They are yellow-red in color and very fragrant. For this reason, honeysuckle is cultivated in gardens. After flowering, a cluster of red berries appears at the tip of the branches.

The leaves of the plant are used medicinally: ⅛ to ¼ cup (6 to 12 grams) per 2 cups (½ liter) water for internal use. This infusion is diuretic. Use externally as a gargle for inflamed tonsils and as compresses for leg sores. This infusion also greatly stimulates the appetite. On application of the bruised herb, skin complaints are cured. The decoction of flowers, ¼ cup (10 grams) per 2 cups (½ liter) boiling water, is very beneficial for lung catarrh: use 1 tablespoon every two hours.

HOPS

Humulus lupulus　　　　　　　　　　　Fam. Urticaceae

Hop is a perennial, herbaceous plant with coarse, hard, quadrangular stems. It is commonly found in the wild and is widely cultivated in Belgium. The leaves are rather large, serrated and rough. The female flowers are a greenish-yellow and form a spike; the male flowers are much smaller and in the form of racemes. The flowering period is July to September. The female flowers are gathered in September. They have a strong, intoxicating smell, a very bitter, pleasant taste, and are used medicinally. There is also a medicinal use for the lupulin, a yellow powder found under the leafy scale of the hop fruit. Lupulin has a sedative effect, particularly on the stomach, without weakening it. The dose is 1 tablespoon (20 centigrams), mixed with an equal quantity of sugar. The infusion of the flowers contains ¾ to 1 cup (6 to 7 grams) per 2 cups (½ liter) boiling water. Hops are an excellent remedy for many illnesses: for weak digestion, abdominal blockage, worms, dropsy, scrofula, rickets, rheumatism, gout. Hops are frequently used as an antiseptic and a stomachic in the preparation of beer.

The consumption of young sprouts in the spring is highly depurative and recommended for blockage of the spleen and liver, jaundice and bronchitis. As a remedy for dropsy, boil hop leaves and flowers in wine and take a liqueur glassful three times a day. Use 1¾ cup (15 grams) to 2 cups (½ liter) wine. Lupulin is highly recommended for involuntary seminal discharge. Use 1 tablespoon (20 centigrams) with an equal quantity of sugar, and take before retiring.

HOREHOUND (BLACK)

Ballota nigra　　　　　　　　　　　　　　　　Fam. Labiatae
Stinking Horehound

This perennial plant with an erect stem and branches which stand right out, has petiolate, heart-shaped or ovate, serrated leaves; the pale purple flower with red and white veins appear in the leaf axils; the roots are fibrous. It has an unpleasant smell and the sap is hot and bitter. The flowering period is from June to September. This herb is frequently found in hedgerows, on wasteland and rough places. Medicinally, the leaves are used for hysteria, hypochondria, and worms. The infusion contains

½ to ¾ cup (15 to 25 grams) per 2 cups (½ liter) boiling water. For scurf (rash on the scalp), apply compresses of this infusion.

HOREHOUND (WHITE)

Marrubium vulgare   Fam. Labiatae

This perennial, herbaceous plant grows on sandy soil and on hills beneath old hedges. It attains a height of 2 feet (60 centimeters) and is much branched. The leaves are ovate, serrated or dentate, and wrinkled; the flower whorls are spherical, appearing in the leaf axils of the ordinary stem leaves. The stem and leaves are covered with white wool; it has a strong, aromatic smell, bitter sap and white flowers. Flowering period is May to October. The leaves and soft stems are used medicinally. White horehound should be gathered during the flowering period. The infusion consists of ⅓ to ½ cup (10 to 15 grams) per 2 cups (½ liter) boiling water and is used for nervous disorders, green sickness and blocked menstruation. It is an efficacious remedy for phlegm in the chest, abdominal blockage, has a particularly solvent effect in cases of liver and lung complaints, asthma and coughs, and is also highly recommended for jaundice. The decoction of the leaves with the addition of a little honey is very beneficial for all these complaints.

Leaves cooked in lard can be applied to scrofulous tumors, and the sap which has been extracted, mixed with honey, can be applied to ulcers and swellings. White horehound boiled in wine with the addition of honey, cleanses the womb and heals internal sores, cures suppressed menstruation, stones, gravel and wind. For skin complaints, the tea or the infusion is highly recommended in the form of compresses. The decoction mixed with honey is still most efficacious for the internal treatment of piles, blockage of the liver and spleen, asthma, consumption, womb disorders, blood-spitting, hysteria, menstrual complaints, general chronic dysentery, pituitous fever, intermittent fever, scrofula, scurvy, especially chronic catarrh, chronic pneumonia, stubborn coughs, glandular disorders, general weakness and particularly for hysteria, hypochondria and green sickness. It improves the gastric juices and stimulates the appetite. The infusion consists of ½ to ¾ cup (15 to 20 grams) per 2 cups (½ liter) water. Or, take 2 to 3 tablespoons (4 to 6 grams) of powder per day: 3 to 5 tablespoons (30 to 50 grams) of extracted sap. For internal use: use 1 to 2 cups daily.

HORSE CHESTNUT

Aesculus hippocastanum   Fam. Sapindaceae

This is an attractive, commonly known tree with a robust trunk and beautiful foliage. The branches grow opposite and decussate; the leaves are seven-lobed palmate; the flowers grow in the form of a pyramid and are pink or white, followed by the fruit called horse chestnuts. These horse chestnuts and the flowers are used medicinally. The freshly plucked flowers, steeped in 75% alcohol, are an excellent remedy for rheumatic pain; the affected area should be rubbed twice a day with this tincture. Chestnut powder, carried in a linen bag over the heart, is to be recommended for cramps; very finely powdered chestnut is an excellent snuff; this powder is also most efficacious internally for colic and cramps. The dose is 2 to 3 pinches per day. Chestnut powder, mixed with vinegar and barley meal, cures hardened breasts and dissolves the clotted milk. The powder alone is an excellent remedy for headaches and eye complaints; it should be sniffed up the nose.

HORSEMINT

Mentha sylvestris   Fam. Labiatae

This is a perennial plant, greatly resembling applemint, but distinguished by its leaves, which are oblong, acute and irregularly dentate. The pale pink flower blooms July to September. The plant can be found near water. It has a strong smell and bitter, hot sap. The leaves should be gathered before the flowering period and used medicinally in the same way as other varieties of mint.

HORSERADISH

Cochlearia armoracia   Fam. Cruciferae

Horseradish is an herbaceous, perennial plant which is frequently grown in gardens and may occasionally be found in the wild on wasteland. It has long, large leaves that are covered with stiff hairs, and attains a height of approximately 3 feet (1 meter). The numerous white flowers form racemes on the stem terminals; the root is white, long and thick; the sap is bitter and hot. The root has both culinary and medicinal uses. The root decoction contains 2 teaspoons (15 grams) per 2 cups (½ liter) water. It is highly praised as a stomachic and is useful for dropsy, chronic catarrh and gravel. Let 4 teaspoons (30 grams) fresh horseradish root seep for twenty minutes in 4 cups (1 liter) of boiling water. Take 2 cups of this daily for asthma, glands and the complaints mentioned above.

HORSETAIL

Equisetum arvense   Fam. Equisetaceae
Snake Pipes

This is an herbaceous plant, commonly found on moist, sandy farmland; its roots reach so deep down into the ground that it is a weed that is almost impossible to eradicate. It is commonly found in apple orchards; this variety deserves preference. The fertile stem, which appears early in April, is hairless, brown-red; the sterile shoots appear in May and grow to a height of 20 inches (½ meter), sometimes growing singly, at other times in dense clusters. This plant deserves an honorable place in the household medicine cupboard, and cannot be recommended highly enough. The decoction contains ¾ to 1 cup (15 to 25 grams) per 2 cups (½ liter) water.

The decoction is excellent when used internally for bladder complaints, painful bladder conditions, gravel and stones; a hot compress should also be applied to the lower part of the body. In cases of difficult urination, hot hip-baths may be taken instead of compresses. For heavy bleeding or vomiting blood, take 1 or more cups of tea. This tea can also be taken in spoonsful;

begin, for example, with 1 tablespoon every five to ten minutes and then decrease the dose gradually according to the condition of the patient. For nosebleeds, the tea should be sniffed up the nose. Externally, compresses of horsetail decoction are highly recommended for all kinds of ulceration, suppuration, or cancer sores. Horsetail is a very astringent, solvent remedy.

Hound's Tongue (poison)

Cynoglossum officinale   Fam. Boraginaceae
Rats and Mice, Gypsy Flower

This biennial, herbaceous plant is found on sandy ground and rubbish tips. The flowering period is May through July. Its thick, hairy, branched, grooved stem with long cymes are covered in leaves. The gray-green, first year radical leaves are long-petiolate, lanceolate, broad and large; those from the second year are sessile, narrow, lanceolate and much smaller. The root is brown, spindle-shaped, thick, branched, white inside and odorless. The fresh bruised leaves can be successfully used for sores, inflamed sores, ulcerations, etc. The decoction of this plant can be used externally in the form of poultices on burns, ulcers, goiter, scrofulous sores, swollen glands, and on scrofulous swellings in general. As this plant is poisonous, I shall for safety's sake say nothing about its internal use.

Houseleek

Sempervivum tectorum   Fam. Crassulaceae

This perennial, herbaceous plant is found on old walls and roofs; it is also used in gardens as an edging to flowerbeds. Houseleek is commonly found growing among stones. The red flowers appear on the stem terminals. The leaves are thick, ovate-round, hairless, form a rosette and are used medicinally; they are truly excellent for bed-wetting in children. Take a handful of houseleek leaves, boil them in 1 quart (1 liter) of sweet milk, then add sufficient tartar for the milk to begin to curdle. This decoction should be taken in cupfuls throughout the day. Children are sometimes cured of this complaint after taking 1, 2, or 3 quarts (liters). They should also be given dry food in the evening for several days. A few drops of freshly extacted houseleek sap placed in the ears every day helps deafness.

Crushed houseleek applied to damaged nipples is an excellent pain reliever and recovery soon follows. The same remedy can be successfully used for painful piles; the pain here also disappears almost immediately. Houseleek sap is always a comfort to burning eyes. The following gargle is recommended for throat complaints and inflammation of the throat. Take 1 tablespoon houseleek sap mixed with ⅓ cup (100 grams) water and 1 tablespoon honey. Houseleek mixed with walnut oil is a good remedy for burns, scurf and corrosive ulcers. Houseleek sap mixed with vinegar is very good for inflammation of the liver; it should be applied in the form of compresses. Houseleek sap mixed with lard is very good for eczema and chapped hands. The sap alone, in the form of a mouthwash, cures thrush. Mix 3 tablespoons (30 grams) houseleek sap with ¼ cup (60 grams) blessed thistle sap. Add 1 tablespoon (8 grams) sugar. Take 1 tablespoon every two hours for high fevers.

HYSSOP

Hyssopus officinalis   Fam. Labiatae

Hyssop is an herbaceous, perennial plant that grows wild in the south of France and is cultivated in our gardens on account of its good properties. The leaves are oblong and acute, the flowers form a spike on the stem terminals; it is interesting to note that the flowers all grow on one side of the stem. The flowering period is July to September. The flower heads should be gathered during this period. The infusion contains 2 to 4 tablespoons (5 to 10 grams) per 2 cups (½ liter) boiling water. Hyssop is an excellent remedy for various illnesses and is particularly used for chronic catarrh, humid asthma, abdominal pain, leukorrhea, green sickness, fever, lack of appetite and stomach cramp. The infusion strengthens the brain, is a diuretic, a stomachic, strengthens the heart, and is very efficacious for fatty degeneration of the heart, intestinal blockage, epilepsy, cold urine and suppressed menstruation. Take 1 cup of tea daily. For asthma and chronic coughs, take 1 tablespoon of the following decoction every two hours: 4 to 5 tablespoons (10 to 12 grams) hyssop, 3 figs and 2 spoons of honey boiled in 2 cups (½ liter) water.

Ivy

Hedera helix   Fam. Araliaceae
Common Ivy, English Ivy

Ivy is a very well-known shrub, found everywhere, especially on dilapidated buildings, ruins, old hedges and in woodlands. It fastens itself by means of fine roots and climbs to a height of 39 feet (12 meters). It has glossy, dark green, hairless leaves; those on the lower branches are usually heart-shaped, three to seven lobed; the higher leaves are smooth-edged, ovate. In September to October it is enhanced by greenish flowers in dense racemes. These are followed by green berries that only ripen to a seed in the spring. The leaves only have an external medicinal use. The nauseating sap can be dangerous. When boiled, the leaves can be successfully used for ulcers, burns and cuts, skin complaints and eczema. If the juice extracted from the leaves is smeared inside the nose, it destroys polyps and drives any foul smell from the nose. Mix 2 parts ivy sap with 1 part lily oil. This mixture is also of use in treating running ears; 5 drops should be dripped in the affected ear every other day. Scurf on the scalp can be cured by washing the scalp twice a day with a handful of ivy boiled in 2¼ cups (500 grams) of white wine; headlice are also killed by this. Callouses disappear if they are covered with ivy leaves boiled in vinegar. The berries act as a purgative; an adult my be given 1 to 2 tablespoons (6 to 8 grams) daily.

Toadflax, Ivy-leaf

Linaria cymbalaria   Fam. Scrophulariaceae
Wandering Jew

This beautiful, perennial, creeping plant can be found along the banks of rivers and on old, damp walls. Its smooth, long, round, purplish, creeping stems bear heart-shaped round, hairless, five to seven lobed leaves and pale blue, long-petiolate, single flowers. The flowering period is May through September. The infusion of this plant can be used externally as a remedy for sores; it is useful internally for heavy bleeding and gravel; a handful of ivy-leaved toadflax should be boiled for eight minutes in 1 quart (liter) water and strained; 1 cup should be taken every now and then.

Juniper, Common

Juniperus communis   Fam. Coniferae

The common juniper bush is abundantly found on sandy ground and heath. It is very strongly branched and often grows in the form of a pyramid shaped shrub. The narrow, oblong leaves are very pointed and prick on contact. This shrub is evergreen. The green berries ripen for the first time in the second year and turn black. The whole plant, including the berries, has a strong smell and a bitter, spicy, sweet taste. The berries and the young twigs are used medicinally. The berries principally have diuretic, diaphoretic, warming and wind-breaking properties and promote digestion. They are especially used for ascites, gastric weakness, accompanied by wind, acid, accumulation of mucus, etc. They are also recommended as a protection from intermittent fever, rheumatism and gout pain. The young twigs, mixed with woodruff and wild strawberry leaves, make a delicious, healthy drink, which can take the place of Indian tea and is certainly much healthier; milk and sugar can be added according to taste.

One of the preparations is juniper oil, which has excellent diuretic properties. The dose is 2-10 drops. You can use 10 to 15 berries for 1 cup of tea. Anyone with a weak stomach should try the following Kneipp juniper berry cure: on the first day, begin with 4 juniper berries; on the second day take 5 juniper berries; then every day take one more berry to a total of fifteen. Then take one berry less every day.

Juniper berries strengthen the nerves, cleanse the blood and the stomach; are also used for kidney, lung and liver complaints, gravel, stones, bladder catarrh, diarrhea and migraines. The decoction of twigs and berries is ½ cup (15 grams) per 2 cups (½ liter) water. The decoction of young twigs and wood: ⅔ to 1 cup (20 to 30 grams) per 2 cups (½ liter) water, which can be taken for gout, rheumatism, syphilis, chronic coughs and phlegm in the chest.

Or, use 3 tablespoons (15 grams) of berries ground to a powder and cooked with 2 tablespoons (30 grams) lard as an excellent remedy for scurf in children; the head should be smeared with it twice a day. As a remedy for phlegm in the chest and coughs, 3 tablespoons (15 grams) juniper berries should be boiled in 2 cups (½ liter) barley water until reduced by half, add a little sugar-candy and drink this quantity throughout the day.

KNOTGRASS

Polyganum aviculare   Fam. Polygonaceae
Swine's Grass

Knotgrass is a widespread plant; it can be found abundantly almost everywhere along country roads, on wasteland and farmland. The stem is either ascendant or, especially along roadsides, decumbent and completely covered with oval, lanceolate, short-petiolate leaves. The flowers are pink-white. The entire plant is used medicinally and gathered throughout the summer. The infusion contains 1 to 1¾ cup (15 to 25 grams) per 2 cups (½ liter) water. Take 2 to 3 cups daily. Knotgrass is highly recommended for stones and gravel; it cleanses the chest, stomach, liver and kidneys and is most efficacious in cases of diabetes, lung disease, heavy bleeding, colic, diarrhea, dysentery, gastric and intestinal ulcers. In cases of fever it is an excellent remedy for thirst. For diarrhea, blood-spitting and heavy menstruation, a decoction should be made with wine; 1 spoonful to be taken every two hours.

The freshly bruised herb heals wounds. When mixed with sweet butter, it can be applied three times a day to painful, swollen breasts. The infusion of the herb in water is highly recommended for epilepsy, complaints of the windpipe, lung catarrh, coughing, constriction of the chest, hoarseness, or coughing blood (especially in consumptives). Nosebleeds are cured in the most amazing manner by the patient simply drinking the tea.

LADY'S BEDSTRAW

Galium verum   Fam. Rubiaceae

Lady's bedstraw can be found quite commonly on dry, sandy soil. It is a perennial, herbaceous plant, with thin, coarse, branched, ascendant stems, the upper part of which is hairy. The yellow flowers grow in racemes on the stem terminals. The long root is brown on the outside, white inside. It has a slightly aromatic smell and a bitter, astringent sap. The flowering period is May through September. The flowers are used for epilepsy, hysteria, nervous and gastric pain. The infusion contains 4 to 5 tablespoons (8 to 10 grams) per 2 cups (½ liter) boiling water. It can also be used in powder form, 2 to 5 teaspoons (3 to 6 grams) daily. The freshly bruised leaves can be poked into the nostrils to staunch nosebleeds.

LADY'S MANTLE

Alchemilla vulgaris   Fam. Rosaceae

This is a perennial, herbaceous plant with a strong rootstock and a rosette of long-petiolate, round, serrated leaves. The ascendant flower stems attain a height of 12 inches (30 centimeters) and bear very small, green flowers in racemes. The flowering period is May to June. This plant preferably grows on dry, sandy soil; it is very rare here [in Europe]. The leaves greatly resemble those of the cultivated geranium. The whole plant is used medicinally. It is gathered during the flowering period. The relatively thick root is black, fibrous and has an unpleasant smell.

The infusion contains ½ to 1 cup leaves (10 to 15 grams) per 2 cups (½ liter) boiling water for internal use, and 2½ cups (50 grams) for external use. It has astringent properties and is used for heavy bleeding, vomiting blood and leukorrhea. It is used externally to cleanse wounds and knit the tissues together again. A decoction of the whole plant, 1 cup (15 grams) per 2 cups (½ liter) water can be used in the form of compresses on sores, ulcers, ruptures and prolapse of the rectum.

Lady's mantle is also used for involuntary seminal discharge, ulcerated lungs, consumption, dysentery, painful bleeding, fistulas, internal and external sores. The powdered leaves cure ruptures in children; it can be taken in wine or bouillon. For leukorrhea and swollen breasts, compresses of the plant decoction should be applied.

LARCH

Pinus larix   Fam. Coniferae
Pine

The larch is an attractive tree with light green needles; it grows very tall with foliage in the form of a pyramid; the short twigs, on which bundles of needles grow, die off in the winter. A fungus, called larch fungus, grows all over the trunk of old larch trees. The white, loose substance inside this fungus is very useful in curbing the excessive perspiration of consumptives if given every evening in a dose of ½ to 1 gram. A dose of 2 to 4 grams has a purgative action.

LAVENDER

Lavendula officinalis   Fam. Labiatae

This is an aromatic plant grown in gardens. It has a pleasant smell, a little like camphor; it is a perennial, woody plant or shrub with narrow, ash-gray leaves and blue, fragrant flowers which are used medicinally; they form spikes on the stem terminals. The flowering period is June to September. Spike oil, or lavender oil, is extracted from these flowers and used for the treatment of several illnesses, including the promotion of menstruation. Take 5 drops on sugar twice a day. It is also beneficial for accumulated wind, colic, congestion of blood in the head, dizziness, headaches, hypochondria, lack of appetite. The well-known, fragrant lavender water is prepared by steeping 2½ cups (60 grams) of freshly picked lavender flowers in 4 cups (1 liter) of 32% alcohol for several days and then filtering it.

LEEK

Allium porrum   Fam. Liliaceae

Leeks are grown in every garden as a nourishing item of food; they are very refreshing and good for the digestion. They have diuretic properties and stimulate the appetite. In cases of bee or wasp stings, leek, like onion, is an excellent remedy to stop the pain and swelling; a bruised leaf should be rubbed to and fro over the affected area. Leeks, boiled and applied as a poultice to swollen legs is efficacious for rheumatic swellings. Where all else has failed, this poultice will help within a few days. In addition, take 1 to 2 cups of the decoction daily.

LEMON BALM

Melissa officinalis   Fam. Labiatae

Lemon balm is a perennial, herbaceous plant that grows one or two feet tall; it grows wild in France and is frequently cultivated in gardens. It contains a fragrant oil and much camphor; the sap is hot and aromatic. The leaves, which resemble those of a nettle, are dentate, a little wrinkled and hairy. The flowers are small, pink or white, growing in axillary racemes along the stems. It blooms from May to June. During this period, the flower heads are gathered for medicinal use, for indigestion, headaches, migraines, convulsions, gastric weakness, a languishing stomach, cramps and nervous twitches, and chronic catarrh; it is especially good for mucus complaints; in addition, for nausea, flatulence, hysteria and menstrual disorders.

The infusion contains ¾ to 1 cup (10 to 15 grams) per 2 cups (½ liter) boiling water and is good for jaundice. Take 1 cup tea daily with sugar. Freshly bruised lemon balm, placed on the heart region, stops palpitations. The dried flowers soaked in rosewater, then pounded together, can also be applied in the same way.

LEMON TREE

Citrus medica (citrus limon)   Fam. Rutaceae

The lemon tree is indigenous to Assyria and Persia, but is also cultivated in Spain and Italy. The well-known fruit from this tree contains a great deal of pure, refreshing juice which, when mixed with sugar and some kind of liquid, may be given as an ordinary lemonade drink for fever. It can be given both internally and externally for scurvy. Consumptives can take the so-called "lemon cure."

LETTUCE

Lactuca sativa   Fam. Compositae

Lettuce, with its smooth stem, uncut, soft, smooth leaves, of which the lowest are oval-round and the upper heart-shaped, with its yellow, raceme-shaped inflorescence, is a well-known vegetable. It has no smell, its sap is a little bitter, but pleasant. The flowering period is July and August. Lettuce is refreshing; it is a mild, sleep-inducing remedy, increases mother's milk, has a beneficial effect on the stomach, is a good nourishing food and softens the sharpness in the blood. Those who suffer from hydrothorax, breathlessness, asthma and who are constantly spitting blood should not eat lettuce. It is recommended for hysteria, hypochrondria, nervous and liver complaints. For seminal discharge, take a grain of powdered seed daily.

LICORICE

Glycyrrhiza glabra   Fam. Leguminosae

The root of this plant is the well-known and commonly used licorice. The plant is native to the south of France, is at home in the southern regions of Russia and is occasionally cultivated here in gardens. The root is woody, wrinkled, yellow-brown on the outside and pale yellow inside; it has a pleasant, sweet, rather slimy taste, leaving a bitter taste behind. This root can also be used medicinally. The decoction consists of 3 to 3½ tablespoons (12 to 15 grams) per 2 cups (½ liter) water, is recommended as one of the mildest phlegm dissolving remedies and can be fruitfully used for burning fevers and for the treatment of chronic conditions of the respiratory organs. It is a very famous remedy for lung complaints, chills, coughs, hoarseness, mucous lungs and consumption, especially for measles, dry coughs, painful or difficult urination, stones, gravel, etc., for gout and rheumatism. This root is also added to any medicine which has a bad taste.

LILY OF THE VALLEY

Convallaria magalis   Fam. Liliaceae

This can be found in woodland and shady spots. Its leaves, usually two or three, are a glossy green color, oblong at the bottom, gradually tapering to a point at the top. The flowers are in the form of small, white, fragrant bells drooping on long stems, facing in one direction. After flowering, these are followed by red berries. This plant winters with a creeping branched rootstock. The flowers are gathered in May, dried and ground to a powder. This is excellent as a snuff and for the treatment of headaches; a little should be sniffed into the nostrils. This will also cure continued nosebleeds. Half a gram of dried flowers is recommended for palpitations.

LIME

Calcium oxide

Unslaked lime is extracted from limestone by means of repeated heating; a white or gray substance is obtained which, when mixed with water, effervesces, generating a considerable amount of heat. The lime can be dissolved in a small quantity of water and this water is used medicinally. It is used internally for acidity, ulceration of the intestines and the urinary organs; externally as a dessicant for certain scrofulous skin complaints, scurvy and constantly gnawing ulcers. To use internally, take 4-30 grams daily in milk. Externally, it should be used in the form of compresses and washes. For inflammation of the throat, mix 2 parts slaked lime with 1 part lard, smear fairly thickly on a linen cloth and place around the neck; as soon as it begins to dry, it should be removed. To heal burns, mix 1 part lime water, 1 part olive oil, and 1 egg yolk; brush this on the burns several times a day with a feather and cover with a fine linen cloth.[6]

LIME TREE

Tilia europoea   Fam. Tiliaceae

This tree is one of the most common sights on walls and in parks. The blossom of the lime tree is used medicinally for dizziness, migraines, indigestion, chills, nervous complaints; this tea is highly recommended for old people in particular. The infusion contains ⅛ to ¼ cup (10 to 15 grams) per 2 cups (½ liter) boiling water. Hot lime blossom baths are highly recommended for convulsions in children. Charcoal powder from lime wood is the best for internal use (see charcoal). A cup of lime blossom tea every evening with ½ to 1 spoon of honey is very depurative, strengthens the heart, is good for the nerves, and promotes sleep. In addition, lime tea is recommended for

---

[6]In modern pharmacopoeia, calcium hydroxide has replaced lime. *Calcii Hydroxidum* or slaked lime is now used as a non-systemic antacid in American allopathic medicine.

nervous complaints in general; also for hysteria, hypochondria, migraines, epilepsy, indigestion, colic, coughs, chills, shivering and to avoid strokes. A handful of young twigs, with or without leaves, drawn in 1 quart (liter) boiling water for twenty minutes, can be highly recommended for dropsy; 3 cups should be taken daily. Lime leaves, dried and used for tea, are diuretic.

LINSEED

Linum usitatissimum   Fam. Linaceae
Common Flax

Flax is an annual plant, blooms from June to August, and is widely cultivated in many parts of the country; it provides flax, linen and linseed. The stem of the plant is ascendant, pale-green and round, branched higher up. The leaves are oblong-acute. The seed, from which a valuable oil is extracted, is flat, very smooth and pointed and is also used medicinally. Flaxseed meal is commonly used to make poultices for ulcers, swellings, stomachaches, etc. and, like fenugreek, has a palliative, solvent effect. Flaxseed is used, above all, for inflamed, painful, cramp-like complaints of the intestines; for intestinal inflammation, cramp colic, gravel and difficult urination. Use 2 to 3 table-spoons (10 to 15 grams) per 2 cups (½ liter) water for both an infusion and a decoction.

Flax or linseed oil is used for rubbing rheumatic com-plaints. Instead of the seed decoction, fresh linseed oil can al-ways be used: 1 to 3 tablespoons daily. A doctor from Neuenahr writes that a daily cup of linseed tea is highly recommended for expectant mothers, six weeks before the confinement. Lin-seed ground to a powder is efficacious in the treatment of chest complaints and dropsy; 1 sugarspoon mixed with honey should be taken four to six times a day.

For pain in the side, abdominal pain and gravel, 2 to 3 spoons of fresh oil should be taken. Boil 1 tablespoon linseed for fifteen minutes in 1 quart (liter) water, strain through a cloth, add 2 spoons honey and you have an excellent remedy for a stubborn cough, blood-spitting, coughing blood, bladder complaints, stones, intestinal and other internal inflammation: take 2 cups daily. Take 1 tablespoon linseed oil every morning and evening to treat piles.

The mixture of linseed powder with honey is highly recommended for constipation, lack of appetite, heartburn, acid stomach, vomiting, intermittent fever, insomnia. For colic (miserere), an enema of the following mixture should be given: 3 tablespoons (40 grams) linseed oil and 3 tablespoons (40 grams) rapeseed oil. This is a most efficacious remedy. For piles and tears in the anus, smear three times a day with linseed oil.

LONG-STALKED CRANESBILL

Geranium columbinum   Fam. Geraniaceae

The long-stalked cranesbill is an annual, herbaceous plant, with fairly long, decumbent stems, long flower stems that stand well above the leaves and hairless fruit capsules. The lower leaves are circular and consist of five or six cut sections with widely spaced, straight lobes. The purple flowers appear in May and June. The plant sap is astringent and salty. The decoction contains 2 tablespoons (20 grams) per 2 cups (½ liter) water and is used for dysentery, dropsy, kidney disorders, and gout. It is especially recommended for gout and dropsy. Drink 1-2 cups daily.

LOUSEWORT (COMMON)

Pedicularis sylvatica   Fam. Scrophulariaceae

Common lousewort is annual and herbaceous, with short stems and a rosette of wide-spread branches which are often larger than the main stem. The petiolate leaves have sharply dentate side-lobes. The flowers, which bloom from May to July, are pink, sometimes yellowish-white. It grows in woods and meadowland. This herb has astringent properties and is used medicinally for heavy bleeding, or externally on sores in the form of compresses. For internal use, an infusion of about 4 tablespoons (8 to 12 grams) per 2 cups (½ liter) boiling water. For external use, take double the quantity.

LOVAGE

Levisticum officinale   Fam. Umbelliferae

This herbaceous, perrenial plant with its hollow, very branched stem, has large, glossy-green, two to three pinnate leaves and yellow flowers in umbels on the stem terminals. The seed is yellow and oblong, the root thick and fleshy. Both herb and roots have a sharp, pleasant, celery-like smell. It grows wild in Italy and is cultivated here in gardens. The flowering period is June to July. The leaves, roots and seed are used medicinally; the powdered root promotes digestion and warms the stomach.

Lovage is commonly recommended for disorders of the stomach, spleen and liver, wind, green sickness, stomach and intestinal pain, menstrual blockage, womb disorders, breathlessness, phlegm in the chest, blockage of the liver and spleen, jaundice, bladder complaints, stones. Take 2 teaspoons (3 grams) powdered dried root or an equal quantity of seed in wine. A decoction of the root, leaves and seed in water or wine may also be taken. The seed is used, above all, for gas, abdominal pain, ulceration of the throat and throat complaints. The oil can also be highly recommended for this purpose; 3 to 4 drops should be taken on sugar twice a day or a little more according to circumstances. Use 3 tablespoons (15 grams) leaves, roots and seeds per 2 cups (½ liter) water for the decoction. Take 2 cups of tea daily with a spoon.

LUNGWORT

Sticta pulmonaria   Fam. Lichenes
Jerusalem Cowslip, Spotted Dog

Lungwort is a perennial, herbaceous plant, with a creeping rootstock. It grows in shady places on the edge of woodland, but is only seldom found. It can be recognized by its oblong, spotted leaves; the flowers, which appear early in April, are red, but soon turn violet-blue and grow in curved or dropping racemes; at a short distance they resemble violets. Both leaves and flower heads can be used medicinally, 1½ cups (15 grams) per 2 cups (½ liter) boiling water. They are useful for treating chest complaints, lung disease, blood-spitting and consumption. Drink 1 cup of tea daily.

MADONNA LILY

Lilium candidum   Fam. Liliaceae

This commonly known plant is grown in most gardens on account of its beautiful flowers and pleasant fragrance. It is perennial, herbaceous, with a fine, ascendant stem which attains a height of 3 feet (1 meter); the leaves are long and glossy; the beautiful, large, pure white flowers, in the shape of a chalice, exude a pleasant fragrance. The root is a bulb. The petals, steeped in gin, are good on sores. If they are bottled in olive oil for a few months, lily oil is obtained. This is recommended for rheumatism and wind; the abdomen should be rubbed with this oil twice a day for the latter, and in cases of rheumatism the affected joints should be treated. This oil is also recommended for wasp or bee stings.

MALLOW

Malva rotundifolia   Fam. Malvaceae

Common mallow is a perennial, herbaceous plant with an erect, branched stem, scattered, almost circular, petiolate, serrated leaves and mauve-purple flowers, which grow in twos or more in the leaf axils. The whole plant is covered in hairs. The flowering period is from June to August. Mallow is used medicinally for inflammation of the mucous membranes. The infusion of the flowers contains 2 to 4 tablespoons (6 to 12 grams) per 2 cups (½ liter) water; that of the leaves, ¼ to ⅓ cup (10 to 15 grams). The herb, boiled with its flowers in milk, is efficacious for the treatment of consumption. Excellent palliative poultices and enemas are made from mallow leaves; they are highly recommended for any kind of inflammation. The flowers are recommended for all complaints of the respiratory organs.

MARIGOLD

Calendula officinalis   Fam. Compositae
Garden Marigold

This annual plant is very well-known. It is grown in many gardens for its beautiful flowers. The stem is thick, quadrangular, soft, a little sticky, pale-green in color and attains a height of 6 to 8 inches (15 to 20 centimeters). The leaves are attached to the stem without a leaf-stem; they are oblong and covered with silky hair. The flowers are large, single and orange-yellow in color. Flowers and stems are used medicinally; they are gathered throughout the summer. They must always be used fresh as they lose their beneficial properties during the drying process.

The infusion contain ¼ to ⅓ cup (8 to 10 grams) per 2 cups (½ liter) boiling water, is diaphoretic, promotes menstruation, is anti-convulsant, febrifugal, and is also used for jaundice, green sickness, general weakness, hysteria and nervous complaints. The infusion of the flowers is a good remedy for dropsy and jaundice; take 1 cup daily. The bruised herb is very efficacious on sores and wounds.

MARJORAM (WILD)

Origanum vulgare   Fam. Labiatae
Oregano

This perennial, herbaceous plant is commonly found on the edge of woodlands, old hedgerows and on dry, sandy soil. It has an ascendant stem and branches covered in soft hairs. The leaves are ovate and serrated; the red flowers grow in racemes on the stem terminals. Wild marjoram attains a height of 1½ feet (40 centimeters) and the flowering period is May to September. The plant's flower heads are gathered. The sap is bitter, strongly resembling that of mint, is used in the same cases, and can replace it. The infusion contains ⅓ to ½ cup (10 to 15 grams) per 4 cups (liter) boiling water. Drink 1 cup per day.

MARSH CUDWEED

Graphalium uliginosum   Fam. Compositae
Life Everlasting

Yellow-white marsh cudweed has an ascendant, usually un-branched stem, covered with white silk. The leaves are long-narrow, the white flowers are clustered in balls on the branch terminals. The flowering period is July to September. The plant may be found on sandy soil and along roadsides. It is an excellent remedy for diarrhea, dysentery and heavy menstruation. The decoction contains 4 to 5 tablespoons (6 to 12 grams) per 2 cups (½ liter) water. Take 1 cup of tea daily with a spoon. The freshly crushed plant cures old ulceration.

MARSHMALLOW

Althaea officinalis   Fam. Malvaceae
Sweetweed, Schloss, Tea Althaea

Marshmallow is a perennial, herbaceous plant that grows in the damp regions of Europe. It attains a height of about 5 feet (1½ meters), is as soft as velvet, gray-green, with short hairs. The leaves are ovate, serrated or crenate. Relatively large white or pink flowers appear in the axils. The flowering period is June and July. The flowers are picked as soon as they appear and then dried in the shade. The root is gathered in the autumn. The outer rind is peeled off, the root is then cut in pieces and dried in the oven. Flowers, leaves and root are used medicinally. The infusion of leaves and flowers consists of ⅓ to ½ cup (15 to 20 grams) per 2 cups (½ liter) boiling water; that of the roots only 2 to 3 tablespoons (10 to 12 grams) per 2 cups (½ liter) water. The root decoction is recommended for bladder complaints, painful urination, chest complaints, stubborn coughs, sore throat and heavy bleeding; also at the onset of pneumonia, inflammation of the stomach, diarrhea, dysentery and other intestinal complaints. Marshmallow is palliative and can be used in any case of inflammation. Hands which have been rubbed by the sap of this plant will not be stung by any wasp or bee.

Meadow Saxifrage

Saxifrage granulata   Fam. Umbelliferae
Fair Maids of France

This perennial, herbaceous plant can be found in meadows and wet places, sometimes quite abundantly but usually scattered. The leaves are long-petiolate and kidney-shaped; the lower ones are cut or lobed, the upper sessile. The white, long-petiolate flowers grow clustered in a raceme. Small, fig-like excrescences grow on the root. The flowering period is May to June. Meadow saxifrage is recommended for swelling of the spleen and liver, kidney stones, gravel and bladder complaints. It is usually mixed with small quantities of chervil to increase its strength. The infusion should consist of ½ to ¾ cup (10 to 15 grams) per 2 cups (½ liter) boiling water.

Meadowsweet

Spiraea ulmaria   Fam. Rosaceae

This beautiful plant is commonly found in marshy areas close to running water; it is also cultivated in gardens for the pleasant smell of its flowers. It is a perennial, herbaceous plant with a red, branched stem which attains a height of more than three feet (1 meter); the leaves are greenish, simple pinnate. It flowers in June and the white, fragrant flowers form branched cymes on the stem terminals. The whole plant (stem, leaves and flowers) is used medicinally. The leaf decoction consists of 3 to 5 tablespoons (10 to 15 grams) per 4 cups (liter) water. The plant is an astringent, diuretic medicine and can be successfully used in the treatment of dropsy, difficult urination, and piles. Take 2 or 3 cups of decoction daily. In addition, it is a sound remedy for those who find urination difficult or impossible; also for scurf, scrofulous rash in children, skin rash, fever, dysentery, diarrhea, blood-spitting, heavy bleeding, hematuria, general loss of blood, ascites and dropsy, heavy menstruation. Take 1 to 2 cups of tea daily, or use 4 teaspoons (3 grams) of powdered root in wine. To staunch bleeding and to heal fresh wounds, apply freshly bruised roots. The leaves and roots can also be mixed together to make a powder.

Micralium Mixture

This remedy cannot be praised highly enough for gastric disorder, for foul stomach, pain in the loins, impure blood, scurvy, and for all kinds of fever. It is a mixture composed of the following:

1⅔ cup (10 grams) mint
4 teaspoons (10 grams) rhubarb
½ cup (10 grams) horsetail
⅓ cup (5 grams) oak leaves
4 tablespoons (5 grams) buckbean
1 tablespoon (5 grams) orange rind
1 tablespoon (5 grams) unripe oranges
1 tablespoon (5 grams) genetian
3 teaspoons (5 grams) calamus
4 teaspoons (5 grams) marshmallow
½ cup (5 grams) Aaron's rod leaves
1 teaspoon (5 grams) horseradish root
1 tablespoon (5 grams) polypody root

Let 1 tablespoon of this mixture steep for twenty minutes in 1 cup boiling water. Take 2 to 3 tablespoons three times a day, before meals.

Milk Thistle

Silybum marianum   Fam. Compositae

This annual plant is found in grassy places of mountainous regions and sometimes on rubbish tips. It has large, glossy, cut, white-spotted, veined leaves, edged with firm prickles. The reddish flowers are followed by large, dark-spotted shiny fruits with a hairy pappus. The flowering period is July and August. The bitter, invigorating, leaf decoction is used for leukorrhea, pain in the side, pleurisy, gravel, jaundice, dropsy and pneumonia. The infusion should contain ¼ cup (10 grams) dried flowers to 2 cups (½ liter) boiling water; 1 cup should be taken daily.

The seed, steeped in wine, can also be used instead of the decoction and is an equally effective remedy; 2 teaspoons (4 grams) should be taken daily. The seed, in particular, is better than the leaf decoction and highly recommended for liver complaints as well as spleen problems and gall stones. The decoction can be replaced by ½ a sugarspoon powdered milk thistle seed taken four times a day.

MILKWORT

Polygala senega   Fam. Polygalaceae
Senega

Common milkwort is a perennial, herbaceous plant with thin stems and is frequently found in both wet and dry meadows and woodlands. The leaves grow opposite in pairs; the upper leaves are lanceolate and longer than the lower ones which are small and oblong-round. From May through July, the stem terminals bear pink or blue flowers in the form of a spike. The plant has a bitter taste; it is used for chronic chest complaints, pneumonia, tuberculosis of the lungs, blood-spitting, catarrh, dropsy and rheumatism. The decoction consists of ¾ to 1 cup (20 to 25 grams) per 2 cups (½ liter) boiling water; take 1 tablespoon every two hours. Or, take 2 teaspoons (1 gram) of the powdered, dried plant daily for the above mentioned complaints.

MISTLETOE

Viscum album   Fam. Loranthaceae

Mistletoe is a parasitic plant which, in some areas, is frequently found on apple trees and poplars, less on oaks. The plant draws its nourishment from these trees but it is of no advantage to them; this is the reason why it is removed as often as possible. The leaves are thick, oblong, sessile; the flowers appear in the leaf axil and give way to white, round berries, which are poisonous. The leaves are used medicinally. Mistletoe should be gathered in autumn or winter, thoroughly dried and preserved in well-corked glass pots. Take 1 cup daily for watery gall, acid stomach, phlegm in the chest, liver, jaundice, lung sores and other internal sores. The infusion, ¼ to ⅓ cup (15 to 20 grams) per 2 cups (½ liter) boiling water, is recommended for convulsions, epilepsy, hysteria, St. Vitus' Dance and whooping cough. The infusion of mistletoe is excellent for bleeding; 1 or 2 cups is usually sufficient to stop heavy bleeding.

MONEYWORT

Lysimachia nummularia   Fam. Primulaceae
Creeping Jenny

Moneywort is a perennial, creeping plant. It frequently grows along the edges of ditches, between the grass, on the edge of ponds, in wet meadows and woodlands. It has circular leaves, hence the name moneywort. The beautiful, yellow flowers grow over the whole length of the stem in the leaf-axils. The flowering period is June to July and it is gathered throughout these months. The infusion contains ¼ to ⅓ cup (10 to 15 grams) per 2 cups (½ liter) boiling water and is recommended for heavy bleeding, diarrhea, dysentery, leukorrhea, blood-spitting, scurvy, ulceration of the lungs, gastric ulcers, internal sores and injuries. Take 1 cup of tea daily and, in addition, an application of the bruised herb.

Motherwort

Leonurus cardiaca   Fam. Labiatae

This perennial, herbaceous plant grows to a height of 3 feet (1 meter). The leaves are long-petiolate, standing wide away from the stem, drooping a little, and are dark green in color; the lower leaves are palmate, the upper ones three-lobed. The flower whorls are sessile, the corolla is pale-pink. The flowering period is July and August. It grows on dry, sandy ground and is very common.

The infusion consists of ⅓ to ½ cup (10 to 15 grams) per 2 cups (½ liter) boiling water. It is useful for palpitations, cramps, gout, constipation, promotes menstruation, is diuretic, cleanses the chest and kidneys, has dissolvent properties, dilutes thickened fluids and kills worms. In addition, it is beneficial for the treatment of rickets, humid asthma, abdominal swelling, green sickness, and illness in children caused by worms and heat complaints. Take 2 teaspoons (3 grams) of powder in wine for intestinal blockage and suppressed menstruation. In cases of abdominal pain or pain in the womb, apply leaves fried in butter. For sores, apply fresh, bruised leaves. For internal use, take 1 cup of the infusion daily.

Mouse-Ear Hawkweed

Hieracium pilosella   Fam. Compositae
Common Hawkweed

Mouse-ear hawkweed is an herbaceous, perennial plant[7] commonly found on grassy, sandy ground. The leaves are covered with long hairs; they are coarse, oblong, green on the upper side, white beneath. They resemble the ears of a mouse; hence the name. The plant is propagated not only by seeds but also by runners. The dirty-yellow flowers bloom from May to September. The plant, which can be gathered throughout the summer, is used medicinally. The decoction, ¼ ounce (15 to 20

---

[7]We were unable to locate this herb.

grams) per 2 cups (½ liter) water, is used for various complaints, such as heavy bleeding, seminal discharge, internal ulceration, chronic diarrhea and gravel, and especially for rheumatism and gout. It is, in particular, an excellent remedy for gravel. The following mixture is a good gargle for ulceration of the throat and tonsillitis: one part hawkweed, 1 part sage and 1 part selfheal; this can be used as a gargle several times a day. A handful of the mixture should be drawn for twenty minutes in 2 cups (½ liter) boiling water.

MUGWORT

Artemisia vulgaris   Fam. Compositae
Felon Herb, St. John's Herb

Mugwort is a widely spread, herbaceous, perennial plant. It is found on sandy soil, in hedgerows and on roadsides; it grows three feet high (1 meter), and has erect, reddish, striped stems, the upper part bearing light green leaves and the lower part bearing gray leaves that are coarsely serrated. Mugwort has many small flower heads which cluster in a spike on the stem terminals. It blooms from July to August. The flower heads should be collected during this period. The root is gathered in September; it must be dried with care so as to avoid mold. The best mugwort is found on dry ground; that found on rich soil is not so potent. Only the root fibers and the root rind are used medicinally; the inside of the root has no value.

The infusion of flower heads contains ¼ to ½ cup (8 to 15 grams) per 2 cups (½ liter) boiling water. Take 2 to 4 teaspoons (2 to 4 grams) of the root powder in hot beer, wine, or water. Or take 3 to 6 tablespoons (4 to 8 grams) of the powdered leaves. Mugwort is used for several nervous disorders such as hysteria, St. Vitus' Dance, nervous vomiting, and nerve pains. The quantity used is 4 teaspoons (4 grams). This same quantity may be taken in some kind of liquid to avoid an epileptic fit. The patient is advised to stay in bed after taking a dose: it will cause sweating, and while the patient is sweating, it is important to remain in bed. There is sometimes an improvement after the first dose. After taking one dose, it is wise to miss a day.

Powdered mugwort can also be used successfully for diarrhea and dysentery. It should be kept in well-corked jars. Bruised mugwort leaves mixed with fresh butter is a good remedy for sprains and dislocations. Boil 1 tablespoon mugwort in wine and water, and take every two hours for gravel and bladder complaints. The infusion may be prepared in water, beer, or wine.

MUSTARD (WHITE)

Sinapis alba   Fam. Cruciferae

White mustard is an annual plant which grows in gardens as well as in its natural state on stony wasteland. The plant attains a height of 3 feet (1 meter); the stem and leaves are hairy; the yellow flowers grow on the stem terminals; they are followed by pods which contain the mustard seed. This is yellowish or white and is used medicinally. The dose is 5 to 6 tablespoons (30 to 40 grams) whole grains, taken with water. White mustard seed is used for constipation and indigestion, also for gout and podagra.

I have recommended this little seed for thirty years for constipation, congestion, stomach, liver and bladder disorders, nervous complaints, dropsy and especially to prevent strokes. A gentleman who suffered for years from intolerable stomachache, indigestion and lack of appetite, who was tormented by heartburn, wind and insomnia, was helped by this. He was radically cured by taking 1 tablespoon daily without any other medicine. Since then I have prescribed it with great success for a number of illnesses including chest complaints, asthma, kidney complaints, general weakness, scrofulous complaints, gout, etc. I advise the reader to try it; there is no need to be afraid of harmful consequences. I usually prescribe 1 sugarspoonful two or three times daily, seldom more.

MYRRH

Commiphora   Fam. Burseraceae

Myrrh is a gum which occurs as a dried, gumlike sap in the
form of pieces of varying size, red or yellow-brown color. It has
a spicy smell and a bitter taste. Myrrh is used medicinally for
weakness of the stomach and intestines, mucous stomach, indigestion, irregular menstruation and leukorrhea, also for
chronic chest complaints. The dose is ½ teaspoon (1 gram) in
pills or powders. Myrrh is beneficial for fevers, inflammation,
indigestion, mucous stomach and intestines, gas, piles, swollen
liver, poor circulation, mucous lungs, thick, bad pus, mucus in
the womb and bladder. It is also an excellent mouthwash for
rotten teeth and gums, ulceration of the throat and other throat
complaints. For a mouthwash or gargle, take 20 to 30 drops of
the tincture in a glass of cold water and add a little honey.

To make myrrh ointment: dissolve 2 teaspoons (4 grams)
powdered myrrh in a little 50% alcohol, 7 teaspoons (12 grams)
charcoal powder, and enough lard to make a soft ointment.
Tincture of myrrh is prepared by letting 2 teaspoons (4 grams)
myrrh steep in a liqueur glass of good gin; 6 drops should be
taken two or three times a day with a spoon of wine or water.
This tincture should not be used during menstruation and pregnancy. People with congestion of blood in the head and nursing
mothers should also refrain from taking it.

NARROW-LEAVED WATER PARSNIP

Berula augustifolia   Fam. Umbelliferae

Narrow-leaved water parsnip is a perennial, herbaceous plant
often found in pools, ditches, or brooks. It has a round, striped,
branched stem; the leaves are unevenly pinnate, sessile, oblong-
ovate and serrated. The umbels are white and short petiolate;
the fruits are densely clustered and provided with five ribs. The
infusion of the dried plant, containing about ½ cup (10 to 20
grams) per 2 cups (½ liter) boiling water, it is used for difficult
urination, scurvy, and also stimulates the appetite.

Nasturtium

Tropaeolum majus   Fam. Tropaeolaceae
Indian Cress

This is an annual climbing plant which originally came from Peru and is frequently cultivated in gardens on account of its beautiful flowers. There are several varieties of this plant, but all have the same properties and can all be used medicinally. The plant has a penetrating smell which greatly resembles that of watercress and has the same hot sap. The dried fruit of the garden nasturtium, ground to a powder, is a good purgative which causes no pain; ½ teaspoon (50 centigrams) may be taken when necessary in some kind of fluid. The leaves are eaten with ordinary garden lettuce as salad, while the fresh fruit may be preserved in vinegar in August. The fresh flowers and leaves, bruised together, are good on sores. The sap is an efficacious remedy for scurvy.

Stinging Nettle (greater)

Urtica dioica   Fam. Urticaceae
Common Nettle

The stinging nettle is notorious as a large weed. It is commonly found on rough wasteland. It is a perennial, herbaceous plant with a quadrangular, hairy stem and opposite and decussate leaves. The stems sometimes reach a height of three feet (1 meter) and shoot up in spring. The leaves are relatively large and hairy. Contact with the hand instantly causes a burning pain followed immediately by a rash. The flowers are almost colorless and grow in the leaf axils. Leaves, seeds and roots are used medicinally. The infusion of the leaves contains ¾ to 1¼ cup (20 to 25 grams) per 2 cups (½ liter) boiling water and is recommended for blood-spitting, vomiting blood and hemorrages. In these cases, 2 or 3 cups of the decoction should be given daily. The same quantity may also be given for skin complaints, since it is an excellent depurative.

In spring, young nettles can be eaten like spinach; they are very nourishing, with a pleasant taste and, in addition, purify the blood. Stinging nettles boiled in equal quantities of water and vinegar are a good hair remedy. When used to wash the hair every day, they prevent hair from falling out and encourage strong growth. A daily dose of stinging nettle tea cures dropsy. The stinging nettle is excellent for gravel, kidney and bladder stones, fever, asthma, coughing, lung ulcers, chronic pleurisy, measles, smallpox, gout, rheumatism, piles and epilepsy. For throat complaints, the powdered seed, mixed with an equal quantity of honey, is highly recommended. Take 1 sugarspoon every two hours. The infusion can also serve as a gargle.

NETTLE (LESSER)

Urtica urens   Fam. Urticaceae

The small nettle is an annual plant commonly found in gardens. It has long-petiolate, coarsely serrated, small, hairy leaves of pale green. The stem is quadrangular, the leaves opposite and decussate. The greenish flowers grow in the leaf axils and, like the large stinging nettle, cause a burning pain on contact. Fresh nettles pounded with a little salt are recommended for cancer sores. For rheumatism, the affected place should be brushed with nettles, causing a rash to appear on the skin.

NIGHTSHADE (WOODY)

Solanum dulcamara   Fam. Solanaceae
Bittersweet

Nightshade, like all Solanaceae, contains a little poison, but so little that it has never been known to have a harmful effect. This perennial shrub-like plant is found in moist shady places. The woody stem can grow four feet high (1½ meters), entwining itself around other plants. The single leaves are heart-shaped, with a short or long point. The violet flowers have a green fleck at the base of the calyx and are followed by glossy, red berries. In May and September the stem tops are gathered with the soft stems and the top leaves. The stems should be split down the middle.

An infusion of the plant should contain 1 tablespoon (4 to 5 grams) per 2 cups (½ liter) boiling water for the first week; 2 tablespoons (5 to 6 grams) for the second week; 3 tablespoons (7 to 8 grams) for the third week; 4 tablespoons (9 to 10 grams) for the fourth week; 5 tablespoons (11 to 12 grams) for the fifth week; 6 tablespoons (15 to 16 grams) for the sixth week. The dose should then be decreased each week down to 1 tablespoon (5 grams). Eczema and skin complaints are cured in this way. It is also used for chronic colds, phlegm tuberculosis, mucous complaints of the lungs, syphilis, scrofula, gout and particulary venereal diseases.

NIPPLEWORT

Lapsana communis   Fam. Compositae

It is found on farmland, alongside roads, hedges, and woods. It is an annual plant, with ascendant branched stems, coarsely serrated, petiolate leaves; the radical leaves are lyre-shaped and pinnate; at the top of the plant they are heart-shaped. The yellow flowers, which form a large flower, appear June to August. The boiled plant can be applied as a poultice to inflamed limbs, old sores, split or sore nipples, and breasts which are swollen through an accumulation of milk.

NOLI-ME-TANGERE

Impatiens Noli-me-tangere   Fam. Geraniaceae
Touch-me-not

Noli-me-tangere is an annual, herbaceous plant with a smooth, ascendant, branched, pale-green stem, rich in sap. The delicate leaves are very pale-green, oval or ovate, and serrated; the flowers are lemon yellow, speckled with red inside, growing in loose racemes and hanging on rather long, very fine stems. The flowering period is July to September. Noli-me-tangere (wild impatiens) is only found on wet, shady ground and in woodlands. It is considered poisonous and has burning, hot sap. If the leaves are crushed or boiled with linseed oil, they can be applied to dissolve the nerve swelling in cases of gout (podagra). A few leaves boiled in a glass of wine immediately alleviates the pain in cases of difficult urination and cold urine. Alternatively freshly bruised leaves can also be applied.

Oak Tree

Quercus robur   Fam. Cupuliferae

The oak is one of the finest trees in the forest; it grows very tall, has strong, spreading branches and thick leaves; the bark is rough and deeply grooved. It flowers in May and bears fruit which ripen in October (acorns). These acorns, together with the bark and leaves, are used medicinally. The acorns are gathered in the autumn, burned and ground to a powder; when steeped in boiling water (acorn coffee), they are highly recommended for scrofula and many indispositions which stem from it, such as diarrhea and abdominal swelling, anemia and leukorrhea. Use 1 sugarspoon powdered acorn in a cup of water.

The bark can be removed from two to three year old branches. It has no smell, but a very astringent taste, and is used externally in the form of compresses, baths, washes, syringes, gargles, etc. For a gargle, take 2 to 4 teaspoons (5 to 10 grams) bark per 2 cups (½ liter) water; for compresses, ⅔ to 1 cup (15 to 20 grams) of leaves or bark per 2 cups (½ liter) water. Internally, 1 to 2 teaspoons (2 to 4 grams) of powdered bark should be taken in syrup, honey, etc., to control heavy menstrual bleeding, blood-spitting, and blood in the stools. The bark is also used externally in the form of compresses for lupus, soft, rotten ulcers, sores, etc.

An excellent remedy for leukorrhea is to boil a handful of oak bark for fifteen minutes in 4 cups (1 liter) water, strain and syringe with this quantity every evening.

Drink 1 cup of oak bark tea daily for blood-spitting, heavy bleeding, painful bleeding, urinary incontinence, chronic dysentery and excessive mucus.

OATS

Avena sativa   Fam. Graminaceae
Groats

Oats originate from Asia and are widely cultivated in this country because they provide one of the best kinds of fodder for horses. They are also used medicinally for a number of illnesses. The grain contains a large quantity of sugar and starch. Oat decoction, ⅛ cup (15 grams) per 2 cups (½ liter) water, is especially recommended for stomach complaints, diseases of the chest and intestines, neck complaints, kidney disease, gout and stones. Oats must be boiled for half an hour. A good quantity of oatstraw, boiled and sweetened with sugar, is very efficacious for coughs, gout and stones. In addition, hot oatstraw baths are highly recommended for rheumatism. After the hot bath, one should always take a cold wash.

OLIVE OIL

Olea Europaea   Fam. Oleaceae

This oil is obtained from the ripe fruit and the best comes from Italy and France; it is white, transparent, with a slightly sweet taste. Rancid oil is not advisable, nor is thick, yellow, opaque oil. Olive oil is frequently used for medicinal purposes, for example: gallstones, cramp-like disorders of the intestines, inflammation of the intestines and stomach, constipation, pleurisy, difficult and painful urination, asthma, blood-spitting, gout, a burned mouth, throat or intestines caused by too hot drinks or food. For ascites, rub the whole abdomen four times a day with hot olive oil and, in addition, cover with a woolen cloth soaked in this oil. Internally, take 1 tablespoon or more according to circumstances. (See, for example, article on gallstones.) Olive oil is the principal ingredient of many ointments described in this book.

ONION

Allium cepa   Fam. Liliaceae

The onion is extensively used in cooking. It is nourishing and
good for the digestion. It also has medicinal uses. It is recommended for dropsy, difficult urination and various complaints
of the respiratory organs. The onion, fried and applied in the
form of a poultice, brings ulcers to a head and encourages
suppuration. The best remedy for a sting by a bee or a wasp is
to rub the sting with an onion. Take 3 to 4 tablespoons (20 to
30 grams) of the extracted sap with sugar daily to cure the most
chronic chest catarrh, likewise podagra. Onion promotes digestion, expels gas and is diuretic. A tincture that can be used with
success for several complaints can be prepared by placing extracted sap with an equal quantity of 45% alcohol in the sun or
near a warm fire for 14 days, after which it should be filtered.
Sniff 4 drops of this tincture diluted with 1 sugarspoon water
two to four times a day for catarrh and a running nose. This
is also good for headaches and ringing in the ears.

Internally, 2 to 3 drops should be given in water three to
five times a day for lack of appetite, abdominal pain, pain in
the chest, bladder complaints, headaches, colic, cramps caused
by wind or piles. Onion sap dripped in the ear cures ringing
in the ears and earache. Onion sap with sugar is recommended
for asthma, coughing, and hoarseness. Dosage: ½ sugarspoon
four to six times a day. You can also fry 3 white onions and 3
egg yolks together to a paste; apply this hot between two linen
cloths on the bladder region for urinary incontinence. Repeat
after three hours if necessary. Raw onions eaten on bread are
recommended for intestinal complaints; 1 tablespoon (15
grams) a day is sufficient.

ORANGE RIND

Cortex aurantium   Fam. Rutaceae

Orange rind is the peel of the orange, the fruit of the orange
tree. This tree originated in India and is cultivated in Italy. The
leaves are hairless, glossy and firm; the flowers are white, fra-

grant and form a raceme. The fruit contains a pleasant, refreshing sap. The rind of this fruit is a stomachic and antifebrile; the flowers act as a stimulant and cure cramps; the leaves expel wind and strengthen the stomach and are highly recommended for hysteria. Use 2 to 3 teaspoons (2 to 3 grams) flowers per 2 cups (½ liter) boiling water. You can also use 4 to 8 teaspoons (3 to 7 grams) leaves per 2 cups (½ liter) boiling water.

ORPINE

Sedum purpureum   Fam. Crassulaceae
Live Forever

Orpine is a powerful, perrenial plant, quite different from other varieties of sedum. It has erect, smooth stems the thickness of a ordinary pencil; the leaves are thick, smooth, glossy green, obovate, either with a smooth edge or lightly dentate. The flowers are pale purplish-red and bloom from July to September. This herb is found in woods on sandy ground, on the edge of woodlands, in hedgerows and bushes. It contains a slimy sap that can be used with success for blood-spitting and bleeding. The fresh sap is good for burns and callouses. The leaves should be applied to sores and swellings.

PARNASSUS GRASS

Parnassia palustris   Fam. Saxifragaecae

This perennial plant is fairly abundantly found in wet marshlands, meadows, fens, and swamps. The angular, ascendant stem attains a height of 12 inches (3 decimeters). A single beautiful white flower and also a single leaf grows on each stem terminal. The leaves, which grow from the knotty rootstock, are long-petiolate, heart-shaped, smooth-edged and bright green. The flowering period is June to September. The plant should be gathered during the flowering period. The brown colored fruits are ovate. The whole plant has a medicinal use. The decoction, ¼ to ⅓ cup (10 to 15 grams) per 2 cups (½ liter) boiling water, is used for heavy bleeding, blood-spitting, diarrhea, and leukorrhea.

PARSLEY

Apium petroselinum   Fam. Umbelliferae

Parsley is a biennial plant, grown in almost every garden. It blooms June and July with green-yellow flowers. It has a strong, aromatic smell; the triangular, three-pinnate leaves with oblong, cut, terminal lobes grow on a grooved stem. The long, thick, fibrous root, white inside, yellow outside, has a sweet taste and a strong, aromatic smell. The small ovate seed is green, has a penetrating smell and a bitter, spicy taste.

The seed infusion, 4 to 5 teaspoons (4 to 5 grams) per 2 cups (½ liter) water, is used internally for difficult urination. The infusion of the green herb, 1½ to 1¾ cup (40 to 50 grams) per 2 cups (½ liter) water, is good for dropsy; an infusion of 4 tablespoons (20 grams) per 2 cups (½ liter) water is used for stomach complaints. The root decoction, 2 to 4 tablespoons (15 to 20 grams) per 2 cups (½ liter) water, is also beneficial for dropsy, gravel, bladder, spleen and liver complaints, and jaundice.

Parsley is a good remedy for glands in the abdomen, neck or elsewhere, and for scrofula in general. Take a handful of leaves and briefly boil in milk without cream; as soon as it boils, it should be removed from the fire and 2 teaspoons of tartar should be added. It should then be left to stand for fifteen minutes, strained through a cloth; then add 1 heaping tablespoon purified flowers of sulphur, 2 tablespoons sugar, and 1 tablespoon magnesia. An adult can take this quantity with a spoon, for example, 3 spoons every hour. Children should be given less.

Bruised parsley leaves can be placed on swollen glands; when laid on the breast, they dry up the milk. Take 2 drops parsley oil daily as an excellent remedy for hematuria, inflammation of the prostate, renal and bladder stones, or difficult urination. The decoction of leaves and stems is very highly recommended for asthma, pain in the chest, phlegm in the chest and stomach. Take 1 cup daily in spoonsful.

PARSNIP

Pastinaca sativa   Fam. Umbelliferae

The parsnip belongs to the family of cultivated umbelliferae and is commonly found in meadows, on farmland and waste-land. The wild parsnip has a thin, woody root; the cultivated variety, on the contrary, has a fleshy root with an aromatic taste and is used in cooking. The stem is angular and has single-pinnate leaves with nine to eleven lanceolate, cut leaflets and many rayed umbels with yellow flowers. The parsnip is a bien-nial plant, blooms in July and August, and is recommended as an excellent medicinal remedy for chronic hoarseness and coughing. Grate 2 parsnips, boil in 4 cups (1 liter) sweet milk, strain, add 3 tablespoons sugar. Take 1 tablespoon of this de-coction every half an hour. The roots boiled in milk are of great benefit to consumptives.

PEA

Pisum sativum   Fam. Papilionaceae

This herbaceous, annual plant has a climbing, pale-green, smooth stem. The leaves are evenly pinnate with two to three pairs of leaflets which produce branched tendrils by means of which the plant attaches itself to surrounding objects. The flow-ers are white or reddish, growing in individual pairs; the fruits (peas) are round or angular and grow in the familiar pods. Flowering period is June to July. There are several varieties which are commonly cultivated. The yellow pea has cleansing, palliative, softening, stimulating and dessicative properties. The decoction of the yellow pea is a recommended remedy for kid-ney complaints, jaundice and accumulation of mucus; it easily dissolves the mucus, kills worms and is generally very beneficial to the health. Weak people sometimes cannot digest the peas themselves, but they can safely take the decoction; it is very potent and wholesome, especially for patients who suffer from dropsy, and for those who are weak.

PEACH TREE

Persica vulgaris   Fam. Rosaceae

The peach comes from Persia and is cultivated in our gardens for its delicious fruit which is well-known for its pleasant taste. The leaves are used medicinally. The infusion should contain ¼ to ⅓ cup (10 to 12 grams) per 2 cups (½ liter) water and is recommended for constipation; it has a mild purgative action. One should never take more than the prescribed dose; more would be dangerous and even fatal.

PELLITORY-OF-THE-WALL

Parietaria officinalis   Fam. Urticaceae
Wallwort

This is a perennial, herbaceous plant, only rarely found on old walls and ruins. It has erect, round stems, reddish on one side; the leaves are small, ovate, glossy green on top, pale green beneath. The small, greenish flowers grow in the leaf-axils in the form of racemes. The flowering period is July. The whole plant is gathered. It has little smell; the sap is salty and contains a large quantity of saltpeter.

Take 1 cup daily of 5 tablespoons (10 to 15 grams) of the dried plant in 2 cups (½ liter) boiling water for all bladder complaints, chronic coughs, kidney disease, gravel, cold urine, ascites, or as a gargle for throat complaints. External use as follows: pellitory boiled in vinegar with houseleek is very efficacious when applied to gangrene. The freshly bruised herb applied to wounds, or a little powdered plant sprinkled on a wound, heals and prevents infection.

PENNYROYAL

Mentha pulegium   Fam. Labiatae

This perennial plant is less commonly seen than other varieties of mint; it is found alongside water and in wet meadows. Its runners creep above the ground and take root; the stems are soft-haired, the leaves are short-petiolate, small, oblong-round, lightly dentate and noticeably decrease in size higher up the stem. The pink flowers grow in round axillary whorls. The flowering period is June to September. Leaves and stems, gathered before the flowering period, are especially used for the treatment of asthma; they facilitate the discharge of phlegm and take away nausea and sickness; jaundice, leukorrhea, gravel and dropsy can also be cured. Take 1 tablespoon dried, finely chopped herbs for 1 cup tea and add, as with all mint teas, a little honey or sugar.

PEPPER SAXIFRAGE

Silaus pratensis   Fam. Saxifragaceae
Meadow Saxifrage

This perennial plant has grooved, branched stems, tri-pinnate leaves with narrow, lanceolate leaflets which are usually found on the lower part of the stems. The flowers, which appear from June to September, are pale yellow. The fruit is oblong, ribbed and hairless. The plant is found on moist ground and fertile meadows. The decoction is a good diuretic, efficacious for bladder and kidney complaints.

PEPPERMINT

Mentha piperita   Fam. Labiatae

Peppermint originated in England and is cultivated in gardens in Europe. It is a perennial, herbaceous plant with a strong, pleasant smell, attaining a height of 20 inches (50 centimeters). The quadrangular, hairy stem is ascendant. The oblong, acute, dentate leaves are hairy underneath; the blue flowers grow in a spike on the stem terminals. The pungent, camphor-like sap is fresh and pleasant in the mouth. The heads are gathered for medicinal use at the beginning of the flowering period. Use ¼ to ⅔ cup (2 to 5 grams) per 2 cups (½ liter) boiling water. Peppermint has a stimulating action, strengthening the heart and stomach; it is especially good for indigestion and mucous catarrh where it dissolves and prevents the further formation of phlegm. It may be used with favorable results for palpitations, shaking and nervous vomiting. It is excellent for worms in children; it increases and thickens the milk for nursing mothers. Take 2 to 5 drops peppermint oil on sugar for migraines, wind, cramps and to calm the nerves.

PERIWINKLE

Vinca minor   Fam. Apocynaceae

This pretty, perennial plant is evergreen; it has many decumbent and ascendant stems. The leaves are oval or ovate, glossy, hairless, leathery; the flowers grow singly at the end of long, pliant stems. The plant is found in shady places, on the edge of woodlands and under old hedges. The leaves are used medicinally for consumption. The infusion of the dried leaves should contain ⅓ cup (15 grams) per 2 cups (½ liter) boiling water. Fresh leaves: use ⅔ cup (30 grams) per 2 cups (½ liter) boiling water.

Periwinkle is depurative, useful for pleurisy, blood-spitting, diarrhea, dysentery, lung ulcers, leukorrhea, milk or sucking sickness, and a deficiency of milk. It is recommended as a gargle for throat infections; it is a most efficacious remedy for the prevention of suffocation and is recommended for all throat complaints. Take 1 cup per day. Vinca major has the same properties.

Peruvian Balsam

Myroxylon balsamum   Fam. Papilionaceae

A brown-yellow aromatic balsam, smelling a little like vanilla, comes from the trunk of a Central American tree, *Myroxylon Balsamum var. pepeirae*. It has been used as a fixative in the soap and perfume industry and as a remedy for healing wounds.

Plantain (Greater)

Plantago major   Fam. Plantaginaceae

This is a very well-known, perennial plant commonly found along roadsides, dykes and on wasteland. It has broad, ovate leaves which are sometimes dentate. The yellow-white flowers form a long, cylindrical spike. The threadlike roots are numerous and the sap is bitter and astringent. The flowering period is May to September. The entire plant is classified for medicinal use. The leaf infusion, containing ½ to ¾ cup (15 to 25 grams) per 2 cups (½ liter) boiling water, is excellent for coughing, accumulation of mucus, diarrhea, blood-spitting, leukorrhea, heavy bleeding of any kind, bleeding piles, involuntary seminal discharge. Fill ⅔ of a bottle with ripe seed, top up with gin and let steep for some time; this will produce a good remedy for dysentery. Take 1 tablespoon three times a day. Or boil 2 teaspoons (4 grams) seed in milk and take throughout the day. The decoction of dried leaves, 1¼ to 1⅔ cup (30 to 40 grams) per 2 cups (½ liter) water, is an excellent gargle for a sore throat; it is also used for thrush.

Plantain (Ribwort)

Plantago lanceolata   Fam. Plantaginaceae

Narrow-leaved plantain is a perennial, herbaceous plant with acute, lanceolate leaves, some hairy, some not. The flower stems have four to six deep grooves; the flowers are first white, later a brownish color, and form a spike on the stem terminals. This plantain is found along roadsides and in meadows, but is particularly abundant in clover fields. The leaves are used medicinally. The infusion contains ½ to 1¼ cups (15 to 30 grams) per 2 cups (½ liter) boiling water and is recommended for diarrhea, dysentery, leukorrhea, blood-spitting, coughing and accumulation of mucus. The leaf infusion is used externally with good result in the form of compresses for inflammation of the eyes.

PLOUGHMAN'S SPIKENARD

Inula conyza   Fam. Compositae

This biennial plant with hairy, erect stems, branched at the top, attains a height of about 3 feet (7 to 9 decimeters). The tops of the bracts are reddish, the leaves lightly hairy, narrow or broad-ovate, slightly dentate, the top leaves petiolate and the lower ones sessile. The numerous yellow-red flowers form an umbel-like raceme. The rather thick roots have a nauseating smell that kills flies. The sap is a little bitter, sour and aromatic. An infusion of the flowers and roots is used medicinally for heavy bleeding. To make, use 3 tablespoons (10 to 12 grams) of the flowers per 2 cups (½ liter) boiling water. For an infusion of the roots: Use 4 tablespoons (15 grams) per 2 cups (½ liter) boiling water.

POLYPODY ROOT (FERN)

Polypodium vulgare   Fam. Filices
Brake Root

Polypody root commonly grows on sandy, shady woodland, on the moldy wood of the pollard willow, and on old walls. The root is used medicinally and is gathered in April. It has very many root fibers which attach themselves to the object on which they grow. Polypody root has no stem. The leaves, which resemble ferns, but which are smaller, have a long stem. The plant does not bear flowers; the fruit is found under the leaves, as in ferns. It is also commonly regarded as a fern. The root decoction contains ¼ to ⅓ cup (40 to 50 grams) per 2 cups (½ liter) water, and is an excellent remedy for a chronic cough and to stimulate the appetite. In the early stages of consumption, it is given for its dissolving and strengthening powers; it also acts as a purgative. Take 2 cups daily.

Take ½ cup (60 grams) polypody root and 2 teaspoons (3 grams) peeled raisins and boil them in 2 cups (½ liter) barley water until reduced by half; this is an excellent remedy for chest complaints, asthma, lung catarrh, phlegm in the chest, fever, intestinal blockage. Take a wineglassful twice a day. The decoction of the leaves, ¾ cup (15 grams) per 2 cups (½ liter) water, is good for coughs, mucus, spleen and lung complaints, liver and scrofula. The powdered root, mixed with honey, is highly recommended for polyps. Polypody root as a tea is conducive to the heart, forms good blood and purifies the blood. For melancholy, sorrow, depression, or nightmares, take 1 cup of tea every morning and evening.

POPLAR TREE

Populus alba   Fam. Salicaceae

This tree, with its long trunk, wide-spread, strong, pliant branches, is found in areas rich in woodland. The young branches are white and woolly, the leaves broad-oval, oblong-oval or oval-round ruggedly dentate; those of the suckers are palmate, five-lobed, hairless and glossy, dark-green above, white and woolly beneath. The male catkins are woolly. The flowering period is March to April. The leaf decoction is used externally in the form of compresses for sciatica; internally, ¾ to 1 cup (10 to 15 grams) per 2 cups (½ liter) water for difficult urination.

PRIVET

Ligustrum vulgare   Fam. Oleaceae

This well-known shrub is found growing wild in thickets and hedges and particularly in parks; privet hedges can be seen everywhere. It reaches a height of about 6 to 7 feet (2 meters), has opposite and decussate, short-petiolate, leathery, hairless, glossy, uncut, narrow-elliptical leaves, which are usually evergreen. The flowers, which appear from June to July, are white, fragrant and form densely clustered racemes on the twig terminals. Like the leaves, the black, round berries, the size of a pea, stay on the plant until the spring. Leaves and flowers are used medicinally, but only externally, for inflammation, and as a gargle for an ulcerated throat and mouth, ulceration of the gums and scurvy.

PSYLLIUM

Plantago Psyllium   Fam. Plantaginaceae
Plantain

Psyllium is a perennial gray-green plant, 1½ feet (½ meter) tall; the leaves are white and woolly underneath, irregularly dentate, oblong and petiolate. The ligulate ray flowers protrude far above the involucre, and are a reddish-yellow; the corolla around the fruit-pappus is dentate. Flowering period is July to August. This plant is sometimes found in large numbers in moist meadows, swampy places and on the verges of ditches. The root, which has filaments, is oblong and thick, brown on the outside and white inside, slimy, slightly aromatic and has a bitter taste. The decoction, consisting of 5 teaspoons (15 grams) of the plant in 2 cups (½ liter) water, is used for diarrhea: take 1 cup daily.

PURPLE Dead-NETTLE

Lamium purpureum   Fam. Labiatae
Red Dead-nettle

This is an annual plant with an erect stem, and ovate, heart-shaped, with irregularly crenate leaves hanging from the top. The flowers, which bloom from March to September, are purplish; the corolla tube has a ring of fine fibers and the lower lip bears two teeth on either side. The creeping roots are fibrous, hairy and small; it has an unpleasant smell and the sap is rather salty and astringent. This plant grows on both farmland and wasteland and in hedgerows. The flowers and leaves are used medicinally.

The infusion is ½ to ¾ cup (10 to 15 grams) per 2 cups (½ liter) boiling water; take 1 to 2 cups daily for renal colic.

An oil can be prepared from the flowers for external use: a bottle should be half-filled with flowers and then filled to the top with olive oil. This should be allowed to stand in the sun or near a fire for a month. This oil can be fruitfully used on burns and old sores, gangrene, ulcers, etc. The herb can also be boiled and made into poultices. The leaves and flowers, fried in fresh butter, produce an efficacious remedy for scrofulous tumors and piles. For scrofulous tumors, a plaster of this ointment should be applied twice a day. Piles should be smeared with it three times a day.

Purple Loosestrife

Lythrum salicaria   Fam. Lythraceae

This perennial plant is quite commonly found in pastures, marshlands and on the water's edge; its ascendant, four or six-sided, single or branched stem grows to a height of three feet. The oblong, lanceolate leaves grow opposite and decussate or in whorls. The attractive purple flowers appear in clustered whorls, two by two, which are separated from each other lower down the spike. The flowering period is June to September, and should be gathered during the flowering periods. Flowers, leaves and stems are used medicinally for dysentery and diarrhea—especially chronic diarrhea. Take 1 cup (30 grams) per 2 cups (½ liter) water. Externally, the decoction, 1¾ cup (50 grams) per 2 cups (½ liter) water, can be used in the form of compresses on fresh wounds and ulcers. Take 1 to 5 teaspoons (1 to 5 grams) of the powdered plant daily for diarrhea. This is highly efficacious for chronic diarrhea.

PURSLANE

Portulaca oleracea   Fam. Portulacaceae

This is a commonly known, annual vegetable with fleshy, hair-less, obovate, glossy green leaves and sessile, yellow flowers in the forks and tops of the branches. The decoction is used me-dicinally—4 to 5 tablespoons (15 to 25 grams) per 2 cups (½ liter) water—or the sap extract for the treatment of internal inflammation, especially for bladder and kidney complaints, impure blood and scurvy, heartburn and blood-spitting. Take 1 sugarspoon or 2 cups of tea three times a day.

QUASSIA

Lignum quassiae   Fam. Simarubeae

Quassia wood comes from Surinam and Brazil; it is a very tall tree which grows in the West Indies and is also found in South America. The wood from the trunk and root is used medici-nally; it has no smell and tastes bitter. It surpasses gentian root in medicinal properties and is used in the same illnesses. It is recommended for intermittent fever, dysentery and jaundice caused by weakness of the intestines. Convalescents (from se-vere illnesses) can tolerate quassia wood better than any other bitter medicine. The infusion consists of ½ teaspoon (1 to 2 grams) per 4 cups (1 liter) water. Tincture of quassia wood may be prepared by letting one part quassia steep in 6 parts gin for three days. The dosage is 10 to 15 drops three times a day in a spoonful of water. For thread worms: briefly boil 4 table-spoons (30 grams) quassia in 4 cups (1 liter) water and syringe it into the rectum or, if necessary, the vagina.

Quassia is also a fortifying remedy for mucus, weak intes-tines, weak stomach, general weakness, heartburn, stomach oppression, fever, gall, worms, congestion of blood in the head, seminal discharge.

RAMPION BELLFLOWER

Campanula rapunculus   Fam. Campanulaceae

Rampion bellflower is an annual plant with an erect, hairy, single or branched stem. It is found on roadsides, hedges and in woodlands. The hairy leaves are lightly dentate; the radical leaves oblong-acute. The beautiful, blue flowers grow along the stem in the leaf axils and droop downwards in the form of bells. The thick root is very good and refreshing to eat. Warts will disappear if bruised leaves are applied.

RAGGED ROBIN

Cardamine pratensis   Fam. Cruciferae
Red Campion, Lady's Smock

This is a perennial plant; very early in the spring, it delights us with its attractive purple flowers which enhance moist meadowlands in abundance as early as April. It has smooth, round, lightly branched stems, which grow from a root rosette of pinnate leaves and nearly round leaves which are reddish-green in color. The plant's taste and smell and all its properties greatly resemble those of watercress. The decoction, ⅓ to ½ cup (15 to 20 grams) per 2 cups (½ liter) water is useful for St. Vitus' Dance, hysteria, epilepsy, nervous cramps and scurvy. Take 1 to 2 cups daily as necessary.

RASPBERRY

Rubus idaeus   Fam. Rosaceae

Raspberry bushes are frequently found in the wild on the edge of woodland and in woods; they are also often cultivated in gardens for the sweet fruit. It has erect, thin stems, covered in prickles; the leaves are three-lobed with a long-petiolate terminal leaflet; the underside is covered in white felt. The white flowers are gathered in racemes and produce red, white, or yellow fruit with a pleasant smell and taste. Maggots are fond of living inside the hollow fruit. The flowering period is May. A popular lemonade can be prepared from the raspberries. Medicinally, raspberry syrup is used for measles, fever and scarlet fever. The infusion of the leaves is a famous remedy for diarrhea and dysentery, especially if these complaints occur in the summer. This tea is also highly recommended for abdominal pain in children and for menstrual disorders.

RED CLOVER

Trifolium pratense   Fam. Leguminosae

Red clover is perennial and grows almost everywhere it is sown. It has a central root rosette from which grow several thin, round stems which are sometimes a little hairy. The leaves are oval or ovate, smooth-edged, soft-haired and usually have a white or black fleck. The flowers are usually dark red and grow on the stem terminals in the form of ovate, thick spikes or heads. The red clover is also commonly found growing wild in meadows and in marshy areas; it makes very good animal fodder. The fresh dried flowers are used medicinally for chronic coughs, lung ulcers, colic, leukorrhea, irregular menstruation and asthma. The infusion of fresh flowers is 2½ cups (50 grams) per 2 cups (½ liter) boiling water. Take 1 to 1½ cups (20 to 25 grams) of dried flowers per 2 cups (½ liter) water or 6 teaspoons (3 grams) of powder in wine or water. The tea should always be taken hot. Boiled flowers, placed on the eyes lukewarm, are highly recommended for inflammation of the eyes.

RED POPPY

Papaver rhoeas   Fam. Papaveraceae
Corn Poppy

This commonly known, annual plant has an erect, branched stem, lanceolate, pinnate leaves and numerous, beautiful scarlet flowers. The flowering period is from June to July. It can be found in abundance on farmland, especially among the corn and wheat. The infusion of the dried flowers consists of 1 sugar-spoon per cup of tea. The red poppy is usually mixed with flowers of the common mallow, marshmallow, Aaron's rod, and lime blossom as a remedy for chest complaints, coughs, dry coughs, whooping cough, spitting blood, and lung diseases. Take ¾ cup (15 grams) of this mixture to 2 cups (½ liter) boiling water; when it has steeped for twenty minutes, add a little honey and take 1 tablespoon every two hours.

RED RATTLE (POISON)

Pedicularis palustris   Fam. Labiatae

This biennial, perennial plant has an ascendant stem with slant-ing branches and lanceolate, pinnate leaves with short, crenate side lobes. The flowers are pink, short-petiolate, growing in the leaf-axils and appear from May to June. The white, wrinkled fibrous roots have an unpleasant smell; the sap is sour, bitter and hot. The plant is found in marshland and wet meadows. The powdered dry leaves get rid of lice.

RED SANDALWOOD

Santalum rubrum   Fam. Santalaceae

Sandalwood grows in the mountains of the East Indies. It is ground to a powder which is used as paint, but also has a medicinal use. Dr. Kneipp recommended this powder, mixed with mistletoe, for heavy bleeding; it can also be added to stom-ach herbs. Sandalwood has a beneficial effect on the blood ves-sels and mucous membranes. Use 1 teaspoon (1 gram) sandalwood powder and add ⅓ cup (10 grams) of the stomach herb.

REED MACE

Typha latifolia   Fam. Typhaceae
Cattail, Bulrush

This plant, with its high stem and broad, erect, leathery leaves can be found alongside canals and pools, ditches and marshes. Dark brown, cylindrical male and female spikes appear on the stem terminals. The flowering period is June to August. The root of this plant is used medicinally; it has astringent properties and is used for chronic diarrhea, bleeding from the womb, and leukorrhea. Externally, an ointment, made by frying the flower heads in lard, is applied to ruptures in children.

RHUBARB

Rheum officinale   Fam. Polygonaceae

Various varieties of rhubarb are available. True rhubarb is still grown in Asia. It is used to treat weakness of the stomach and intestines, poor digestion, acid, wind, jaundice, inflammation of the intestines, internal hardening and cancer, and foul-smelling air accompanying bowel movements. For children, it is recommended for the treatment of rickets, swollen, soft abdomen, very foul-smelling bowel movements, accumulation of mucus, etc. Rhubarb should be given in the form of powder or mixtures in the dose of ½ to 1 teaspoon (½ to 1 gram) as a laxative and a decoction of 1½ to 2 teaspoons (2 to 3 grams) per 2 cups (½ liter) water. The tincture is obtained by steeping 1 part chopped rhubarb in 8 parts gin for several days. Dose: take 1 to 3 grams per day.

ROSEMARY

Rosmarinus officinalis   Fam. Labiatae

This evergreen shrub is native to southern countries and is grown here in pots. The plant has gray-green, very narrow leaves, a whitish color underneath, with lightly curled edges and white or blue flowers; its sap is bitter and aromatic; the whole plant has a pleasant fragrance. Rosemary is an excellent medicine for numerous stomach disorders. The decoction contains ⅓ to ½ cup (15 to 25 grams) per 2 cups (½ liter) water; it promotes digestion and stimulates the appetite, cleanses the stomach, is a recommended remedy for fainting, dizziness, stroke, diarrhea and mucus. When steeped in wine, rosemary is very efficacious in the treatment of heart complaints, hydrothorax and dropsy in general.

Rosemary wine can be prepared by steeping 1 part rosemary in 8 parts white wine for 48 hours: take 2 wineglasses daily. This wine is recommended for asthma, weak stomach, gas, fever; for the same complaints take 3 tablespoons rosemary and steep in 1 cup (¼ liter) hot white wine: take 1 tablespoon hot or cold every two hours. Rosemary oil strengthens the nerves, expels gas and is diaphoretic; the tea has the same properties. Leukorrhea is cured by boiling ¾ cup (30 grams) rosemary with a bottle of white wine and taking 1 spoonful every two hours. Rosemary may also be recommended for kidney and liver disorders, rheumatism, ascites and anasarca (edema).

ROUND-LEAVED MINT

Mentha rotundifolia   Fam. Labiatae

This perennial plant is completely covered with a woolly, gray-green down. The leaves are either sessile or short-petiolate, almost entirely round or ovate, broad dentate, wrinkled, with thick ribs and more hairy beneath than above. The purple-red flowers form a spike on the stem terminal. The flowering period is July through September. The leaves, which have a medicinal use, must be gathered before the flowering period. The plant can be found on wet ground, alongside canals and ditches; its smell is stronger than that of the other varieties. This mint is a stimulant; it strenghtens the heart and stomach. It can be highly recommended for those who suffer from nerves or problem stomachs; it stimulates the appetite, aids digestion, calms vomiting and hiccups, expels water, staunches leukorrhea and heavy bleeding, is recommended for stomachache, diarrhea, colic, wind, nervous headache, migraine, blockage of the liver, spleen and kidneys, abdominal pain, hysteria, hypochondria, palpitations and asthma. In children it can be used for the treatment of worms. Mint is an excellent stomach remedy and one of the most commonly used medicines. The application of the crushed herb on the breasts dries up the milk. The decoction of dried leaves is made from 1⅔ to 4 cups (10 to 25 grams) per 2 cups (½ liter) boiling water.

ROWAN

Sorbus aucuparia   Fam. Rosaceae
Mountain Ash

This is a well-known wild tree with an upright trunk; it is extensively cultivated in parks and has reddish, very hard wood and oblong, serrated leaves. The flowers, which bloom in May, are small, white and grown in racemes. As soon as they fall off, the fruit appears from the flower calyx; it ripens in late August into beautiful red racemes. Thrushes and blackbirds are very fond of them and do not leave a single berry hanging. Rowan berries are astringent. The sap was formerly recommended for vomiting and heavy bleeding.

RUE

Ruta graveolens   Fam. Rutaceae

Rue is a perennial, branched plant which is grown in gardens; in southern Europe it grows in the wild. The leaves are pale-green, very numerous and divided; the yellow flowers appear on the stem terminals. This plant is used medicinally. The decoction contains 1 to 2 teaspoons (1 to 2 grams) per 2 cups (½ liter) water. It is used for hysteria, epilepsy, nervous headache, wind, congestion of blood in the head, dizziness, delayed menstruation due to cramps. For external use, the decoction contains ½ to ¾ cup (25 to 30 grams) and is used in the form of compresses for convulsions. This remedy cannot be praised highly enough. Rue is rather poisonous, so one should never take more than the prescribed dose. Palpitations are soon cured by taking a little rue decoction. Rue oil is made from rue. Take 2 to 5 drops on sugar.

SAGE

Salvia officinalis   Fam. Labiatae

Sage is a commonly known shrub and highly valued for its beneficial qualities. It can be found in most gardens either for medicinal use or as an ornamental plant. The numerous stems are quadrangular and a grayish color; the rather long leaves are opposite, oval-round and gray-green; the flowers are blue-white or pink. The plant has a pleasant, aromatic smell. The leaves are used medicinally for various complaints. The decoction of the dried leaves, ⅓ to ½ cup (10 to 15 grams) per 2 cups (½ liter) water, is for internal use. For external use, as a gargle or on sores, the decoction contains ⅔ to 1⅓ cup (20 to 40 grams) per 2 cups (½ liter) water. Sage should not be taken internally by pregnant women. For internal use, sage is recommended for sweating at night, asthma, chronic coughs, indigestion, diarrhea, lung catarrh and heavy bleeding. Sage is an excellent external remedy as a gargle for hoarseness; sage cannot be recommended highly enough in the form of compresses for old sores and bed sores.

When boiled in milk, with the addition of sugar, sage, taken hot, is one of the best remedies for hoarseness. Sage is an efficacious remedy for paralysis, epilepsy, rheumatism, dizziness, shivering and shaking of the limbs, catarrh, stroke, congestion of blood in the brain, nervous complaints, weak stomach, gas, colic, asthma, worms, indigestion, chronic coughing and gout. Externally, it is used as a gargle for scurvy, thrush and throat complaints. For mouth disorders, boil sage in wine and rinse the mouth with this several times a day. Dried sage leaves smoked every morning and evening enlighten the brain.

SANICLE

Sanicula europaea   Fam. Umbelliferae

This perennial, herbaceous plant is highly recommended, although rare. It is found on the edge of woodland, especially near beech trees. Sanicle has a rosette of long-petiolate, three-lobed radical leaves, a bare flower stem on which several pale pink flowers appear. The leaves are glossy green, like the leaves of celery. From a distance, it resembles young celery. These leaves are used medicinally. The decoction contains 1 to 1⅓ cups (15 to 20 grams) per 4 cups (1 liter) water. For use, add 1 spoon of honey. Especially recommended for gastric ulcers, blood-spitting, hematuria and diarrhea. It must be gathered before it flowers in April.

Sanicle boiled with honey and water heals internal sores and lung complaints such as blood-spitting, bleeding, side and abdominal pain, chest, intestinal and gastric complaints, ulcers in the chest and stomach, heavy menstrual bleeding, rupture, fistulas, bleeding of the kidneys, thrush, scurvy, and purifies the stomach. In serious cases, 1 cup of tea should be taken every morning and evening. An efficacious remedy for all kinds of blood loss, such as kidneys, bladder, womb, lungs, stomach etc. is 2 tablespoons sanicle steeped in a glass of white wine for twelve hours and taken in the mornings on an empty stomach.

The extracted sap taken with rose-sugar is highly recommended for those who suffer from diseased lungs and blood-spitting; 3½ tablespons (30 grams) of sap should be mixed with 1½ tablespoons (15 grams) of rose-sugar and this quantity should be taken every morning and evening. Infusion of sanicle should contain 1⅓ cups (20 grams) per 2 cups (½ liter) boiling water with the addition of 2 or 3 tablespoons of honey; 3 to 6 tablespoons should be taken every morning and evening as an excellent remedy for internal sores, intestinal and chest complaints.

Powdered sanicle, 2 to 4 teaspoons (1 to 2 grams) taken four times a day with some kind of fluid or honey, is very beneficial for St. Vitus' Dance. Or, 3 teaspoons (3 grams) powder taken with honey every evening dissolves mucus in the chest, stomach and intestines. The decoction of the plant has the same effect if 1 cup is taken every evening mixed with honey and licorice.

If an equal quantity of goldenrod is added to sanicle and 2 cups (30 grams) is steeped in 2 cups (½ liter) boiling water, it is an excellent gargle for throat infections, throat tuberculosis, mouth disorders, rotting gums, scurvy, etc. In addition, 1 tablespoon tea should be taken every two hours, with the addition of a little honey.

Sanicle powder sprinkled in bleeding sores staunches the bleeding; in the case of nosebleeds, a little powder can be sniffed up the nose with good results. For complaints of the womb, boil 2 handsful sanicle in 4 cups (1 liter) water until reduced by half, strain and use this quantity daily. Ruptures, fistulas, bleeding, blood-spitting, dysentery, kidney bleeding, hematuria and ulcerated kidneys are cured by taking a wineglass of the following infusion every morning and evening: 2 cups (30 grams) sanicle steeped for half an hour in 2 cups (½ liter) boiling white wine. Since goldenrod has the same effect, this plant can be mixed with sanicle.

SARSAPARILLA

Smilax ornata   Fam. Liliaceae

Sarsaparilla grows in warm countries: Spain, Portugal, Brazil, etc. The root of this shrub is used medicinally for the treatment of venereal disease, old chronic skin complaints, gnawing ulcers, cancer, chronic gout and rheumatism. For the decoction, take ⅓ to ⅔ cup (30 to 50 grams) per 2 cups (½ liter) water and allow to reduce by half; if used in any other way, it has no potency. It should boil for ten minutes and 1 to 2 cups should be taken daily.

SASSAFRAS

Lignum sassafras   Fam. Lauraceae

Sassafras is a tree that grows in North America. The bark and the wood are used medicinally and have stimulating, diuretic, diaphoretic properties. Sassafras is recommended for catarrh, rheumatism and gout, scrofulous skin conditions, scurvy and dropsy. The decoction contains 1 tablespoon (7 grams) per 2 cups (½ liter) water. Dosage: 1 cup daily.

SCARLET PIMPERNEL

Anagallis arvensis   Fam. Primulaceae
Poor Man's Weatherglass

Scarlet pimpernel is an annual, herbaceous plant, commonly found in gardens and fields, particularly on clay soil. It has small, quadrangular, half decumbent and half ascendant stems; oblong, acute, or ovate leaves with perfectly smooth edges and no stems. The star-shaped flowers are the color of red lead and grow in pairs on the stems and branches. The flowering period is from July to August.

The decoction of this plant was formerly used for epilepsy, melancholy, liver complaints and fever, but it is no longer used medicinally.

SKULLCAP (COMMON)

Scutellaria galericulata   Fam. Labiatae
Madweed

Skullcap is a perennial plant to be found alongside waterways and ponds. It has ascendant or decumbent stems 1 to 2½ feet (20 to 60 centimeters) high, and short-petiolate, oblong, acute, serrated leaves. The flowers are blue-violet, rather large, and only grow in the leaf axils, all facing in one direction. The calyx is usually hairless; the roots are yellow and fibrous and smell like garlic; the sap is bitter and salty. The flowering period is June to September. The decoction of the plant, containing ⅓ to ½ cup (10 to 15 grams) per 2 cups (½ liter) boiling water, is used for intermittent fever, throat infections, dysentery and difficult urination. Take 1 cup daily taken with a spoon.

Scurvy Grass

Cochlearia officinalis   Fam. Cruciferae

Scurvy grass grows in the wild in the sand by the sea and is cultivated in gardens for its medicinal properties. It also has a culinary use in salad. It is an annual plant, 1½ to 2 feet (40 to 60 centimeters) high, pale-green in color; the leaves are round and hollow, the white flowers grow in racemes on the stem terminals. Scurvy grass is recommended, as the name suggests, for scurvy; it is also taken for asthma and chronic catarrh. The infusion contains ¼ to ½ cup (10 to 25 grams) per 2 cups (½ liter) cold water. Boiling water should *not* be used or the plant will lose its potency. This infusion is excellent for scrofulous complaints, dropsy, and swollen liver.

Sea Holly

Eryngium maritimum   Fam. Umbelliferae

Sea holly[8] is a perennial plant with pale green, strongly branched, round stems, 1½ feet high. Its numerous flowers are spherical, white or pale green. The prickly lower leaves are broad, double-pinnate and hard. The upper leaves are deeply cut and have much smaller lobes. The stems between the flowers are smooth. This plant grows in sandy fields; the seed is oblong-round, the root long, whitish and with a bitter taste. The flowering period is July and August. The root is used for difficult urination, gravel, dropsy, to stimulate the appetite, promote menstruation and is recommended for liver, kidney and spleen complaints, jaundice and abdominal pain. Steep about 1 ounce (20 to 25 grams) in 2 cups (½ liter) boiling water.

---

[8]We were unable to locate this herb.

SELFHEAL

Prunella vulgaris   Fam. Labiatae

This perennial, herbaceous plant is commonly found in meadows, on roadsides and in woodlands. It has creeping, lightly hairy side-stems, which grow roots and later separate from the mother plant. The long-petiolate, oblong-ovate, smooth-edged leaves are single. The flowers are violet, white, or purplish, and form an almost spherical spike on the stem terminals, with a few leaves at the base. The flowering period is May to September. During these months, the whole plant with roots is gathered and dried. It has little scent and the sap is bitter. Medicinally, the decoction of the plant is used for diabetes, for which it is most efficacious; in addition: for blood-spitting, hematuria, throat infections, sore throat, inflammation of the gums, mouth, and tongue, and especially the tonsils (for which it is used as a gargle). For internal and external sores, and to make clotted blood fluid again, it is boiled in wine and drunk. The decoction, ⅔ to 1 cup (15 to 25 grams) per 2 cups (½ liter), is recommended for lung complaints and heavy bleeding.

SENNA LEAVES

Cassia acutifolia   Fam. Leguminosae

Senna leaves come from various kinds of cassia, shrubs native to Asia Minor, Egypt and Arabia. They are one of those mild, drastic purgatives and are used in cases where one wishes to ensure bowel movement. It often causes cramps and severe abdominal pain, especially if the leaves are boiled; they should preferably be steeped in boiling water with the addition of a little aniseed to prevent the pain. Use 3 to 4 teaspoons (3 to 4 grams) per cup of boiling water and a good spoonful of aniseed. A strong purgative can be prepared by mixing 3 tablespoons (10 grams) senna leaves, ¼ cup (20 grams) star anise, ½ cup (30 grams) marshmallow, and ¾ cup (90 grams) fennel. Take ½ cup (20 grams) of this mixture and boil in 2 cups (½ liter) water until reduced by half.

Shepherd's Purse

Capsella bursa-pastoris   Fam. Cruciferae
Shovelweed

Shepherd's purse cannot be recommended highly enough. No
home should ever be without it on account of its excellence. It
is an annual plant with a thin stem, branched. A raceme of little
white flowers grows on the stem terminal and shortly afterward
makes way for fruit in the form of a heart or shepherd's purse—
hence the name. The leaf edges are sometimes smooth, sometimes dentate. Both hairy and hairless leaves are found. Shepherd's purse is commonly found on the verges of country lanes,
in meadows, etc. The whole plant is gathered in the summer
for winter storage. But it should be used fresh as far as possible
since it loses much of its strength during the drying process.

The infusion consists of 1⅓ cups (50 grams) per 2 cups (½
liter) boiling water and should be left to steep for two hours.
It should be taken in cupfuls. For example, 3 cups daily in the
case of very heavy bleeding, during the change of life. Shepherd's purse is one of the best remedies for dysentery, blood-
spitting, severe bleeding, scurvy, nosebleeds, hematuria, heavy
menstruation, change of life, etc. In all of these cases, it is usual
to take a mixture of shepherd's purse with an equal quantity
of horsetail. Drink 1 to 3 cups of tea daily. For nosebleeds,
drink 1 cup of the infusion and sniff a little into the nose.

The fresh herb is even more effective if it is chewed, the
sap swallowed, and a pellet of it placed in the nostrils.

Silver Birch

Betula alba   Fam. Betulaceae

The birch is a well-known tree or shrub with spirally placed
leaves and stipules which soon fall off. The flowers are catkins
consisting of an axis with spiral scales. The flowering period is
April and May. The leaves are diamond-shaped, with long
points, double-serrated, smooth or with a little hair; the ripe
catkins are elliptical. The birch grows in regions rich in woodland, on heaths and dunes; it has a white trunk. The bark is

bitter and astringent; the leaves are bitter, hot, dessicative, solvent, and stimulate the appetite. It is recommended for dropsy. The decoction of the leaves, bark and thin twigs is ½ to 1 cup (15 to 30 grams) per 2 cups (½ liter) water. People who suffer from nerves or dropsy should take 1 to 2 cups per day.

SLOE

Prunus spinosa   Fam. Rosaceae
Blackthorn

The sloe is found on high, dry ground; it is a much-branched, thorny shrub; the leaves are broad, lanceolate and serrated. The flowers are white and open before the leaves; each bud contains a single flower so that the flowers have a scattered appearance. The flower stems are hairless, and the upright fruits are round and the size of a small marble, blue-black in color; they have a tart, very astringent taste. The flowering period is April to May. The flowers, boiled in milk or taken as a tea, are an excellent purgative and are recommended for scurvy and dropsy; 3 to 4 teaspoons (3 to 4 grams) of the powdered, ripe fruit taken in white wine dispels gastric acid and urine which has been left behind.

SOAPWORT

Saponaria officinalis   Fam. Caryophyllaceae

Soapwort is commonly found along the banks of the Meuse. It is a perennial, herbaceous plant with green, lanceolate leaves and an ascendant, knotty, round stem, lightly branched, which attains a height of four or five feet. The flowers are white or violet colored and grow in racemes on the stem terminals. It bears the name soapwort because the water in which it is boiled becomes as soapy and greasy as soap and water. The whole plant has a medicinal use. The infusion contains ½ cup (15 grams) per 2 cups (½ liter) boiling water and is especially used for eczema, for skin disorders in general, blockage of the urinary organs, syphilis, impure blood, jaundice, gout and rheumatism, venereal disease and asthma. Take 1 to 2 cups daily. It can be used externally in the form of compresses and washes for itching and ulceration.

SOLOMON'S SEAL

Polygonatum officinale   Fam. Liliaceae

This plant is to be found in dry woodland; it is perennial, has a thick, white rootstock and an angular stem. Its leaves are short-petiolate, oblong, blunt or acute and alternate. The flowers are white, tubular and hang to one side of the leaf-axils; they give way to red berries which later turn black. The flowering period is May to June. Both flowers and berries are poisonous. The sweet, slimy, scentless rootstock is used medicinally for gravel. The root decoction cures scurf and skin disorders and clears the flecks left by ulcers or sores. The affected areas should be washed twice a day with the decoction. It can be applied in the form of compresses for sores, bruising and inflammation. For internal use 2 tablespoons (15 grams) per 2 cups (½ liter) water. For external use ½ to ⅔ cup (40 to 50 grams) per 2 cups (½ liter) water.

SORREL

Rumex acetosa   Fam. Polygonaceae

This perennial, herbaceous plant can be found abundantly in meadows and is grown in gardens for culinary use. The stem has beautiful green sagittate leaves. The flowers are red and grow in oblong racemes on the stem terminals. The root is brown, long and fibrous. Sorrel can cure those who suffer from chest and stomach complaints. It is recommended for scurvy; it is a diuretic and stimulates the appetite.

SOUTHERNWOOD

Artemisia abrotanum   Fam. Compositae
Old Man, Lad's Love, Maiden's Ruin

Southernwood is a bushy, perennial plant with erect reddish stems, attaining a height of three feet (80 to 90 centimeters). The small, narrow, oblong leaves are numerous and ash-green in color. The yellow flowers grow in racemes on the stem terminals. The plant's pleasant fragrance very much resembles that of lemon. Southernwood sap is sour and bitter. Only the leaves are used medicinally, and these must be gathered before the flowering period. The plant does not grow wild here; it is frequently grown in gardens on account of its pleasant smell.

The infusion contains 2 to 3 tablespoons (8 to 10 grams) per 2 cups (½ liter) boiling water; it is recommended as a stomachic, for blockage of the liver and kidneys, for jaundice, and to cure housemaid's knee. Use 1 tablespoon every two hours.

SOW THISTLE

Sonchus oleraceus   Fam. Compositae

Sow thistle is an annoying weed which spreads rapidly; animals are fond of eating it on account of the large quantity of sap it contains. It can be found on farmland and wasteland, as well as in gardens. It is an annual plant with smooth, ascendant, sometimes hairy stems, gland-shaped at the top. Its leaves are smooth, oblong, dentate, lyre-shaped and rather prickly. The flowering period is June to September. The decoction of the plant is used for inflammation of the liver, jaundice, gravel, inflammation of the stomach and the chest, asthma, sugar in the urine, painful urination. It increases mother's milk and is depurative. Freshly bruised leaves can be applied to gout. The infusion is made from ¼ to ⅓ cup (15 to 25 grams) per 2 cups (½ liter) boiling water. Take one or two cups per day. The sap extracted can also be taken in wine. Take ⅛ cup (50 grams) daily.

Speedwell (common)

Veronica officinalis   Fam. Scrophulariaceae

Speedwell is a perennial, herbaceous plant frequently found in Germany in woods and on dry ground. The stems, which are usually decumbent, are thickly covered in hair. The leaves grow in opposite pairs; they are short-petiolate, ovate or oblong, and finely serrated. The flowers are light-blue and form a spike on the stem terminals. A spike of flowers grows in almost every leaf axil. Speedwell blooms throughout a large part of the summer. The sap is bitter. The infusion contains ⅓ cup (15 grams) per 2 cups (½ liter) boiling water; take 1 to 2 cups daily for indigestion, migraine, congestion of blood in the head, asthma, spitting blood, and a dry cough.

It can also be used internally for cancer, chronic chest complaints, chronic catarrh, consumption, lung ulcers, eczema, itching, mucus, dizziness, foul stomach, stomachache, stomach cramps, bladder complaints, hematuria, gravel, kidney pain, blockage of the liver and spleen, scabies, difficult urination, and especially for mucus in the respiratory organs, sores, ulcers, congestion, chronic skin complaints. Instead of speedwell alone, an equal quantity of yarrow can be added, or yarrow alone, or *Verbena officinalis* with an equal quantity of yarrow, or verbena alone.

Spignel

Meum athamanticum   Fam. Umbelliferae
Baldmoney

This perennial, herbaceous plant, with a twisted, many-headed rootstock, brown on the outside, white on the inside, has a branched stem about 2 feet high (30 to 40 centimeters) that produces up to three flower stems with the same number of leaves which are long-petiolate and double-pinnate. The flowers are yellow-white, with a little pink. The flowering period is from June to August. This plant is found in the Alps and in the meadows of the Eifel. Spignel strengthens the stomach, is useful for asthma, hysteria, fever, and is a diuretic. The root is used medicinally; the infusion contains 5 teaspoons (5 grams) per 2 cups (½ liter) boiling water. Take 4 to 5 teaspoons (4 to 5 grams) of the root powder.

Spindle Tree (poison)

Euonymus europoeus   Fam. Celastraceae

This is a widely spread shrub which can grow to a height of 13 feet (4 meters). It has a smooth, greenish rind and oval, finely serrated leaves. In the spring it sports racemes of greenish-white flowers. The small four-lobed fruit later turns red. This shrub is found in woods, hedges and thickets. Steep 4 table-spoons (8 to 10 grams) of rind in 2 cups (½ liter) boiling water to make a strong purgative. In view of the fact that it is highly poisonous, care should be taken in its use.

Spiny Rest-Harrow

Ononis spinosa   Fam. Leguminosae

Two varieties are found growing in the wild. Both are shrublike, usually armed with thorns and sporting beautiful pink, occasionally white, flowers which bloom in May. The stems are erect, usually with stiff, sharp thorns. The leaves are narrow, oblong, usually three-lobed, sometimes single on the upper branches, but always sharply dentate. The flowers on the ends of the branches, one or two in the leaf axils, are roughly in the form of racemes, occasionally broken off. The pods are as long as or longer than the calyx. Spiny Rest-Harrow particularly grows along dykes, sunken roads and meadowlands. The root is strong, long and has an unpleasant smell; the sap is bitter and nauseating. It is used for stones, gravel, and bladder complaints. The decoction of the leaves and roots is ⅓ to ⅔ cup (15 to 30 grams) per 2 cups (½ liter) water. This decoction is also used as a gargle for scurvy, sore throat and swollen gums. The rind is an efficacious remedy for gravel, jaundice and inflamed piles. The decoction of the rind is ⅓ to ½ cup (15 to 20 grams) per 2 cups (½ liter) water.

Spotted Dead-Nettle

Lamium maculatum   Fam. Labiatae

This is a perennial plant that grows in moist places, in woodland and hedgerows. The rather tall, erect stem is usually decumbent at the base. The leaves are petiolate, heart-shaped, long-acute, irregularly crenate and bear white spots or stripes. The flowers, which appear from March to September, are purplish, with a dark-spotted lower lip and a fine tooth on both sides. The plant has astringent qualities and is used medicinally for sores. It is commonly used for the same complaints as the purple dead-nettle.

Spotted Orchis

Orchis maculata   Fam. Orchidaceae

This is an attractive, perennial plant, commonly found in moist meadowland. Its erect stem is 8 to 10 inches (20 to 25 centimeters) high. The leaves, which only number four to six, are oblong and spotted with black or gray; the beautiful flowers form a spike and are light or dark red. The root is a globular tuber the size of a hazelnut. The dried, powdered tubers are very nourishing; use 1 tablespoon powder mixed with milk and sugar daily. This powder is also used for several different illnesses such as dysentery, diarrhea, consumption, chest complaints, dry cough, blood-spitting, paludal fever, and for convalescents.

SPRUCE

Picea abies   Fam. Pinaceae
Norway Spruce

The spruce tree is one of the most beautiful conifers to be found
and as such is frequently planted in parks as an ornamental
tree. The branches grow in horizontal whorls, giving the crown
a beautiful pyramid shape. The long, stiff needles are a glassy
green color and end in a thorn. The cylindrical fruits are sessile,
yellow-brown and have winged seeds. The flowering period is
May and June. In the spring, the young shoots, covered with
brown scales, are gathered and made into tea to cleanse the
blood; this tea is also useful for eczema, skin rashes and phlegm
in the lungs. Boil 1 cup (30 grams) of dried, finely chopped
shoots in 2 cups (½ liter) water; take 1 to 2 cups daily. For
seminal discharge, take 3 teaspoons (3 grams) of powder from
the finely ground, dried needles with red wine or a fresh egg.

SUNFLOWER

Helianthus annuus   Fam. Compositae

The sunflower is the largest flower to be found in our gardens
here. The seed is used medicinally and is an excellent remedy
for coughing caused by a chill. A decoction of the bruised seed
should contain 2½ teaspoons (5 grams) per 2 cups (½ liter)
water.

SWEET CICELY

Myrrhis odorata   Fam. Umbelliferae

Sweet cicely grows wild in the Alps and is cultivated in gardens
where it rapidly spreads due to its abundant seed. It is a perennial plant with a long taproot and erect, strong, branched
stems. The leaves are large, soft-haired, three-lobed, soft and
smell of aniseed. The flowers are white and appear from May

to June in erect umbels on the stem terminals. The fruits are blackish and glossy with protruding ribs; they are partly hollow inside. The leaves can be eaten like lettuce. They are used medicinally as a remedy for strengthening the stomach and against consumption, chest complaints, bad humors, epilepsy, and asthma. The dried leaves have a greatly palliative effect on asthma when smoked. The infusion of the plant consists of ¾ to 1 cup (15 to 20 grams) per 2 cups (½ liter) boiling water. Take 1 to 2 cups daily.

SWEET CLOVER

Melilotus officinalis   Fam. Leguminosae
Yellow Melilot

Sweet clover, called after its sweet smell and taste, grows in old buildings, alongside canals, roads and in meadows. It is a biennial plant with fine, erect, very branched stems. The leaves are divided into three and resemble the varieties of clover. The flowers are golden, very small and form a spike on the stem terminals. Sweet clover blooms throughout the summer. The flower heads should be gathered before the flowers open; they are used in the form of compresses for inflammation of the eyes. The infusion contains ½ to ¾ cup (10 to 15 grams) per 2 cups (½ liter) boiling water. The infusion of the flower heads, ⅓ cup (8 grams) per 2 cups (½ liter) water, is a very good remedy for colic, wind, bladder complaints, gravel, abdominal pain, leukorrhea, inflammation of the abdomen. Take 1 spoon every two hours. White sweet clover has the same action.

SWEET VIOLET

Viola odorata   Fam. Violaceae

The violet is a commonly known, perennial, herbaceous plant. It is commonly found under old hedges and on the verges of woodland; it is also cultivated in gardens on account of the pleasant fragrance of the flowers. It blooms in the spring and has violet-blue flowers; the rather large leaves have a long stem and are hairless. The dried flowers are used medicinally for lung disorders, measles, scarlet fever and smallpox. Take 1 sugarspoon violets per 2 cups (½ liter) boiling water. The root is an emetic. The leaves of the plant are also used externally as a gargle for throat infections. The infusion consists of 1 cup (15 grams) per 2 cups (½ liter) boiling water. The decoction of the leaves (boiled in vinegar) and used in the form of compresses is an efficacious remedy for podagra. The infusion consists of 6¼ cups (100 grams) per 4 cups (1 liter) vinegar.

TANSY

Tanacetum vulgare   Fam. Compositae

Tansy is found in mountainous, sandy soil, and abundantly along the banks of the Meuse; it is occasionally even grown in gardens. It is a perennial, herbaceous plant that has gold-colored flower heads which cluster in umbel-shaped racemes on the stem terminals; they are as round as buttons. The lower leaves are petiolate, the upper sessile, deeply cut, serrated and dark green. The whole plant has a strongly aromatic smell. All parts of the plant are used medicinally: leaves, flowers and seed; they all have the same properties.

The infusion contains ¼ to ½ cup (10 to 20 grams) per 2 cups (½ liter) boiling water. It is used for irregular menstruation, hysteria, dizziness, cramps and colic. Tansy can also be steeped in wine, 2½ cups (100 grams) of the plant to 1 quart (1 liter) white wine; 6 spoonsful should be taken daily; take 1 tablespoon every two hours. A very good external remedy for eczema, chapped hands, scurf and rheumatism is ⅔ cup (25 grams) flower heads steeped in a bottle of gin; the joints or affected areas should be rubbed with this twice a day. The infusion is also of benefit in the treatment of worms, jaundice and dropsy. Crushed fresh leaves, mixed with fresh butter, are an excellent remedy for sprains and dislocations.

TEASEL

Dipsacus sylvestris   Fam. Dipsaceae

This annual or biennial plant may be found on dry, clay soil, areas of wasteland, along dykes, etc. Its erect, branched stems are covered with strong prickles; the sessile leaves which are smooth on the upper side also have prickles underneath. The radical leaves are petiolate, oblong and dentate. The flowers grow on the stem terminals; the ovate flower heads are usually pale red or violet. The flowering period is from July to September. The leaves are used medicinally for heavy menstruation, dysentery, and blood-spitting. The infusion contains ⅓ to ½ cup (10 to 12 grams) of dried leaves per 2 cups (½ liter) boiling water. Instead of this, 2 to 3 teaspoons (4 to 5 grams) of powdered leaves can be taken daily. The application of fresh leaves is an excellent remedy for gangrene; a change for the better will be noticed after a couple of days.

THORNAPPLE (POISON)

Datura stramonium   Fam. Solanaceae
Jimson Weed

This is an annual plant that grows wild in America and some European countries and which is cultivated here in our gardens. The leaves are large, ovate, acute, angular, dentate, smooth and supported by a strong stem; they have an intoxicating smell. The seed is black, kidney-shaped, scentless, but with a nauseating, narcotic taste, enclosed in a thick, ovate, prickly seed capsule. Thornapple is extremely poisonous and must be included among the most narcotic medicines. Externally the following tincture is an excellent remedy for neuralgia:

    1 cup (60 grams) thornapple seed
    2 cups (½ liter) Spanish wine
    2 cups (½ liter) alcohol

The painful area should be rubbed with it by hand; it alleviates the pain most wonderfully.

THRIFT

Armeria vulgaris   Fam. Plumbaginaceae
Sea-pink, Ladies Cushion

This perennial plant has much in common with the *Primulaceae* with respect to the regular shape of its flowers and the number of sepals and petals. Thrift[9] is found on wasteland; it attains a height of about 10 inches (25 centimeters) has oblong leaves of equal width throughout, and pink, sometimes white, flowers on petiolate flower heads. It blooms throughout the summer. The whole plant is used medicinally. It is used internally for dystentery, spitting blood and heavy menstruation; externally as a gargle when the mouth cavity is affected by mucus. The infusion of leaves and flowers consists of ¼ ounce (8 to 10 grams) per 2 cups (½ liter) boiling water. For internal use, 1 tablespoon should be taken every two hours with a little sugar, as the sap is very astringent.

THYME (WILD)

Thymus serpyllum   Fam. Labiatae

This fragrant plant is abundantly found on dry ground, old hills, sandy soil, etc. If thyme is touched or rubbed, it exudes a pleasant smell. It is also grown in gardens for culinary use. It is a perennial, herbaceous plant with numerous, thin stems and small, ovate, gray-green leaves. The flowers form a spike on the stem terminals; they are purple or white. The black ones are of no use. The whole plant should be gathered during the flowering period for medicinal use. The sap is bitter. The infusion contains 2 tablespoons (5 grams) per 2 cups (½ liter) boiling water. It is particularly recommended for a stubborn cough, whooping cough, anemia, worms, excessive gall and bladder complaints. Thyme boiled in wine has a stronger effect. Honey or sugar can be added according to taste. Thyme must be gathered very early in the morning, before the dew is dry.

---

[9]We were unable to locate this herb.

The infusion mixed with honey is a very good remedy for whooping cough, it cleanses the lungs, is excellent for migraines, dizziness, and as a depurative.

TOADFLAX (POISON)

Linaria vulgaris   Fam. Scrophulariaceae

This herbaceous, biennial plant, 1½ feet (30 to 40 centimeters) high, is found along roadsides, on both farmland and wasteland, rubbish tips and especially alongside railways. It has a smooth, round, beautifully green, terminally branched stem, lanceolate, hairless, acute, narrow leaves, lemon yellow flowers in the form of a slipper. The flowering period is June to October. When boiled in milk, the plant kills flies; for this reason and also on account of its unpleasant smell, it is rather suspect. In general it has solvent and palliative properties. For painful piles, ½ cup (20 grams) of the plant should be boiled in 2 cups (½ liter) milk and applied in the form of a poultice. The decoction, 2 to 3 tablespoons (5 to 8 grams) per 2 cups (½ liter) boiling water, is recommended for internal use for skin complaints, eczema, jaundice, swollen liver, bladder stones and dropsy. Never take more than the stated dose as it could have harmful consequences.

TORMENTIL

Potentilla tormentilla   Fam. Rosaceae

Tormentil is an herbaceous, perennial plant with a dark brown rootstock that has no smell. It has a strongly astringent taste. It grows in wet place and heath. The plant stems are very fine, rather branched and covered in leaves. The yellow flowers grow on the terminals of long stems. The flowering period is May, June and July. The root can be used to prepare a red tincture used medicinally for heavy bleeding, chronic diarrhea, blood-spitting, ulcers from scurvy, and to quench the thirst in cases of diabetes; in the latter case it is very effective. Take 3 to 4 sugarspoons daily in cold water. Or, take 1 to 2 teaspoons (1 to 2 grams) of the powdered root daily for the same complaints. The decoction contains 2 tablespoons (15 grams) per 2 cups (½ liter) water. Take 3 teaspoons (3 grams) tormentil powder daily with wine for the treatment of heavy menstruation, hematuria and internal sores. The decoction can be used as a mouthwash for mouth disorders. Tormentil is one of the best remedies for bed-wetting or urinary incontinence in women, for example.

Turnip (rapeseed)

Brassica rapa   Fam. Cruciferae
Bird's Rape

The turnip supplies us with rapeseed for which oil is extracted for burning and for use by the poor in their food instead of butter and fat. Rapeseed oil, mixed with egg white and chalk, is an excellent remedy for scrofulous sores. The turnip has a culinary use but is also an efficacious remedy for old sores; it should be boiled in milk and the resulting paste applied in a very thick layer. Fried turnips can be applied to chapped hands or feet; it will not fail to help. Boil a quantity of turnips with the rind and squeeze them out into the decoction, add 1 pound (half a kilo) loaf sugar to each quart (liter) of juice, leave it to swell. This is a highly recommended drink for consumptives, also for tubercular throats. Take 1 tablespoon every two hours. In cases of tubercular throats, this decoction can also be used as a gargle.

Valerian

Valeriana officinalis   Fam. Valerianaceae

Common valerian is a perennial, herbaceous plant, found abundantly in both mountainous regions and wet places. It is usually found in woodland and meadows. The stem is ascendant, lightly branched, grooved, pale-green; the leaves are dark-green, smooth and deeply cut. The fragrant, pink flowers are small and form a raceme on the stem terminal. The root, which is used medicinally, has a fibrous bud, surrounded by thin brown side-roots, with a singularly unpleasant smell and a nasty, bitter taste. This root is gathered in the spring. The decoction contains 2 to 3 tablespoons (10 to 20 grams) per 2 cups (½ liter) water. Powdered root is preferable; the dose is ½ to 2 teaspoons (1 to 4 grams). Valerian is recommended for chronic nervous disorders and feverish illness, at the onset of epilepsy, St. Vitus' Dance, hysteria, hypochondria, dizziness, stomach cramps, nervous headaches, paralysis and pituitous stroke. Valerian is an excellent remedy for worms, since it kills the worms and cures any resulting nervous condition. In addition, it is used for cramplike asthma, trembling of the limbs, nervous vomiting, stomach and abdominal pain, hoarseness due to nerves, complete loss of voice, palpitations and paralysis of the tongue. Take 10 to 15 drops of Valerian tincture with the addition of a few drops of ether. This should be taken twice a day before meals in a spoon of water. The tincture can be used instead of the tea decoction. Old people suffering from eye weakness can take 1½ teaspoons (3 grams) powdered root with a little honey every morning; it will strengthen the eyes.

VERVAIN

Verbena officinalis   Fam. Verbenaceae

Vervain is an herbaceous, perennial plant with violet florets which form a thin spike on the stem terminal. The oblong leaves are coarsely haired, deeply and irregularly serrated, opposite and decussate. The stems are very hard and difficult to grind to a powder. It is found along roadsides and on wasteland; it flowers from June to October. The sap is astringent and bitter. The infusion contains 1½ to 2 tablespoons (10 to 12 grams) per 2 cups (½ liter) boiling water and is recommended for cramps, and spleen, liver and kidney complaints. It has more strength when taken in wine. Vervain taken as a tea is febrifugal. The dried herb, mashed in hot water, can be applied to the throat to cure severe hoarseness and headache; a little of the tea can also be taken. Mouth ulcers and loose teeth can be cured by rinsing the mouth several times with this tea. The decoction is also an efficacious remedy for the treatment of migraines, liver disorders, jaundice, colic, chest complaints and chronic cough. The dosage is 1 cup per day.

VIPER'S BUGLOSS

Echium vulgare   Fam. Boraginaceae

Viper's bugloss is a biennial plant with a very prickly, thick stem, with narrow, lanceolate, slightly hairy leaves and rather large, funnel-shaped flowers. The latter grow in racemes in the leaf-axils; they are first red and later turn blue or white. Viper's bugloss grows on old walls, wasteland, along the banks of the Meuse, alongside railway lines and in stony woodland. The infusion of leaves and stems is used for the treatment of pneumonia, rheumatism and measles. It contains ⅓ to ½ cup (12 to 15 grams) per 2 cups (½ liter) boiling water. The dried root is used in the form of powder for the treatment of epilspsy; take 2 teaspoons (2 grams) daily in a spoon of wine.

WALLFLOWER

Cherranthus cheiri   Fam. Cruciferae

The wallflower frequently grows on old walls, but is also cultivated in gardens on account of its attractive fragrance. It is a low shrub with a woody stem and lanceolate, acute, dentate, gray-green leaves; the gold-colored flowers are clustered in racemes on the branch terminals. The flowering period is May to June. Young plants only have a rosette of radical leaves. The flowers are used medicinally for nervous disorders.

The infusion is made from 1⅓ to 1⅔ cups (10 to 15 grams) per 2 cups (½ liter) boiling water. Let 2 handsful mixed flowers, leaves, and seed steep together in half a bottle white wine and you will have an excellent remedy for stones, gravel, involuntary seminal discharge, nervous headaches, prevention of strokes, and to fortify the heart and nerves. Take 3 to 4 tablespoons daily. Use 3 to 4 teaspoons (3 to 4 grams) powdered seed daily as a beneficial relief for dysentery. The flowers, steeped in olive oil, are most efficacious in the treatment of nervous and rheumatic pain.

WALL RUE

Asplenium ruta muraria   Fam. Filices

This plant is only found on old walls and rocks, where it grows in small clusters. It remains green the year round; in older plants the rootstock has many heads and has gray-green, triangular oval leaves that grow irregularly in different directions. The infusion is made from ¼ cup (10 grams) per 2 cups (½ liter) water and is recommended for jaundice, pneumonia, coughing, pain in the loins, gravel, bladder complaints, asthma, and scurvy. It is particularly worthy of recommendation for lung disorders and intestinal blockages.

WALNUT

Juglans nigra   Fam. Juglandaceae

The walnut tree is a beautiful tree with gray bark and a fine, broad, round crown; the leaves are pinnate. The male catkins appear in May and June; the female flowers are clustered together and difficult to find. All parts of this tree are useful: the leaves, the bark, the green rind of the unripe fruit, the fruit oil, the septa which can be found in the middle of the fruit, the flowers, etc.; everything has a medicinal use. The leaves should be harvested in mid-June, the bark may be gathered at any time of the year, the flowers during the flowering period, and the fruit rind when the nut has fully grown.

The infusion of leaves contains ½ to ¾ cup (15 to 20 grams) per 2 cups (½ liter) boiling water and is one of the best remedies for scrofulous constitutions. An infusion of flowers contains ⅔ to 1 cup (10 to 15 grams) per 2 cups (½ liter) boiling water, and is used for leukorrhea. The green rind of the unripe fruit, preserved in gin, is a well known stomachic. The fruit septa, ground to a powder, is a commonly known remedy for fleshy excrescences: this powder should simply be sprinkled on the affected area. It can especially be used for gangrene: 1 sugarspoon powder should be taken twice a day in wine, and a little powder should be sprinkled on the wound. The young buds can be used to prepare an excellent ointment to prevent hair from falling out and to get rid of dandruff; a handful of buds should be fried for about half an hour in 1½ cups (300 grams) lard. Take 1 to 2 cups of the flower infusion daily for jaundice, heavy bleeding, or lupus.

WATERCRESS

Nasturtium officinale   Fam. Cruciferae

Watercress is an herbaceous, perennial plant, usually with a decumbent stem, on which racemes of white flowers appear. The roots are white and fibrous. Watercress is found almost everywhere where there is water. It flowers in the summer. The whole plant is used medicinally and is also eaten in salad. Watercress must always be used fresh. It is employed for the treatment of a swollen spleen, eczema, chronic catarrh, Guinea worm and lack of appetite. Take ⅓ cup (100 grams) of the plant sap daily or take it in the form of salad. Watercress is also beneficial for blockage of the spleen and liver, gravel and womb, especially for scurvy, hysteria, hypochondria, melancholy, dropsy and to promote menstruation.

When boiled in wine, it is a good remedy for consumption, catarrh and chest complaints in general. Boil 3 handsful watercress in 1 cup (250 grams) wine; 1 wineglass to be taken every morning and evening. The decoction in water or milk contains ⅓ cup (15 grams) per 2 cups (½ liter). Externally, it is highly recommended as a mouthwash for thrush. Freckles and flecks on the face will disappear upon application of the freshly bruised herb.

WATERMINT

Mentha aquatica   Fam. Labiatae

Watermint is distinguishable from other mints by its long-petiolate leaves; its reddish flowers grow in round whorls. It has long creepers and the branched stem usually bears ovate, serrated leaves. It is commonly seen alongside water, canals and marshes. The flowering period is July to September. The leaves are only gathered for use before the flowering period. Watermint is second only to peppermint as the variety which is most commonly used medicinally.

WHITE DEAD-NETTLE

Lamium album   Fam. Labiatae
Blind Nettle

The white dead-nettle is distinguishable from other nettles in that it does not sting. It is called the white nettle because the flowers are white; this is not found in any other nettle. It is a perennial, herbaceous plant, with a large, quadrangular stem. The leaves are paler than those of other nettles and have one or more small, sharp teeth; the white flowers grow in the leaf axils. It has an unpleasant smell and bitter, astringent sap. It blooms throughout the summer. It is the flower heads which should be gathered.

The infusion contains ½ to ¾ cup (10 to 15 grams) per 2 cups (½ liter) boiling water and is recommended for leukorrhea and diarrhea, heavy bleeding and excessive mucus. Take 1 to 2 cups daily. Externally, the boiled leaves and flowers should be placed on swellings, bleeding ulcers and scrofulous tumors.

WHITE MAGNESIA

Magnesia alba

Magnesia is a white, light, tasteless, powder-like substance which can be dissolved easily in acids but not in water. It is an excellent remedy for nervous complaints, and, through combination with gastric acid, forms a salt which promotes bowel movement; it is excellent in cases where acid causes complaints such as sluggish bowel movements, etc. Magnesia is a good, harmless remedy for gravel and kidney stones. It should be given as a powder or in mixtures: about ½ teaspoon (1 to 2 grams) every two to three hours. Magnesia should not be mixed with acids.

WHITE STONECROP

Sedum album   Fam. Crassulaceae

White stonecrop is a perennial plant with cylindrical, smooth leaves; the petals are three to four times as long as the sepals. The flowers are white or pink and appear in June or July. It grows on old walls, roofs, rocks and dry, sandy ground; the stems are decumbent. The plant sap is used externally in ointments and especially in poplar ointment.

WHITE WATER LILY

Nymphaea alba   Fam. Nymphaeaceae

This beautiful, perennial plant is found in ponds. It can be recognized by the large, green, almost circular, cut leaves, heart-shaped at the base, which lie flat on the water and grow on long, thick, round stems which come from a horizontal rootstock. The white flowers bloom from June to September. The roots are used medicinally for inflammation of the kidneys and bladder, lung catarrh, seminal discharge, heavy menstruation and diarrhea. Dosage: 3 teaspoons (3 grams) powdered root or seed in wine. The decoction of the dried roots contains 1 to 2 tablespoons (12 to 15 grams) per 2 cups (½ liter) water. For pain in the spleen, take 4 tablespoons (30 grams) root to ½ cup (125 grams) wine in two doses.

WHITE WILLOW

Salix alba   Fam. Salicaceae

The tree's name comes from the white, glossy down that covers the leaves and young twigs. It has pliant, gray-green branches with lanceolate, short-pointed, finely serrated leaves. It is commonly found alongside ditches, canals and in wet meadows. Before the flowering period (April), the bark of the two and three year old branches should be gathered and left to dry. The decoction of this is very bitter astringent and can be fruitfully used for the treatment of fever. It is, indeed, one of the best febrifugal remedies, especially for intermittent fever. It is also highly recommended for blood-spitting and is a very potent tonic. Boil 3 to 4 tablespoons (15 to 20 grams) in 2 cups (½ liter) water until reduced by half; add a little sugar or honey as it has a rather bitter taste. Take 1 tablespoon every two hours; 1 tablespoon every hour in cases of fever. It is a most efficacious remedy for heavy bleeding, also for chronic diarrhea, leukorrhea, excessive mucus, stomach cramps, nervous complaints, spleen and liver disorders, foul or mucous stomach.

Powder from the dried bark of willow can also be used for the same complaints; take 2 to 2½ tablespoons (5 to 10 grams), as necessary, per day with a little honey or syrup or in wine. When taken in wine, ½ to ¾ cup (50 to 60 grams) should be steeped in 1 quart (liter) of wine for 14 days. Dosage: 1 tablespoon three times a day. Boil 3 handsful of willow leaves in 1½ cups (350 grams) wine until reduced to two-thirds. This is a beneficial remedy for blood-spitting, vomiting blood, heavy bleeding, heavy menstruation and leukorrhea. Dosage: a liqueur-glassful three times a day. A tincture of willow bark can also be prepared by letting 3 parts powdered willow bark steep for ten days in 10 parts alcohol; it should then be filtered. The dose is 5 drops in a spoon of water one to four times a day.

WILD STRAWBERRY

Fragaria vesca   Fam. Rosaceae
Wood Strawberry

It is unnecessary to describe this plant as even a child knows it.
The wild strawberry is palliative and stimulates the appetite but
is rather indigestible. It is also somewhat too cold for the stomach and is therefore not recommended for weak stomachs. It
is recommended for consumptives, for rheumatic complaints,
gout, liver disorders, gravel and stones, and is also depurative.
Wild strawberries with milk are the best remedy for the complaints mentioned above. Mix 1 part wild strawberry leaves, 1
part young juniper stems, and 1 part woodruff prepared as tea
for a delicious, healthy drink with a pleasant fragrance. Milk
and sugar may be added. This is an excellent alternative to tea
from abroad. Use ⅓ to ½ cup (15 to 25 grams) per quart (liter)
of boiling water.

WINTER CRESS

Barbarea vulgaris   Fam. Cruciferae

This is an annual plant with an erect, branched stem, attaining
a height of 2½ feet (20 to 40 centimeters). The leaves are deeply
cut and are dark green in color. The yellow flowers grow in
racemes on the stem terminals. The flowering period is June.
The plant is usually found on roadsides, and on the edges of
woodland. The plant decoction consists of ⅓ to ½ cup (15 to
20 grams) per 2 cups (½ liter) water and is used for scurvy and
poor appetite; it is also diuretic and depurative. Take 1 cup of
tea daily.

WINTERGREEN

Pyrola rotundifolia   Fam. Pyrolaceae
Wild Lily-of-the-Valley

This is found abundantly in woodland; it is a perennial plant
with a bare, ascendant stem, and a long creeping rootstock with
a rosette of long-petiolate, approximately round, very finely
serrated leaves. The beautiful white, pink colored flowers grow
in pointed racemes on the stem terminals; the stamens are
curved to one side. The flowering period is June to July. The
whole plant should be harvested during this period. The infusion is used for all kinds of bleeding, and both internal and
external wounds. For internal wounds, chronic catarrh and
diarrhea, boil ¼ cup (15 grams) of the dried plant in 1 cup (200
grams) wine; 1 tablespoon should be taken every two hours.

For a hard, blocked spleen, apply the leaves after boiling
them in vinegar. For earaches and running ears, boil the leaves
in olive oil and put 5 drops in the ears. For gravel and dropsy,
take 3 teaspoons (3 grams) of powdered berries in wine. To
strengthen the brain and cleanse the head, wintergreen sap
should be sniffed up the nose.

WOOD AVENS

Geum urbanum   Fam. Rosaceae
Herb Bennet

Wood avens is an annual plant which is commonly found in
shady, damp places, under old hedges, etc. The stem grows to
a height of one to two feet, is ascendant, hairy, a reddish color
and covered with branches; the leaves are divided, dentate and
hairy; the yellow flowers can be seen on the stem terminals and
appear from May to September. Wood avens root is used medicinally; the roots must be gathered in April. The decoction
should consist of ⅛ cup (10 grams) per 2 cups (½ liter) water.
This decoction is recommended for intermittent fever, dysentery, nervous headaches and fevers. It strengthens the heart,
stimulates the appetite, improves digestion, strengthens the
stomach, promotes menstruation and is good for blood-spitting,

heavy bleeding, palpitations and leukorrhea. The whole plant, boiled in wine, promotes menstruation, strengthens the brain, dissolves clotted blood in the body and cures pains in the stomach and side, and liver and heart complaints. Boil ½ cup (40 grams) of dried wood avens root and ⅔ cup (40 grams) leaves in 4 cups (1 liter) wine or water until reduced by half. Take 3 tablespoons three times a day; this is also efficacious for the treatment of internal and external piles, chest complaints, indigestion and cramps.

Wood Sorrel

Oxalis acetosella   Fam. Oxaliaceae

This perennial plant is well-known. It grows abundantly in shady, moist places and in woods. It has a crimped rootstock with thin runners from which glossy green, oblong, long-petiolate, soft-haired leaves grow. The white, red-veined flowers bloom from April to May. The decoction of the fresh plant consists of ½ to 1 cup (10 to 20 grams) per 2 cups (½ liter) boiling water and is recommended for scurvy, as a gargle and mouthwash for rotting gums, ulcerated mouth and inflammation of the throat. Add 2 teaspoons aniseed per 2 cups (½ liter) decoction to get a very good remedy for jaundice. The above mentioned quantity can be taken for this complaint. For bilious fever, the decoction of wood sorrel, without aniseed, can be applied as a cooling remedy.

Woodruff

Asperula odorata   Fam. Rubiaceae
Woodward

This is a perennial, herbaceous plant which is very commonly found in Germany in moist, shady places in woodlands. It has a creeping rootstock, with numerous, quadrangular knotty stems. The leaves are pale-green, lanceolate, in whorls of six to eight; the flowers are white, appear on the stem terminals and, like the whole plant, exude a pleasant fragrance which is increased by drying. Woodruff is also grown in gardens on account of the pleasant scent of the flowers and attains a height of about 8 inches (20 centimeters). The flowering period is May and June. The plant is gathered during this period. The infusion contains ⅓ to ½ cup (8 to 10 grams) per 2 cups (½ liter) boiling water. It is used medicinally for jaundice, dropsy, gravel, spleen and liver disorders, epilepsy, paralysis, nervous complaints, hysteria and it strengthens the heart, chest and liver. Take 1 cup of the infusion daily.

WORMWOOD (COMMON)

Artemisia absinthium Fam. Compositae
Absinthe, Green Ginger

Common wormwood is a perennial shrub-like plant and the leaves and flower heads are used medicinally. Common wormwood is very often grown in gardens. The stem is straight, hairy, dark gray in color, branched. The leaves grow all the way down the stem, are pale green, grayish, very divided, a silvery color above, white and silky beneath. The plant attains a height of about 3 feet (80 centimeters). The flowers are abundant, a yellow color, divided into small racemes and grow on the stem terminals. The flowering period is from July to September. Common wormwood must be gathered a few days before flowering. It should be dried in the shade and stored in a dry, draft-free place. It has a very bitter taste and a strong, rather intoxicating smell which is not lost by drying, especially if this is done carefully. Common wormwood can be considered as one of the most valuable indigenous plants. A bag of dried common wormwood tied to the forehead promotes sleep.

It is always recommended for indigestion, heartburn, worms, jaundice, suppressed menstruation, leukorrhea and especially fever and dropsy. The infusion consists of 3 to 5 tablespoons (10 to 15 grams) per 2 cups (½ liter) boiling water, 1 tablespoon every two hours. Additional preparations are: wormwood tincture, obtained by letting one part dried flower heads draw for six days in 6 parts gin; 50 to 70 drops or 1 to 2 sugarspoons should be taken three or four times a day. Wormwood oil is used in attacks of hysteria and cramp colic; 3 to 5 drops every hour. Wormwood wine (absinthe) is prepared by steeping ¾ to 1 cup (30 to 40 grams) of dry wormwood for twenty minutes in 2 cups (½ liter) boiling white wine. It should be given with a spoon; it is especially recommended for intermittent fever and dropsy. It is not advisable to prepare more than 2 cups (½ liter) at a time as this infusion soon spoils. Wormwood powder is used as a febrific in the dose of 2 teaspoons to 1 tablespoon (1 to 3 grams) in some kind of liquid.

The most efficacious preparation of wormwood is the following mixture:

> ¾ cup (2 grams) common wormwood
> ⅓ cup (100 grams) 90% alcohol
> 4 cups (1 liter) white wine

First leave the wormwood to steep in the alcohol for twenty-four hours, then add the wine and let steep for another two days, then strain and filter. Take 3 to 6 tablespoons of this tincture daily. It is especially recommended for indigestion, general weakness, weakness of the digestive organs, heavy bleeding and leukorrhea; it promotes menstruation, stimulates the appetite and is the remedy for gastric weakness, acid stomach, dropsy, scurvy, gout, uterine complaints, kidney disorders, stones, and blockage of the liver. But, here too, it should be taken in moderation.

Monseigneur Kneipp used to say, "Nur des Guten nicht zu viel," which means that good things should not be misused. There are, indeed, people who take a far too strong infusion of wormwood tea every day. This is very injurious, particularly as there is no fixed dose.

YARROW

Achilles millefolium   Fam. Compositae
Milfoil, Woundwort, Carpenter's Weed

This perennial, herbaceous plant is commonly found on wasteland, meadows, roadside verges, etc. It has an erect, grooved stem with few branches and numerous soft-haired, lanceolate, double-pinnate leaves. The white or pale-pink flowers grow in cymes on the stem terminals. Leaves and flower heads are gathered for internal and external medicinal use. The flowering period is June to October.

The infusion consists of ⅓ to ½ cup (10 to 15 grams) per 2 cups (½ liter) boiling water. The leaves and flowers have a strengthening effect on the intestines and mucous membranes, and cure cramp in the former. The infusion is used for weakness and mucus in the digestive organs, for lung complaints and especially for internal cramps, heavy bleeding, piles, irregular menstruation and nervous complaints. It is particularly recommended for the treatment of insomnia: one cup of this infusion to be taken before retiring. If menstruation has ceased due to some temporary cause, such as a chill or a severe shock, yarrow tea is the remedy to use.

It is especially recommended for nervous complaints. For nervous complaints and in order to sleep well, ¾ to 1½ cups (20 to 40 grams) per 2 cups (½ liter) boiling water should be taken instead of the normal ⅓ to ½ cup (10 to 15 grams). Do not prepare too much of this infusion at one time as it spoils rapidly.

Externally, the fresh pounded leaves are excellent for caries. If, in winter, the fresh plant is unavailable, a strong decoction of flowers and leaves may be applied as compresses.

Yarrow is particularly effective in strengthening convalescents; also for the consequences of self-abuse, internal ulcers. It strengthens those who suffer from their nerves. Back pain caused by piles is cured by yarrow tea; furthermore, this tea can be taken by patients suffering from intestinal complaints, colic, stomach cramp, stomachache and leukorrhea; with this last complaint, the area should be washed with the tea twice a day.

I cannot recommend this tea highly enough for lung complaints, bleeding in the lungs, chills and rheumatism; 1 cup should be taken before retiring.

The bruised herb is beneficial for fresh sores, scrofulous sores and fistulas. Compresses of the plant decoction can also be applied. When taking yarrow internally, do not drink any coffee or wine. For any kind of stomach cramp or bleeding, do not fail to try this tea. A better remedy will not be found.

YELLOW DOCK

Rumex crispus   Fam. Polygonaceae

Yellow dock is a perennial, herbaceous plant that is grown in gardens for household use. The stem is grooved and attains a height of at least three feet; it is a reddish color. The leaves are very long and acute; the flowers greenish. The root is yellow-brown on the outside, white inside; the sap is bitter, rather sour. The leaves have a culinary use; the roots a medicinal use. The root decoction should contain 3 to 4 tablespoons (20 to 25 grams) per 4 cups (1 liter) water. It is gathered before the flowering period and dried in the oven. The infusion is highly recommended for skin complaints and eczema; it is an excellent depurative. For optimal results, it should be used over a long period. Take 1 to 2 cups per day.

YELLOW GENTIAN

Gentiana lutea   Fam. Gentianaceae

Yellow gentian grows in both the Swiss Alps and the Pyrenees, and has large, beautiful, golden-yellow flowers. The root is several fingers thick and knobbly; brown on the outside and yellow on the inside. It has a very bitter taste. This root is used medicinally. No home should be without the tincture prepared from it. This is the best stomachic remedy to be found in the dispensary and also a very good nerve tonic and febrifugal.

For the complaints already mentioned, take 20 to 25 drops daily in ½ glass of cold water over a period of time; this will restore a good appetite and also promote digestion. This tincture is one of the best remedies for anyone who suffers from oppression in the stomach or nausea. When traveling, tincture of gentian is a comfort to the stomach; if no water is available, a few drops should be taken on sugar. It is the best possible help in the case of fainting. If you brush redness on scars or the consequence of ulcers, etc., twice a day with this tincture, it will disappear. Gentian can also be steeped in wine or beer.

YELLOW IRIS (FLAG)

Iris pseudacoris   Fam. Iridaceae

This plant is but seldom found. It grows on the verges of ditches, ponds and marshes, has a horizontal rootstock from which a long, flat stem grows with long, ribbon-shaped leaves. The yellow, long-petiolate flowers appear in the leaf axils. The flowering period is June and July. The dried root, which has no smell and a bitter, astringent sap, is not used medicinally because it has an injurious effect of the stomach. The root decoction is very good for itching; the areas that itch should be washed with it. The dried roots can be placed in the linen cupboard: they will give the linen a violet-like fragrance.

YELLOW WATER LILY

Nymphaea lutea   Fam. Nymphaeaceae

The yellow water lily noticeably differs from the white lily with its yellow flowers and smaller leaves. The leaves, which also float on the water, are oval, smooth-edged, leathery, heart-shaped at the base, cut and grow on a leaf stem which is tri-angular at the top and comes from a horizontal rootstock. The unpleasant smelling flowers appear above the water at dawn and close and disappear under the water at dusk, only to open up again the following morning. The flowering period is May to August. The root decoction, containing 1 to 2 tablespoons (12 to 15 grams) per 2 cups (½ liter) water, has the same strength as the white water lily.

HERBAL RECIPES
FOR VARIOUS ILLNESSES

Each mixture to be made using 2 cups (½ liter) water.

1. HEMORRHOIDS (PILES)

Yarrow	3 tablespoons (7 grams)
Aaron's rod	⅓ cup (3 grams)

Drink 1 cup twice a day.

2. BLADDER COMPLAINTS

Horsetail	3 tablespoons (3 grams)
Knotgrass	⅛ cup (2 grams)
Broom	2 teaspoons (2 grams)
Bearberry	4 teaspoons (2 grams)

Take 1 hot cupful twice a day.

3. GREEN SICKNESS

Thyme	4 teaspoons (3 grams)
White Horehound	7 teaspoons (3 grams)
Common Centaury	4 tablespoons (3 grams)

Take 1 cup daily.

4. HEAVY BLEEDING

Mistletoe	3 teaspoons (4 grams)
Knotgrass	¼ cup (3 grams)
Shepherd's purse	5 teaspoons (3 grams)

Drink 2 to 3 cups per day.

5. ANEMIA

Thyme	3 teaspoons (2 grams)
Common Centaury	4 tablespoons (3 grams)
White Horehound	5 teaspoons (2 grams)
Hyssop	5 teaspoons (2 grams)

Take 1 tablespoon every two hours.

6. HEAVY BLEEDING

Mistletoe	3 teaspoons (4 grams)
Knotgrass	¼ cup (3 grams)
Shepherd's Purse	5 teaspoons (3 grams)
Tormentil	3 teaspoons (3 grams)
Sandalwood	3 teaspoons (3 grams)
Oak bark	1 teaspoon (2 grams)
Horsetail	6 teaspoons (2 grams)

Steep for thirty minutes in 4 cups (1 liter) boiling water. Take 1 tablespoon every hour.

7. DEPURATIVE TEA (KNEIPP)

Wormwood (common)	1½ teaspoons (1 gram)
Stinging Nettle	2½ tablespoons (2 grams)
Common Centaury	3 tablespoons (2 grams)
Juniper Berries	1 tablespoon (3 grams)
Yarrow	4½ teaspoons (2 grams)
Rosemary	4 teaspoons (1 gram)
Horsetail	6 teaspoons (2 grams)
Sage	2½ teaspoons (1 gram)
Plantain	3 teaspoons (2 grams)
Common St. Johnswort	2 teaspoons (2 grams)

Take 1 cup daily.

8. DIZZINESS

Tansy	3 teaspoons (2 grams)
Valerian	2 teaspoons (3 grams)
Rue	1 teaspoon (1 gram)
Caraway	2 teaspoons (2 grams)

Take 1 spoon every two hours.

9. DYSENTERY OR DIARRHEA

Comfrey	5 teaspoons (3 grams)
Knotgrass	¼ cup (3 grams)
Plantain seed	1 teaspoon (3 grams)

Take 1 cup twice a day.

10. FALLING SICKNESS (EPILEPSY)

Valerian	1 teaspoon (2 grams)
Mistletoe	2 teaspoons (3 grams)
Horsetail	3 tablespoons (3 grams)
Lady's Bedstraw	1 tablespoon (1 gram)
Wormwood (common)	1½ teaspoons (1 gram)

Take 1 cup per day in three doses.

11. Epilepsy

Hawthorn	¼ cup (5 grams)
Rue	2 teaspoons (2 grams)
Horsetail	6 teaspoons (2 grams)

Take 1 cup per day in three doses.

12. Heart Complaints

Burnet root	1 teaspoon (2 grams)
Rue	1 teaspoon (1 gram)
Cinquefoil	3 teaspoons (3 grams)
Motherwort	2½ teaspoons (2 grams)
Lemon Balm	3 teaspoons (2 grams)

Take 1 spoon every hour.

13. Coughs (chronic coughs)

Coltsfoot	4 teaspoons (2 grams)
Ground Ivy	2 teaspoons (2 grams)
Marshmallow	1 teaspoon (1 gram)
Licorice	1½ teaspoons (2 grams)
Elder flowers	5 teaspoons (2 grams)

Take 1 spoon every hour.

14. Gout

Cowslips	4 teaspoons (2 grams)
Broom	2 teaspoons (2 grams)
Stinging Nettles	2½ tablespoons (2 grams)
Ash leaves	¼ cup (3 grams)

Take ½ cup twice a day.

15. WHOOPING COUGH

Thyme	3 teaspoons (2 grams)
Mistletoe	3½ teaspoons (5 grams)
Honey	3 tablespoons (50 grams)

Take 1 spoonful every two hours.

16. CRAMPS AND COLIC

Cinquefoil	3 teaspoons (3 grams)
Mint	½ cup (2 grams)
Lime blossom	2 teaspoons (2 grams)
Fennel	½ teaspoon (1 gram)
Thyme	2¼ teaspoons (1 gram)

Take ½ cup hot, twice a day.

17. CRAMPS

Chamomile flowers	3 tablespoons (3 grams)
Lime flowers	3 teaspoons (3 grams)
Fennel	½ teaspoon (1 gram)

Take ½ cup hot, twice a day.

18. LIVER COMPLAINTS

Agrimony	6 teaspoons (3 grams)
Woodruff	3 tablespoons (3 grams)
Lady's Bedstraw	2 tablespoons (3 grams)

Take 1 to 2 cups daily.

19. PHLEGM IN THE LUNGS

Violet leaves	4½ teaspoons (1 gram)
Plantain	5 teaspoons (3 grams)
Lungwort	⅓ cup (3 grams)
Coltsfoot	5 teaspoons (3 grams)
Licorice	1 teaspoon (1 gram)

Take 1 spoon every hour.

20. Lung Complaints

Lungwort	⅓ cup (3 grams)
Plantain	5 teaspoons (3 grams)
Fennel	1½ teaspoons (3 grams)

Take 1 spoon every two hours.

21. Measles

Lime blossom	4 teaspoons (4 grams)
Licorice	2½ teaspoons (3 grams)

Take 1 spoon every hour.

22. Stomach Herbs (to stimulate the appetite)

Angelica	1½ teaspoons (2 grams)
Wormwood	2 teaspoons (2 grams)
Sage	5 teaspoons (3 grams)
Juniper berries	1¼ teaspoons (1 gram)
Chicory (wild)	1 teaspoon (1 gram)

Take 1 spoon every two hours.

23. Equally good stomach herbs

Buckbean	4 teaspoons (2 grams)
Common centaury	4 tablespoons (3 grams)
Juniper berries	1¼ teaspoons (1 gram)

Take 1 spoon every two hours.

24. Digestion (to strengthen the stomach)

Fennel	1½ teaspoons (3 grams)
Mint	⅓ cup (3 grams)
Rhubarb	1 teaspoon (1 gram)

Take 1 spoon every two hours.

25. DIGESTION (TO STRENGTHEN THE STOMACH)

Wormwood	1 tablespoon (3 grams)
Horsetail	6 teaspoons (2 grams)
Aniseed	2 teaspoons (2 grams)
Thyme	3 teaspoons (2 grams)

Take 1 spoonful every two hours.

26. DIGESTION (TO WARM THE STOMACH)

Eyebright	⅛ cup (4 grams)
Mint	⅓ cup (3 grams)
Angelica	1½ teaspoons (2 grams)

Take 1 spoonful every two hours.

27. DIGESTION (TO STRENGTHEN STOMACH AND DISSOLVE MUCUS)

Rosemary	2½ teaspoons (2 grams)
Buckbean	2 teaspoons (1 gram)
Sage	3½ teaspoons (2 grams)
Knotgrass	⅛ cup (2 grams)
Fennel	1 teaspoon (2 grams)

Take 1 spoonful every two hours.

28. MELANCHOLY

Speedwell	4 teaspoons (3 grams)
Valerian	1¼ teaspoons (2 grams)
Pennyroyal	6 teaspoons (2 grams)
Agrimony	1 tablespoon (2 grams)

Drink 1 to 2 cups per day.

29. To Promote Menstruation

Burnet root	2 teaspoons (3 grams)
White horehound	7 teaspoons (3 grams)
Lavender flowers	3½ tablespoons (3 grams)

Drink 1 cup daily.

30. To Promote Menstruation

Chamomile	3 tablespoons (3 grams)
Catmint	2½ teaspoons (3 grams)
Coriander	2½ teaspoons (3 grams)

Drink 1 cup daily.

31. Migraines (severe headaches)

Speedwell	4 teaspoons (3 grams)
Cowslip	2 teaspoons (1 gram)
Wormwood	1 tablespoon (3 grams)

Take ½ cup twice a day.

32. Mouthwash for Ulcerated Mouth

Agrimony	6 teaspoons (3 grams)
Horsetail	6 teaspoons (2 grams)
Blackberry leaves	2½ tablespoons (4 grams)

To be used internally and externally as a mouthwash. Take 1 spoonful every hour.

33. Kidney Complaints

Thyme	3 teaspoons (2 grams)
Knotgrass	⅛ cup (2 grams)
Rosehips	1 teaspoon (2 grams)
Oatstraw	1 tablespoon (2 grams)
Plantain	3 teaspoons (2 grams)

Take 1 to 2 cups per day.

34. KIDNEY COMPLAINTS

Shepherd's Purse	5 teaspoons (3 grams)
Knotgrass	⅛ cup (2 grams)
Rosehips	1 teaspoon (2 grams)
Chicory (wild)	2 teaspoons (2 grams)

Take 1 to 2 cups daily.

35. PHLEGM IN THE CHEST

Fennel	1 teaspoon (2 grams)
Plantain	3 teaspoons (2 grams)
Coltsfoot	5 teaspoons (3 grams)
Lungwort	3½ teaspoons (2 grams)

Take 1 spoon every two hours.

36. STONES AND GRAVEL

Horsetail	3 tablespoons (3 grams)
Broom	2 teaspoons (2 grams)
Knotgrass	⅛ cup (2 grams)
Rosehips	1 teaspoon (2 grams)

Take 1 to 2 cups daily.

37. DROPSY

Dwarf Elder	3 teaspoons (3 grams)
Licorice	1½ teaspoons (2 grams)
Rosemary	1 tablespoon (3 grams)

Take 1 to 2 cups daily.

38. DROPSY

Inner rind of Elder	4 teaspoons (4 grams)
Licorice	3½ teaspoons (4 grams)
Horsetail	4½ teaspoons (1 gram)

Take 1 to 2 cups daily.

39. DROPSY

Meadowsweet	4 teaspoons (3 grams)
Dwarf elder	2 teaspoons (2 grams)
Rosemary	2½ teaspoons (2 grams)
Juniper berries	1¼ teaspoons (1 gram)
Horsetail	6 teaspoons (2 grams)

Take 1 to 2 cups daily.

40. SUFFERING FROM NERVES

Lemon balm	3½ tablespoons (3 grams)
Mint	⅓ cup (3 grams)
Pennyroyal	4 teaspoons (1 gram)
Valerian	1¼ teaspoons (2 grams)

Take 2 spoonsful three times a day.

41. GOOD DROPS FOR NERVES

Use equal quantities of valerian and orange peel, and a third as much of rosemary, steeped in gin. Take 25 drops twice a day in a spoon of water.

42. DIAPHORETIC TEA

Chamomile flowers	3 tablespoons (3 grams)
Elder flowers	3 tablespoons (4 grams)
Lime blossom	2 teaspoons (2 grams)

Drink 1 to 2 cups hot.

43. DIAPHORETIC TEA

Hazel Catkins	3 tablespoons (4 grams)
Lime blossom	3 teaspoons (3 grams)
Aaron's Rod	4 tablespoons (2 grams)

Drink 1 to 2 cups hot.

44. INFLUENZA

Mint	½ cup (4 grams)
Hazel Catkins	4 tablespoons (5 grams)

Drink 1 to 2 cups hot per day.

45. DYSENTERY OR DIARRHEA

Tormentil	3 teaspoons (3 grams)
Sherpherd's Purse	6½ teaspoons (4 grams)
Bistort	1 teaspoon (2 grams)

Take 1 spoon every hour.

46. DIARRHEA

Plantain	5 teaspoons (3 grams)
Cinquefoil	4 teaspoons (4 grams)
Knotgrass	⅛ cup (2 grams)

Take 1 spoon every hour.

47. DIARRHEA

Rosemary	2 tablespoons (4 grams)
Sage	5 teaspoons (3 grams)
Comfrey	3½ teaspoons (2 grams)

Take 1 spoon every hour.

48. CONGESTION OF BLOOD IN THE HEAD

Rue	2 teaspoons (2 grams)
Speedwell	6 teaspoons (5 grams)
Lavender flowers	3 tablespoons (2 grams)

Take ½ cup twice a day.

49. JAUNDICE

Woodruff	4 tablespoons (4 grams)
Long-stalked Cranesbill	1 teaspoon (3 grams)
Dandelion	1 tablespoon (2 grams)

Take 1 to 2 cups per day.

50. WIND

Juniper berries	1¼ teaspoons (1 gram)
Chamomile flowers	1 tablespoon (2 grams)
Coriander	1½ teaspoons (2 grams)
Peppermint	¼ cup (2 grams)
Fennel	1 teaspoon (2 grams)

Take 2 spoonsful three times a day.

PRESCRIPTIONS
AND DRAUGHTS

ALMOND MILK

Take ⅓ cup (30 grams) sweet almonds, stew them in boiling water, then peel them and pound them in a mortar, slowly adding 3 cups (¾ liter) water; then squeeze through a cloth and add ⅛ cup (16 grams) fine sugar.

ANGELICA LIQUEUR

Combine the following:

Green Angelica stems . . . . 1¾ cup (100 grams)
Gin . . . . 10 cups (2½ liters)
Water . . . . 6 cups (1½ liters)
Sugar . . . . 4½ pounds (2 kilos)

Steep the finely chopped angelica in gin for six days, then add the sugar and water; let steep for a further ten days; filter and store in well-corked bottles.

BALSAM

This is an excellent remedy for indigestion and stomach pains. Take 1 to 4 tablespoons daily for internal use; this balsam is highly recommended for external use in the treatment of rheumatic and gout pain. Rub it on the affected areas by hand. For internal use, it can also be taken with wine or water, according to choice. For worms: 2 tablespoons should be taken in a little warm water in the morning on an empty stomach.

Ingredients and Preparation:
Combine the flowers and leaves of

Balsam	⅓ cup (100 grams)
Thyme	2½ cups (100 grams)
Sage	.3 cups (100 grams)
Marjoram	1½ cups (100 grams)
Lemon Balm	6 cups (100 grams)
Rosemary	2½ cups (100 grams)
Speedwell	2½ cups (100 grams)
Basil	1½ cups (100 grams)
Hyssop	2½ cups (100 grams)
Wormwood	2 cups (100 grams)
Lavender	8 cups (200 grams)
Juniper berries	1 cup (100 grams)
Laurel leaves	5 cups (100 grams)
Ground Ivy	2½ cups (100 grams)
Gin	10 cups (2½ liters)

Chop the plants very finely; put all the ingredients in an earthenware or stone pot; seal with a linen cloth folded double three times, and place in direct sunlight for two months; then filter and bottle.

BALSAM FOR ULCERATED, CHAPPED HANDS AND FEET

Camphor	2 tablespoons (20 grams)
Red Sandalwood powder	3½ teaspoons (4 grams)
Peruvian Balsam	½ teaspoon (2 grams)
Yellow wax	5 teaspoons (10 grams)
Turpentine	2 tablespoons (12 grams)
Olive Oil	⅓ cup (70 grams)

Melt the wax, turpentine and oil together in a double boiler; as soon as the mixture begins to boil, add the sandalwood powder, stirring continually; then remove from the fire. When it has cooled a little, add the camphor and Peruvian balsam.

HEALTH DRINK

Let the following ingredients steep together for ten days:

Finely chopped Chervil	12¾ cups (275 grams)
Common Centaury	6⅔ cups (225 grams)
White wine.	10 cups (2½ liters)
Then add: honey	3½ tablespoons (60 grams)
water	3 tablespoons (20 grams)

Boil all the ingredients until a good foam can be seen; let stand for another ten days; then strain through a cloth and filter. This wine is an excellent remedy for constipation; it stimulates the appetite and is recommended for stomach complaints in general.

CURRANT WINE

Take 2 to 3 quarts of red and white currants, or of one kind only, finely crush them and leave to stand for a night; then squeeze them out and add 1 pound (½ kilo) sugar, 1 cup (200 grams) Rhine wine and ⅓ cup (100 grams) gin to each 2 cups of juice. Let stand in the sun until it has fermented; then bottle. Gooseberry wine can be prepared in the same way.

REMEDIES TO STIMULATE THE APPETITE

1) Bitter sap from fresh herbs which stimulate the appetite are beneficial for gall bladder complaints. Take half a handful of green angelica stems, 2 handsfuls each of fumitory, wild chicory and dandelion. Pound them all together in a porcelain mortar and squeeze through a cloth. Take 5 to 6 tablespoons twice a day. This should be used immediately as it does not keep.

2) Take 12 drops of sweet almond oil three times a day.

3) Swallow 6 to 8 corns of pepper daily.

4) The following stimulates the appetite: caraway, cherries, white mustard, parsley, asparagus, common wormwood, leek, fennel, etc.

Raspberry Wine

Take a quantity of raspberries, finely crush them and let stand for four days; to each quart (liter) raspberry juice, add 2 pounds (1 kilo) sugar and ¾ cup (180 grams) of 75% alcohol. Place this mixture in the sun for four days with the pot lid loose, pour through a linen cloth and filter; then bottle.

Juniper Berry Wine

Juniper berries	⅓ cup (30 grams)
Young Juniper twigs.	1 cup (30 grams)
White wine.	4 cups (1 liter)

Crush the berries and mix all the ingredients together; let steep for four days and then add:

Sugar	¼ cup (30 grams)
Wormwood	5 tablespoons (15 grams)
Horseradish root	2 teaspoons (15 grams)

This is one of the best appetite stimulants to be found. It is also beneficial for both dropsy and fever. Take 4 to 6 tablespoons daily to stimulate the appetite. More may be taken for dropsy.

White Horehound Wine

White Horehound.	3⅓ cups (90 grams)
White wine.	2 quarts (2 liters)

Let the ingredients steep for fourteen days then filter and bottle. This wine is excellent for the stomach; it also stimulates the appetite and is particularly recommended for anemia.

BITTER WINE

Cinchona, finely chopped.	1 cup (106 grams)
Orange peel, finely chopped	1 cup (100 grams)
Virginia snake root	4 tablespoons (25 grams)
Gentian root, finely chopped	¼ cup (25 grams)
Bitter Quassia wood	2 teaspoons (5 grams)
Saffron	2½ tablespoons (7 grams)
Cochineal powder.	3 teaspoons (5 grams)
Gentian extract	1 teaspoon (2 grams)
Alcohol	4½ cups (1⅛ liters)
Rainwater	4 cups (1 liter)

Let steep for a month, filter and bottle. A normal wineglassful is used per bottle of Bordeaux wine. Take 2 liqueur glasses daily. Bitter wine is an excellent stomachic.

QUINCE WINE

Grate the quinces without peeling them; discard the seeds. After being grated, they should be thoroughly squeezed out through a linen cloth. To each quart (liter) of juice add:

75% alcohol	4 cups (1 liter)
Rainwater	4 cups (1 liter)
Sugar	6¼ cups (750 grams)
Finely pounded bitter almonds . . .	1 tablespoon (4 grams)
Cinnamon	1 tablespoon (5 grams)
Coriander	1½ teaspoons (2 grams)
Mace	1 teaspoon (1 gram)
Cloves.	½ teaspoon (40 centigrams)

The almonds, cinnamon and cloves should be finely powdered. Then steep all the ingredients for two to three weeks. (It may be stirred from time to time.) When it has finished fermenting, add the sugar and then bottle. While fermentation is taking place, the vessel should remain open and should stand in a warm place. Quince wine is one of the finest liqueurs.

CHEST TEA

Speedwell	1¼ cups (50 grams)
Coltsfoot	1½ cups (50 grams)
Ground Ivy	1¼ cups (50 grams)
Devil's Bit Scabious	2 ounces (50 grams)
Lemon Balm	¾ cup (10 grams)
Sage	⅓ cup (10 grams)

Take ½ cup (15 grams) of this mixture per 2 cups (½ liter) boiling water. This tea is very efficacious for coughs and at the onset of consumption.

CHEST HERBS

Knotgrass	13 cups (200 grams)
Speedwell	2⅔ cups (125 grams)
Coltsfoot	3¾ cups (125 grams)
Polypody root	½ cup (60 grams)
Marshmallow root	½ cup (30 grams)
Licorice root	1 cup (60 grams)
Fennel	3 tablespoons (24 grams)

Take ⅓ to ½ cup (10 to 15 grams) of this mixture per 2 cups (½ liter) boiling water. This tea is recommended for coughs, phlegm in the chest and consumption.

BARLEY WATER

Boil a quantity of barley in 4 cups (1 liter) water until the husks split; then strain through a cloth and add 3 to 4 tablespoons honey and 3 tablespoons vinegar. This is a drink which is highly recommended for chest complaints.

COMMON ST. JOHNSWORT OIL

Fill a bottle with Common St. Johnswort flowers and top it up with olive oil; leave for some time in the sun (the longer the better). This is an excellent oil for burns, abrasions, etc.

DRINK (STIMULATING)

Tartar . . . . 5 teaspoons (16 grams)
Sugar Candy . . . . 2 tablespoons (30 grams)
Slice 1 lemon and 1 orange and put them into 4 cups (1 liter) of boiling water. Allow to cool before use.

LAVENDER WATER

Lavender flowers (fresh) . . . . 2½ cups (60 grams)
32% Alcohol . . . . 4 cups (1 liter)

Filter after fourteen days.

LEMON BALM SPIRIT

Lemon Balm (the fresh flowers) . . . . 2 cups (800 grams)
Lemon Peel . . . . 1⅓ cups (130 grams)
Powdered Cinnamon . . . . ½ cup (70 grams)
Powdered Nutmeg . . . . ½ cup (70 grams)
Cloves. . . . . ¾ cup (70 grams)
Angelica root. . . . . ⅓ cup (40 grams)
Coriander seed . . . . ½ cup (40 grams)
90% Alcohol . . . . 18 cups (4½ liters)

Let all the ingredients steep for six days, then place in a double boiler and boil until 2 cups (½ liter) has evaporated. The dose is 1 to 2 tablespoons (4 to 10 grams) and can be used instead of Carmelite Spirit. Lemon Balm Spirit is a very good stomachic.

Stomachic Tincture

Blessed Thistle . . . . ½ cup (15 grams)
Common Centaury . . . . ⅓ cup (15 grams)
Orange Peel . . . . 2 tablespoons (15 grams)
Gentian . . . . 2½ tablespoons (15 grams)
Calamus root. . . . . 2 tablespoons (12 grams)
Wormwood . . . . 4 tablespoons (12 grams)
Wood Avens . . . . .4 tablespoons (8 grams)

Let all the ingredients steep for fourteen days in 4 cups (1 liter) gin and take 2 tablespoons before meals.

Stomach Drops

Tincture of Orange Peel . . . . . . 2 teaspoons (5 grams)
Gentian tincture . . . . 2 teaspoons (5 grams)

Take 15 drops twice a day.

Angelica Tea

Angelica. . . . . .2½ teaspoons (3 grams)
Fennel . . . . .1 teaspoon (2 grams)
Buckbean . . . . 6 teaspoons (3 grams)
Eyebright . . . . .⅛ cup (4 grams)

Let all ingredients steep in 2 cups (½ liter) boiling water and take 1 tablespoon every hour. Or take 4 tablespoons three times a day.

Eye Tonic Water

Take 1 cup (200 grams) rainwater or distilled water, ½ sugar-spoon salt and 1 sugarspoon gin and wash the eyes with this three times a day.

Eye Powder for Weak Eyes

Take ⅔ cup (30 grams) eyebright, 4 teaspoons (7 grams) sweet fennel, 1 teaspoon (1½ grams) loaf sugar, and 1 tablespoon (15 grams) sugar candy. Grind all the ingredients to a powder. Take 1 tablespoon (3 grams) in a little wine before retiring over some period of time.

A Remedy for Bed Sores

Place a large, wide container of cold water under the bed and renew the water twice a day.

To make Birthmarks Disappear on a New Born Infant

Every morning chew some mustard seed and rub the marks with it. The mother should smear the marks twice a day with a little of her milk.

Mussels (poisoning from)

Drink a quart (liter) of cold water and vinegar.

Peppermint Water

Mix together:

> 1 part peppermint oil
> 9 parts strong alcohol
> 990 parts water.

Red Blemishes on the Face

Smear the blemishes with fresh, pounded chickweed in the evenings before retiring.

To Prevent Herb Saps from Spoiling

Add ½% salicylic acid[10] which has been dissolved in 94% alcohol.

To Make Children's Teeth Come Out More Easily

Take a clean, washed marshmallow root, dip it in honey and put it in the child's mouth. Chewing this makes the gums soft and facilitates the extraction of the teeth.

Tar Water

Add 50 parts ship's or wood tar to 1000 parts boiling water. Shake as well as possible for half an hour and then filter.

Tincture of Iodine for Asthma

Put 10 drops iodine tincture in 2 cups (½ liter) boiling water. The vapor of this should be inhaled once a day, perferably in the evening. The inhalation should last fifteen minutes.

Efficacious Remedy for Gangrene

Boil 1½ cups (180 grams) finely chopped oak bark from young wood with 4 quarts (4 liters) spring water until reduced to 1 cup (¼ liter). Strain through a cloth and apply in the form of compresses on cloths folded in four. The compresses should be renewed every half hour. The cloths which have been applied should not be used again until they have been thoroughly washed. The compress cloths should be large enough to cover the black or affected area completely. If the gangrene is wet, the foul smell disappears after only a few hours and the patient begins to improve. The compresses should be continued until the affected area has been dissolved and has begun to ulcerate. Continue to apply the compresses, but renew them only once every hour. If improvement continues, renew every three or four hours. We have the famous Dr. Hahnemann to thank for this remedy.

---

[10]Salicylic acid: available from most pharmacies; not to be taken internally.

A Second Remedy for
Gangrene from the Same Source

Boil ½ cup (60 grams) finely chopped oak bark in 2 cups (½ liter) rain or spring water; while boiling add ½ cup (15 grams) chamomile flowers; leave to boil until reduced to about 1 cup (200 grams); strain through a cloth, leave to cool and add 3 teaspoons (7 grams) myrrh tincture. Apply in the form of compresses and renew when nearly dry.

Sweaty Hands

Wash the hands daily in an infusion of sage and apply compresses of wheat bran on the hands one or more times a day. Take a daily cold armbath for 1 to 3 minutes.

A harmless Remedy
Which Cures Scurf in Two Hours

The patient should take a hot bath for half an hour after which he or she should smear the body well with green soap, and then have another hot bath for an hour, thoroughly washing the body afterward. When dry, he or she should thoroughly apply the following ointment:

Lard	1 tablespoon (21 grams)
Flowers of Sulphur	6 teaspoons (7 grams)
Potassium Carbonate	.2 teaspoons (3½ grams)

He should then take yet another bath in order to wash off the ointment and he can be sure that the scurf will be cured.

Remedy for Liver Spots and Freckles

Let ¼ cup (30 grams) white hellebore steep for eight days in 1 cup (240 grams) alcohol. Brush the liver spots with this three times a day. This tincture should not be filtered.

BURNED MOUTH CAUSED BY HOT FOOD OR DRINK

If the mouth is burned, it should be rinsed several times with cold milk or olive oil. If hot food has been swallowed, take several spoons of cold milk in succession, or take several spoons of olive oil.

UNHEALTHY ULCERATION

Apply constant compresses of the juice extracted from rotten apples. The cloths which have been used should be thoroughly washed before further use. This remedy has a wonderful power of healing and also cleanses the sores.

TO STOP VOMITING AND SPITTING BLOOD IMMEDIATELY

Take 15 to 20 drops spirits of turpentine in a glass of cold water. This immediately stops vomiting or spitting blood (Dr. Baille).

A SIMPLE REMEDY FOR CONSUMPTION

The patient should take a knife-point of grated horseradish root with a sugarspoon of honey every morning on an empty stomach for six weeks. An hour later take 1 sugarspoon olive oil mixed with sugar. Do not eat or drink anything else for the first three hours. After six weeks, if the patient cannot take any more horseradish on account either of weakness or coughing, take 1 sugarspoon olive oil before retiring and continue this treatment until the illness has improved.

A TINCTURE FOR INDIGESTION
ESPECIALLY IN OLD PEOPLE

Melt 5 cups (250 grams) best potash in 4 cups (1 liter) pure water in a new earthenware pot and let stand in a warm place for forty-eight hours. Stir frequently and thoroughly; then pour it slowly through a cloth so that the residue remains in the pot; clean the pot thoroughly, pour in the solution and add:

Gentian . . . . 3 tablespoons (21 grams)
Unripe Oranges . . . . 2 tablespoons (21 grams)
A handful of Tansy flowers
A handful of Blessed Thistle
A handful of Buckbean

Boil for ten minutes, remove from the fire, cover the pot well, place for several hours in a warm place. Then strain the mixture, when cold, through a cloth. This tincture should be stored in a well-corked bottle. It can be stored in this way for years and is especially recommended for indigestion, consequent headache, heartburn, constipation, wind and irregular bowel movements. Take 1 sugarspoon after the midday or evening meal, followed by a glass of water or wine. This tincture is also useful for piles, difficult urination and stones.

HEADLICE

For a child, use 3 drops aniseed oil, for adults 7 drops, and regularly rub this all over the head. They will soon disappear.

SCURVY

1) Combine the following:

Young Fir twigs. . . . . ½ cup (15 grams)
Fumitory . . . . 4 tablespoons (10 grams)
Yarrow . . . . ⅓ cup (10 grams)
Buckbean . . . . ⅓ cup (10 grams)
Calamus. . . . . 4 teaspoons (8 grams)
Young Juniper twigs. . . . . ½ cup (15 grams)

Boil all the ingredients in 6 cups (1½ liters) of water for fifteen minutes; use it as a gargle six times a day and take 1 tablespoon every two hours.

2) Let 1 cup (30 grams) elder flowers steep in 2 cups (½ liter) of boiling water; strain through a cloth and add 1 tablespoon of rapeseed oil, 1 tablespoon vinegar. Wash the mouth with this six times a day.

3) Take 1 tablespoon scurvy grass tea every hour.

4) Wild Strawberries are also good for scurvy.

5) Tincture for scurvy:

Scurvy Grass . . . . ⅔ cup (15 grams)
Sage . . . . ½ cup (15 grams)
Rue. . . . . ¼ cup (10 grams)
Lemon Balm . . . . 1 cup (15 grams)

Put these ingredients in 4 cups (1 liter) gin. A tablespoonful should be held in the mouth for some time twice a day. An improvement will soon be evident. A cup of buckbean tea should also be taken daily or 1 tablespoon of the remedy described above (No. 1) should be taken every two hours.

HERBS FOR THE NERVES

Mix ⅓ cup (6 grams) lemon balm, 1 tablespoon (6 grams) valerian, 1 tablespoon (6 grams) cinquefoil, 6 teaspoons (6 grams) rue, ⅔ cup (6 grams) mint, and 3 tablespoons (6 grams) rosemary; 3 tablespoons (3 grams) arnica and 5 teaspoons (3 grams) cowslip; 2½ teaspoons (½ gram) lavender; 3 tablespoons (3 grams) woodruff; ¼ cup (6 grams) motherwort, 2 tablespoons (6 grams) common St. Johnswort, and 3 teaspoons (6 grams) balsam. Let 1 tablespoon of this mixture steep for twenty minutes in 1 cup boiling water and take 2 or 3 spoons every day.

NERVE OINTMENT

Melt together 1 tablespoon (16 grams) pork fat, 2 teaspoons (8 grams) mutton fat, 2 teaspoons (3 grams) yellow wax and 2 teaspoons (3 grams) nutmeg oil. When it has cooled, add ½ teaspoon (1 gram) each of rosemary oil and juniper oil. Rub with this ointment twice a day in cases of nerve pain. This ointment is also most efficacious in the treatment of rheumatism.

THRUSH

Thrush consists of small spots or blisters which appear along the sides of the tongue, or inside the lips and cheeks; after a few days they burst and cause a great deal of pain.

1) Gargle with a strong infusion of bramble (blackberry) leaves.

2) Gargle with the following mixture: 1 part honey, 1 part houseleek sap, and 8 parts water in which a little alum has been dissolved.

3) Also drink tea made from sage, common wormwood and juniper berries, and take a mild purgative.

BAD BREATH

Take 1 sugarspoon black bonemeal mixed with powdered sugar several times a day.

TOOTHACHE

1) Moisten a piece of wild chicory root in water and place in the ears.

2) Put a few drops oil of cloves on cotton wool and place on the tooth, or put a drop of spirit of ammonia on cotton wool and carefully place on the tooth without touching the gums.

3) Keep a piece of plantain or yarrow root on the tooth, or chew a cinquefoil root.

4) Wash the mouth out with the following mixture: 3½ teaspoons (8 grams) alum, 10 drops oil of cloves, and 1 cup (250 grams) water.

GUMS (LOOSE)

Chew calamus root and drink cinquefoil tea.

ULCERATED GUMS

1) Drink a daily cup of buckbean tea over a long period of time.

2) Boil 3 handsful of mouse-ear hawkweed in 2 cups (½ liter) water until reduced by a third. Wash the mouth out with this at frequent intervals.

LEUKORRHEA

Apply hot compresses of hayseed decoction to the lower part of the body; take upper body washes and whole body washes. Drink 1 cup of tea every day made from mint, watermint or peppermint, or from dead-nettle, or from cross-leaved heath sweetened with sugar. Or drink 2 cups walnut leaf tea daily, or 1 cup haws tea, or 1 cup horsetail and juniper berry tea.

PREPARATION OF SOFT CHEESE

Let sweet milk stand in a clean vessel until cream has formed. Skim this off carefully until none remains. Put the remaining milk on the fire until it thickens and the whey can be seen. Strain it through a coarse linen cloth placed in a sieve, let stand for a while and place a weight or stone on top so that the whey will run out more quickly. When the whey has drained off, the cheese is ready. We have often mentioned soft cheese in this book and since most people are not familiar with the method of preparation, I considered it necessary to describe it here. If buttermilk is available, the soft cheese can soon be prepared and will be just as efficacious. The buttermilk should be warmed (not hot), then the cheese will soon separate, the whey will rise and it can be handled as above to drain off the whey.

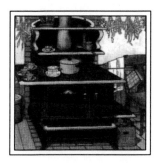

Part III

The Water Cure

INTRODUCTION

Waterings, washes, compresses, etc., have all been repeatedly mentioned in this book in connection with the treatment of various illnesses. It would, therefore, serve a useful purpose to give here a brief description and directions concerning the water cure, all the more since lengthy experience has taught me how little knowledge most people have on the subject. A few general tips are provided and these should be borne in mind for all applications.

1) Cold water should be used unless the contrary is expressly stated.

2) Before taking a watering, the patient must have a normal body temperature; the patient should neither be trembling and shivering nor burning.

3) Undressing and dressing must be done as quickly as possible and the same applies to the watering itself.

4) After the watering, the body should not be dried; the head-hair and the hands alone should be thoroughly dried.

5) Following the watering, the patient should ensure some form of action; i.e., the patient should endeavor to bring the body back to normal warmth by means of vigorous movement, gymnastics, etc. This is a most important requirement.

6) Patients who are not in a state to be able to warm themselves by means of the necessary movement must go to bed and stay there until they are thoroughly dry and warm. The reaction usually takes half an hour.

WATERINGS

1) *Knee Watering*: Water should be poured on both sides of the legs from the feet to just above the knees. One should begin at the back with the right heel, let the water stream slowly upward over the calf to above the back of the knee and then down again to the foot. The other leg should be treated likewise beginning with the heel, and the treatment should continue on alternate legs until the legs are red. Then one should start on the front of the legs, beginning with the toes and ending just above the knee. When the top of the knee is reached, the stream of water should be continued for a moment. A knee watering usually lasts one to two minutes.

2) *Thigh Watering*: Begin at the back with the right heel, move slowly upward as far as the hips, return the same way to the foot and spray the left leg in the same way. The backs of both legs should be treated alternately until the skin is red. The patient should then turn over so that the front of both legs can be alternately treated up to the hips. After having sprayed the back of both legs for some time, it is advisable to direct the stream for a moment on to the kidney area so that the water can run down both legs at the same time. It lasts 2 to 3 minutes and one should count on six cans of water.

3) *Upper Body Watering*: The patient should stand bent over forward with hands resting on a low bench, or in a tub so that the water can run off. The watering begins with the right hand and moves slowly over the arm to the right shoulder. The chest should then be sprayed momentarily and then the shoulder again so that the stream can run over the back. If a chest watering is prescribed, only the upper part of the back should be sprayed. The water should run evenly over that whole area of the back, also over the left side and the neck. If the patient holds the head up a little, the hair usually remains dry; if it becomes wet, it should be thoroughly dried after the treatment. This watering should not last too long at first, especially in the case of a weak patient; later the spraying can continue until the back is red. Use 1 to 3 cans of water. This watering requires a measure of practice.

4) *Back Watering*: The back watering should begin with the right

heel. After spraying both legs, one at a time, up to the hips, one should continue from the right hip, up the right side to the right shoulder. One should ensure that no water flows forward over the shoulder. The stream should now move the same way backward to the right hip and from there to the left hip, so as to reach the left shoulder via the left side. Until now the stream has not been directed on to the spine. One should now move from the left shoulder to the neck and then slowly zig-zag over the spine down to the hips. If the watering has not yet finished, the treatment should be recommended from the front as described. Use 3 to 6 cans of water.

5) *Chest Watering*: The position for this is the same as for the upper body watering. The patient raises one arm and bends sideways a little so that the water can flow evenly over the whole chest. One should start by spraying the arm on which the patient is leaning and then move the stream slowly up to the chest and seek a place where the water will spray the whole chest at once. Use 3 cans of water. The length of treatment is one to two minutes. This treatment should not be given to heart patients.

6) *Whole Body Watering*: As with the back watering, one should begin with the right heel. When the back watering has been applied, the patient should turn round and if strong, one should immediately spray the chest and seek the place from where the water will cover the whole chest like a mirror and run off over the body. In the case of weak patients, after the back watering, the stream should not be directed immediately onto the chest, but below on the legs and slowly climb higher as in the thigh watering, and apply the chest watering as described above last of all.

7) *Quick Watering*: A quick watering, which is actually nothing more than a whole body watering applied with a powerful stream, necessitates some skill in the applicant. Since it is rather complicated and is also seldom used, I shall not describe it further. It is occasionally used on people with good blood circulation and who are sufficiently hardy, in cases such as obesity and corpulence, where excellent results can be obtained.

8) *Arm Watering*: The arm watering begins with the fingers and continues as far as the shoulders. The areas where pain is felt

or which have been affected by illness should be especially well sprayed. Quick arm watering is sometimes prescribed. This is nothing other than an ordinary arm watering, applied with the hose which is used for the quick watering.

9) *Ear Watering*: This watering is applied round the ear and especially behind the earlobe; four times around the ear.

10) *Head Watering*: It can best be applied before an upper body watering. The area of the head which is covered with hair should be sprayed, especially the back of the head. This watering should be applied gently and when it is finished the hair should be thoroughly dried. The length of treatment is thirty seconds.

BATHS

If good results are to be obtained, baths should never last long: five seconds is long enough. The water must be cold, the colder the better. The same general tips given for the waterings should also be borne in mind for the baths. With respect to the number of baths per week, the doctor's recommendation should be strictly followed. There are three principal kinds of baths. These are the hip bath, the half bath and the whole bath.

1) *Hip Bath*: It is necessary to have a tub which is deep enough so that when the patient is sitting in the bath, the water can reach the kidney area and approximately halfway up the thighs. The rest of the body remains out of the water. This bath should last ten to fifteen seconds.

2) *Half Bath*: A tub should be filled with water in such a way that when the patient sits in it the water reaches the navel. It is a good idea to wet the chest with a little water before stepping in the bath so as to be able to stand the cold water all the better. The half bath should only last five to six seconds.

3) *Whole Bath*: A whole bath is a bath in which the water reaches the neck. The whole body, except for the head, must be under the water, the arms also therefore. The whole bath should last five seconds.

4) *Arm Bath*: After the baths that have already been described,

this is the next most important and the best. Its nerve strengthening action is sufficiently well-known. The arms should be placed up to the armpits in cold water for one to two minutes. After the bath, the hands can be dried but not, of course, the arms.

5) *Head Bath*: With the head bath, one should ensure that the scalp and forehead are in the water. Since it is rather difficult to hold the back of the head under water, water can be tipped over by hand or with a sponge. The head should be thoroughly dried after the bath. A cold bath should last approximately one minute and a warm bath five minutes.

6) *Eye Bath*: The forehead should be dipped deep into the water, which should cover the eyes. The eyes should then be opened and closed several times so that the water rinses the eyeballs.

7) *Foot Bath*: The foot bath is usually hot, and the water can be mixed with salt, ash, alum, soda, herbs, etc., according to the nature of the complaint for which the bath is being taken. For congestion of blood in the head, asthma, etc., salt and wood-ash are mixed in the hot bath; this soon draws the blood away. This bath should be taken as hot as possible. The feet should afterward be rinsed in cold water so as to close the pores.

8) *Hot Baths*: Monseigneur Kneipp did not approve of hot baths and so they are rarely applied in his curative method. If they are prescribed, the doctor's recommendation should be strictly followed, especially with respect to the duration and the temperature of the bath. After each hot bath, the patient should take a cold water application in order to close the pores; a cold watering or wash, for example.

Vapor Baths
The vapor bath is never applied alone; it is usually a preparation for a subsequent cold application, so as to increase the effect of the latter. The vapor bath has a solvent, expelling action.

1) *Head Vapor Bath*: The patient should bare the upper part of the body and stand over a container of hot water. In order to

exclude the air and prevent the vapor from escaping, the patient and the tub should be covered with a large, woolen blanket. The patient should remain in this position for at least a quarter of an hour, and should then be thoroughly rinsed with cold water. The patient should take plenty of exercise; this can best be done before retiring.

2) *Hip Vapor Bath*: The patient should sit for fifteen minutes on a night chair or on a rush chair with openings. A container of water in which chamomile flowers or other herbs have usually been mixed should be placed underneath. The patient must naturally first remove clothes but should be well covered so that air is excluded and no vapor can escape. After the vapor bath, the patient should take a cold half bath, a wash, or a thigh watering.

3) *Other Vapor Baths*: From the information given above, one can easily deduce how other vapor baths, which are occasionally prescribed, can be taken: for the ears, neck, etc., for example. The area which has been treated by vapor should always be given a cold application or wash.

WASHES

1) *Whole Wash*: By washing, one does not mean rubbing, but regularly and quickly wetting all the pores. With the whole body wash, every part of the body must be moistened in this way with cold water, even the soles of the feet. Before taking a wash, the patient should have been in bed for some time so that both patient and the bed are warm; after the wash, the patient should remain in bed for at least half an hour. The patient should be thoroughly and quickly washed with a coarse linen cloth, a hand towel for example, which has been dipped in water and wrung out so that it no longer drips. The use of a sponge is not suitable since it is so small that the wash would take longer, while it can in fact be completed in half a minute. A wash can be taken without the help of anyone else: after wetting the towel, one should unfold it, take one corner in each hand, throw it over one's head so that it covers the shoulders and back and then pull it downward. One should then wash the neck, chest, arms and other parts, quickly pull on a shirt and jump into bed.

2) *Upper Body Wash*: As the name indicates, this wash consists of wetting the neck, chest, back, and arms. It is applied in the same way as the whole wash. The patient should also have been in bed before the wash and, following it, remain in bed for at least half an hour.

COMPRESSES

For compresses, wraps, etc., cloths made of coarse linen material are required. After an application, they should be thoroughly washed. Cloths used by one patient should not be used on another. When the cloth has been soaked and well wrung out, it is normally folded in four and placed on the affected part of the body. A dry, unfolded linen cloth should be laid over this wet cloth and a woolen blanket or cloth placed on top of that. The patient should then be well covered with the bed clothes. One should not apply too many bed covers under the pretext that the patient will have more reaction. The patient will almost certainly begin to sweat and that is not the intention. While the compresses are in position, the patient must lie quietly without moving, and when they have been removed, the patient should continue to remain quiet for a few minutes.

Chest Compresses: A coarse linen cloth, dipped in hot water or in hayseed decoction (according to the doctor's prescription) should be well wrung out, folded double or in four and placed on the patient's chest. The wet cloth must be large enough to cover the whole chest, i.e., from the neck to the stomach region. A dry cloth should be laid over everything and a woolen cloth or blanket on top of that, completely excluding the air. The best and most practical method is to spread the woolen blanket under the patient's back before applying the compress in such a way that there is an area left on both sides large enough to wrap over the chest when the compress has been applied. The patient should be covered over and left to lie quietly. Should the patient fall asleep, which would be most beneficial, he should be left until he wakes up; otherwise the compress should be removed after the prescribed time and the patient should be left lying down, well covered. All compresses should be applied in the same way.

THE WRAPS

1) *The Spanish Coat*: The Spanish Coat, which is also sometimes mistakenly called a goose wrap, covers the whole body with the exception of the head. A coarse linen shirt which reaches over the feet and has long sleeves is necessary for this treatment; it is best if it is completely open at the front (like a coat) as it can then be more easily wrapped over the body. Two large woolen blankets should be laid over the breadth of the mattress so that the whole body from the shoulders down to the feet can be fully wrapped, excluding all air. The coat should now be dipped in water and wrung out until it no longer drips; it should be placed on the patient and wrapped right round in front so that it touches as much of the body as possible. The patient should then be laid on the blanket and covered over well, especially around the shoulders and feet, so that the air is completely excluded. The bed covers should then be pulled over and well tucked in, and the patient should remain thus for one and a half hours, according to the prescription of the doctor who will take the patient's strength into account.

2) *The Goose Wrap*: This is so called because it covers almost the whole body. As it greatly resembles the Spanish Coat, only the following points need be noted:

A) Instead of a shirt, one should use a coarse linen cloth which is large enough to wrap round the patient from the armpits to the feet. A coarse bed sheet is ideal.

B) The goose wrap leaves the head, neck, shoulders and arms free and begins under the arms. The treatment is exactly the same as with the Spanish Coat.

3) *The Short Wrap*: It encircles the body from the armpits to the knees. A bedsheet cut across the breadth gives two suitable short wraps. After the bed has been prepared in accordance with the instructions for the Spanish Coat, the wet, wrung out cloth should be wound around the body from the armpits to the knees. The patient should then be firmly wrapped in the woolen blanket, excluding all air. The patient should be lying thus for one hour. It should not be forgotten that after each wrap, as with each compress, the patient may not immediately

leave the bed but should remain there for at least another ten minutes.

4) *The Chest Wrap*: The chest wrap encompasses the whole chest and back. A sleeveless, linen undervest, large enough to go right over the chest, should be used. After it has been soaked and wrung out until it no longer drips, it should be drawn over the patient, then covered with a second, dry linen cloth and finally a third of flannel or wool, to exclude the air. The patient should be firmly tucked in and left to lie there for three-quarters to one hour.

5) *The Head Wrap*: This wrap only leaves the face, i.e., eyes, nose and mouth, free. The rest of the head should be wrapped in a wet, wrung out cloth so that the scalp and hair also become wet. This should be covered by a dry linen cloth and then a woolen cloth. The head wrap should remain in place.

6) *Other Wraps*: Anyone can easily apply neck, knee and foot wraps after reading the instructions given above. Each wet cloth should be covered by a dry linen cloth to exclude the air.

7) *The Wet Shirt*: A coarse linen shirt should be dipped in the fluid prescribed by the doctor: for example, salt or clay water or some kind of decoction such as haystraw, or oatstraw, and then put on. One then refers to a salt-shirt, a clay-shirt, hay-shirt, etc. When the patient has been warmly tucked into bed, he or she should remain there in the wet shirt for an hour and a half.

REMEDIES FOR HARDENING THE BODY

Hot applications are generally injurious; they occasionally have to be given before a cold water application to increase the action of the latter. In all cases, apart from exceptions, they are harmful as they soften the body instead of hardening it. An excellent remedy for hardening is, as experience has taught me, going barefoot.

The so-called "treading water" is also for the purpose of hardening. When this is prescribed by the physician for the first time, the patient should only go in water up to the ankles for the length of time prescribed. When the patient is used to it, the water may be allowed up to the knees. The length of time varies from one to five minutes. One should not stand still in the water but tread it or walk. Streaming water is preferable; in its absence, a tub may be used. A third method of hardening is to walk on grass. This should be done when the grass is still wet with dew and the patient should walk barefoot for ten to fifteen minutes. After both walking in the grass and treading water, energetic exercise should be taken for half an hour.

INDEX

Full discussions of herbs and diseases are referenced in bold type; word definitions are referenced in italics.